Cell Therapy, Bispecific Antibodies and Other Immunotherapies against Cancer

Cell Therapy, Bispecific Antibodies and Other Immunotherapies against Cancer

Editor

Vita Golubovskaya

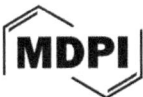

Basel • Beijing • Wuhan • Barcelona • Belgrade • Novi Sad • Cluj • Manchester

Editor
Vita Golubovskaya
Promab Biotechnologies
Richmond, CA, USA

Editorial Office
MDPI
St. Alban-Anlage 66
4052 Basel, Switzerland

This is a reprint of articles from the Special Issue published online in the open access journal *Cancers* (ISSN 2072-6694) (available at: https://www.mdpi.com/journal/cancers/special_issues/cell_therapies).

For citation purposes, cite each article independently as indicated on the article page online and as indicated below:

Lastname, A.A.; Lastname, B.B. Article Title. *Journal Name* **Year**, *Volume Number*, Page Range.

ISBN 978-3-0365-9566-5 (Hbk)
ISBN 978-3-0365-9567-2 (PDF)
doi.org/10.3390/books978-3-0365-9567-2

© 2023 by the authors. Articles in this book are Open Access and distributed under the Creative Commons Attribution (CC BY) license. The book as a whole is distributed by MDPI under the terms and conditions of the Creative Commons Attribution-NonCommercial-NoDerivs (CC BY-NC-ND) license.

Contents

About the Editor vii

Vita Golubovskaya
Editorial on "Cell Therapy, Bispecific Antibodies and Other Immunotherapies against Cancer"
Reprinted from: *Cancers* 2023, 15, 5053, doi:10.3390/cancers15205053 1

Marta Włodarczyk and Beata Pyrzynska
CAR-NK as a Rapidly Developed and Efficient Immunotherapeutic Strategy against Cancer
Reprinted from: *Cancers* 2023, 15, 117, doi:10.3390/cancers15010117 7

Md Faqrul Hasan, Tayler J. Croom-Perez, Jeremiah L. Oyer, Thomas A. Dieffenthaller, Liza D. Robles-Carrillo, Jonathan E. Eloriaga, et al.
TIGIT Expression on Activated NK Cells Correlates with Greater Anti-Tumor Activity but Promotes Functional Decline upon Lung Cancer Exposure: Implications for Adoptive Cell Therapy and TIGIT-Targeted Therapies
Reprinted from: *Cancers* 2023, 15, 2712, doi:10.3390/cancers15102712 35

Elin M. V. Forsberg, Rebecca Riise, Sara Saellström, Joakim Karlsson, Samuel Alsén, Valentina Bucher, et al.
Treatment with Anti-HER2 Chimeric Antigen Receptor Tumor-Infiltrating Lymphocytes (CAR-TILs) Is Safe and Associated with Antitumor Efficacy in Mice and Companion Dogs
Reprinted from: *Cancers* 2023, 15, 648, doi:10.3390/cancers15030648 59

Simona Gössi, Ulrike Bacher, Claudia Haslebacher, Michael Nagler, Franziska Suter, Cornelia Staehelin, et al.
Humoral Responses to Repetitive Doses of COVID-19 mRNA Vaccines in Patients with CAR-T-Cell Therapy
Reprinted from: *Cancers* 2022, 14, 3527, doi:10.3390/cancers14143527 77

Mohamed Shanshal, Paolo F. Caimi, Alex A. Adjei and Wen Wee Ma
T-Cell Engagers in Solid Cancers—Current Landscape and Future Directions
Reprinted from: *Cancers* 2023, 15, 2824, doi:10.3390/cancers15102824 91

Vita Golubovskaya, John Sienkiewicz, Jinying Sun, Yanwei Huang, Liang Hu, Hua Zhou, et al.
mRNA-Lipid Nanoparticle (LNP) Delivery of Humanized EpCAM-CD3 Bispecific Antibody Significantly Blocks Colorectal Cancer Tumor Growth
Reprinted from: *Cancers* 2023, 15, 2860, doi:10.3390/cancers15102860 105

Zhen-Hua Wu, Na Li, Zhang-Zhao Gao, Gang Chen, Lei Nie, Ya-Qiong Zhou, et al.
Development of the Novel Bifunctional Fusion Protein BR102 That Simultaneously Targets PD-L1 and TGF-β for Anticancer Immunotherapy
Reprinted from: *Cancers* 2022, 14, 4964, doi:10.3390/cancers14194964 119

Lijun Wu, Yanwei Huang, John Sienkiewicz, Jinying Sun, Liselle Guiang, Feng Li, et al.
Bispecific BCMA-CD3 Antibodies Block Multiple Myeloma Tumor Growth
Reprinted from: *Cancers* 2022, 14, 2518, doi:10.3390/cancers14102518 133

Vera Rentsch, Katja Seipel, Yara Banz, Gertrud Wiedemann, Naomi Porret, Ulrike Bacher and Thomas Pabst
Glofitamab Treatment in Relapsed or Refractory DLBCL after CAR T-Cell Therapy
Reprinted from: *Cancers* 2022, 14, 2516, doi:10.3390/cancers14102516 143

Sebastian Hörner, Moustafa Moustafa-Oglou, Karin Teppert, Ilona Hagelstein, Joseph Kauer, Martin Pflügler, et al.
IgG-Based Bispecific Anti-CD95 Antibodies for the Treatment of B Cell-Derived Malignancies and Autoimmune Diseases
Reprinted from: *Cancers* **2022**, *14*, 3941, doi:10.3390/cancers14163941 . . . . **155**

Kaitlyn Maffuid and Yanguang Cao
Decoding the Complexity of Immune–Cancer Cell Interactions: Empowering the Future of Cancer Immunotherapy
Reprinted from: *Cancers* **2023**, *15*, 4188, doi:10.3390/cancers15164188 . . . . **169**

About the Editor

Vita Golubovskaya

Dr. Vita Golubovskaya is the Vice-President of Research and Development at *Promab Biotechnologies* leading research on novel anti-cancer immunotherapies including CAR-T cells, bispecific antibodies, and CAR-NK cell therapy. She has more than 20 years of experience in cancer research, oncology, and immunology. Previously, Dr. Golubovskaya was a Research Associate Professor at Roswell Park Cancer Institute and Research Professor at University of Buffalo, SUNY, Buffalo, NY. Dr. Golubovskaya is a Volunteer Clinical Associate Professor at the University of Oklahoma Health Sciences Center. Dr. Golubovskaya has authored more than 100 publications, 20 patents, and several book chapters, and has presented data at National and International meetings. Dr. Golubovskaya served as a Guest Editor in *Frontiers in Bioscience*, *Vaccines*, *Anti-Cancer Agents in Medicinal Chemistry* and *Cancers*. She is an Active Member of AACR.

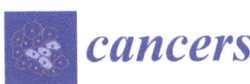

Editorial

Editorial on "Cell Therapy, Bispecific Antibodies and Other Immunotherapies against Cancer"

Vita Golubovskaya

Promab Biotechnologies, 2600 Hilltop Drive, Richmond, CA 94806, USA; vita.gol@promab.com

Citation: Golubovskaya, V. Editorial on "Cell Therapy, Bispecific Antibodies and Other Immunotherapies against Cancer". *Cancers* 2023, *15*, 5053. https://doi.org/10.3390/cancers15205053

Received: 13 October 2023
Accepted: 17 October 2023
Published: 19 October 2023

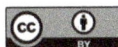

Copyright: © 2023 by the author. Licensee MDPI, Basel, Switzerland. This article is an open access article distributed under the terms and conditions of the Creative Commons Attribution (CC BY) license (https://creativecommons.org/licenses/by/4.0/).

This Special Issue in *Cancers*, "Cell Therapy, Bispecific Antibodies and other Immunotherapies Against Cancer", includes interesting reports and reviews on cell therapies and bispecific antibodies. The authors showed that cell therapy, bispecific antibodies, vaccine and immunomodulator approaches, combined with checkpoint inhibitors, are effective in improving anticancer therapies. The immunomodulators and immune checkpoint players, PD-1, PD-L1, CTLA-4, TIGIT and LAG-3, activate immune cells in the tumor microenvironment and increase immune response. The main approaches, challenges and future directions from this Special Issue are discussed.

Recently, a chimeric antigen receptor, CAR-T, cell therapy has revolutionized hematological cancer treatment. The FDA approved several CAR-T cell agents such as Kymriah, Yescarta, Tecartus and Breyanzi, which target CD19, and Abecma and Carvykti, which target BCMA antigens [1–4]. While the first round of treatments was successful, several challenges persist, such as low efficacy against solid tumors, cytokine release storm, the exhaustion of CAR-T cells, patient relapse, and the high cost of manufacturing. Novel generations of CAR-T cells are developed, such as bi-specific or tandem CAR-T cells [5–10], CAR-T cells with silenced checkpoint inhibitor pathways [11,12], CAR-T cells with different secreted cytokines (IL-15, IL-18, IL-12) to increase cell persistence and overcome a repressive tumor microenvironment, CAR-T cells with different switches to increase their safety. CAR-T cell therapy efficacy increased using different checkpoint inhibitors, such as PD-1, PD-L1, TIGIT, LAG-3, CTLA-4 and TIM-3 antibodies [11,13,14]. The disruption of PD-1 in CAR-T cells with Crispr/Cas-9 technology enhanced the functional activity of CAR-T cells [12]. Future combinations of CAR-T cells and other immunotherapies must be developed in clinical studies [15].

Another highly promising immunotherapy approach is CAR-NK cell therapy [16–20]. The advantage of using the NK cell for therapy is the absence of a GvHD (graft-versus-host disease) response applied to the generation of allogenic CAR-NK cells. CARs can be delivered into NK cells using lentiviruses, retroviruses, or mRNAs [21]. NK cells can be generated from different sources: blood PBMC, umbilical cord blood, induced pluripotent stem cells (iPSC) or the NK-92 cell line. There are several challenges for CAR-NK cell therapies: the low efficiency of expansion and genetic modification in vitro. CAR mRNAs can be embedded into lipid nanoparticles (LNPs) for increased stability and used for an efficient transfection of NK cells. Recently, an efficient encapsulation of BCMA and CD19-CAR mRNA into LNP and delivery to >500-fold expanded NK cells has been demonstrated, resulting in the generation of highly functional CAR$^+$CD56$^+$ NK cells against cancer cells and tumors [22]. The increased persistence of CAR-NK cells via a combination of CAR-NK cell therapy with other therapy approaches will be developed in the future.

Different immune cells, such as macrophages, T cell-infiltrating lymphocytes (TILS) [23], and gamma-delta T cells [24–27], can be used for the expression of CAR to target tumor cells. More clinical studies on these CAR-T cells are needed to understand their safety and efficacy against different types of cancer.

The application of T or NK cell-engaging bispecific antibodies is an alternative and promising approach to immunotherapy against cancer. BITE (blinatumomab), a CD19-CD3 antibody, is successfully used against B-cell malignant tumors in a clinical setting [28–31].

This year, the FDA granted accelerated approval for glofitamab, a CD20-CD3 bispecific antibody [32], against relapsed or diffuse large B-cell lymphomas (DLBCL). Many different designs of bispecific antibodies are developed with one domain binding to T/NK cells and another domain binding to cancer cell antigens: BITEs, Fc-containing, CrossMab, knob-hole, uni-, bi-valent and others [33,34]. There are several advantages of bi- and tri-specific T cell engagers versus cell therapy, such as off-the-shelf availability, easier logistics of administration and more economical manufacturing [35]. Several challenges exist for this approach, such as toxicity or repressive tumor microenvironment, that will be addressed in future pre-clinical and clinical studies. The improved engineering of antibodies and combination with inhibitors of tumor microenvironment can be applied to design these therapies.

Cancer vaccines (cell-based, peptide/protein-based, or gene-based) are another promising approach developed by several groups [36–39]. The goal of cancer vaccines is to target cancer cells via antigen-specific effector T cells. Activated T cells recognize MHC (major histocompatibility complex) I-peptide complexes, effector T cells target tumor cells and memory T cells prevent tumor relapse. The dendritic vaccine is a promising approach that stimulates T cells against tumor antigens [40]. The pulsing of DC with tumor cell lysate, tumor antigen or mRNA is a widely used approach for antigen delivery and the stimulation of an immune response. Dendritic cells are antigen-presenting cells and can be divided into several groups: conventional dendritic cells (cDC), plasmocytoid (pDC) and monocyte-derived DC (MoDC) [40]. The benefit of cancer vaccines is that they can target intracellular antigens versus CAR-T cells or bispecific antibodies, which target extracellular tumor-specific antigens [40]. Although conventional dendritic vaccines encounter limitations due to the low immunogenicity of cold tumors, the induction of immunogenic cell death (ICD) can convert cold tumors into hot tumors and improve DC vaccine potential. Immunogenic cell death can be achieved via chemotherapy, radiotherapy, photodynamic or photothermal therapy [40]. The local delivery of immunostimulants can increase the effect of immunogenic cell death of tumors and lead to the activation of DC and effector T cells.

The combination of cell therapy, bi-, tri-specific antibodies, CAR-NK, immunomodulators, checkpoint inhibitors and vaccines will be developed in future pre-clinical and clinical studies [41–43]. In addition, a personalized medicine approach will be used when patient tumors are sequenced to detect neoantigens that can be used for dendritic vaccine, bispecific antibody, and cell therapy development [35]. The combination therapy targeting several tumor antigens will be used to better target heterogeneous solid tumors. All discussed linked approaches are presented in Figure 1. For example, bispecific antibody (EpCAM-CD3 Ab is shown in Figure 1) can be delivered into tumors using mRNA [44], embedded into LNP [45] and attract T cells to kill tumor cells. The lysed tumor cells can release tumor neoantigens, serve as a cancer vaccine for attracting dendritic cells and, in combination with co-stimulants (cytokines, chemokines, receptor ligands and other immuno-stimulants), can target distant circulating tumor cells [37,46,47]. While EpCAM-CD3 mRNA-LNP was delivered intratumorally, future studies will expand the tumor-specific delivery of mRNA-LNP and the intravenous delivery of mRNA with tumor-specific expression of proteins. The proteins and antibodies can be produced inside tumors representing factories of proteins or antibodies, and secreted proteins will attract immune cells in the case of bispecific immune-engaging antibodies. Combination therapy with immunomodulators and checkpoint inhibitors will increase the efficacy of bispecific antibody and cell therapy to target distant metastatic tumor cells [48–50].

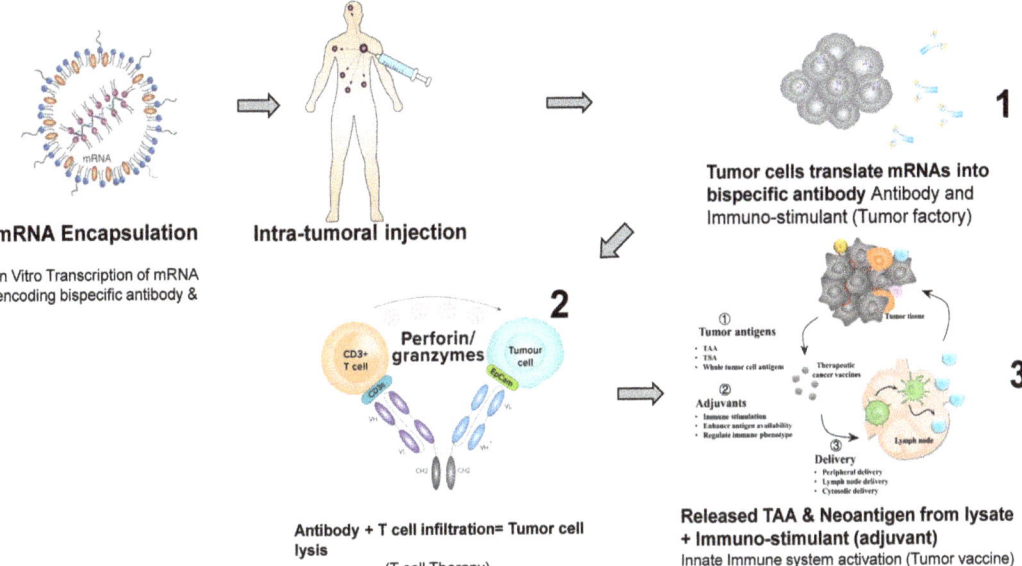

Figure 1. Bispecific antibody, immune T cell, immunostimulant and vaccine approaches. mRNA-LNP is shown for intratumoral delivery of bispecific antibodies. Secreted bispecific antibody attracts T cells to tumor and kills tumor cells. Tumor is lysed and serves as a tumor vaccine for stimulating further immune response in combination with immunostimulants.

Conclusions

Novel immunotherapy approaches, including bispecific antibodies, cell therapies, checkpoint inhibitors, vaccines and immunomodulators or their combination, must be developed and tested in future pre-clinical and clinical studies. The mRNA-LNP is a novel approach to deliver bispecific antibodies locally by enhancing immunomodulators to target distant tumor cells. The personalized medicine approach with a high-throughput sequencing of tumor antigens, detecting novel antigens and targets for immunotherapy, will be developed for more effective anticancer therapies. Dendritic, peptide and protein vaccines will be improved via novel tumor targets. The reports from this Special Issue in *Cancers* provide a basis to further develop novel immunotherapies.

Funding: This research received no external funding.

Acknowledgments: I would like to thank Lijun Wu and Phoebe Hsukeim for the design of Figure 1.

Conflicts of Interest: The author declares no conflict of interest. V.G. is an employee of Promab Biotechnologies.

References

1. Abrantes, R.; Duarte, H.O.; Gomes, C.; Walchli, S.; Reis, C.A. CAR-Ts: New perspectives in cancer therapy. *FEBS Lett.* **2022**, *596*, 403–416. [CrossRef] [PubMed]
2. Maus, M.V.; June, C.H. Making Better Chimeric Antigen Receptors for Adoptive T-cell Therapy. *Clin. Cancer Res.* **2016**, *22*, 1875–1884. [CrossRef] [PubMed]
3. Gross, G.; Eshhar, Z. Therapeutic Potential of T Cell Chimeric Antigen Receptors (CARs) in Cancer Treatment: Counteracting Off-Tumor Toxicities for Safe CAR T Cell Therapy. *Annu. Rev. Pharmacol. Toxicol.* **2016**, *56*, 59–83. [CrossRef] [PubMed]
4. June, C.H.; O'Connor, R.S.; Kawalekar, O.U.; Ghassemi, S.; Milone, M.C. CAR T cell immunotherapy for human cancer. *Science* **2018**, *359*, 1361–1365. [CrossRef]
5. Cronk, R.J.; Zurko, J.; Shah, N.N. Bispecific Chimeric Antigen Receptor T Cell Therapy for B Cell Malignancies and Multiple Myeloma. *Cancers* **2020**, *12*, 2523. [CrossRef]

6. Hegde, M.; Mukherjee, M.; Grada, Z.; Pignata, A.; Landi, D.; Navai, S.A.; Wakefield, A.; Fousek, K.; Bielamowicz, K.; Chow, K.K.; et al. Tandem CAR T cells targeting HER2 and IL13Ralpha2 mitigate tumor antigen escape. *J. Clin. Investig.* **2016**, *126*, 3036–3052. [CrossRef]
7. Martyniszyn, A.; Krahl, A.C.; Andre, M.C.; Hombach, A.A.; Abken, H. CD20-CD19 Bispecific CAR T Cells for the Treatment of B-Cell Malignancies. *Hum. Gene Ther.* **2017**, *28*, 1147–1157. [CrossRef]
8. Shah, N.N.; Johnson, B.D.; Schneider, D.; Zhu, F.; Szabo, A.; Keever-Taylor, C.A.; Krueger, W.; Worden, A.A.; Kadan, M.J.; Yim, S.; et al. Bispecific anti-CD20, anti-CD19 CAR T cells for relapsed B cell malignancies: A phase 1 dose escalation and expansion trial. *Nat. Med.* **2020**, *26*, 1569–1575. [CrossRef]
9. Zah, E.; Lin, M.Y.; Silva-Benedict, A.; Jensen, M.C.; Chen, Y.Y. T Cells Expressing CD19/CD20 Bispecific Chimeric Antigen Receptors Prevent Antigen Escape by Malignant B Cells. *Cancer Immunol. Res.* **2016**, *4*, 498–508. [CrossRef]
10. Zah, E.; Nam, E.; Bhuvan, V.; Tran, U.; Ji, B.Y.; Gosliner, S.B.; Wang, X.; Brown, C.E.; Chen, Y.Y. Systematically optimized BCMA/CS1 bispecific CAR-T cells robustly control heterogeneous multiple myeloma. *Nat. Commun.* **2020**, *11*, 2283. [CrossRef]
11. Rafiq, S.; Yeku, O.O.; Jackson, H.J.; Purdon, T.J.; van Leeuwen, D.G.; Drakes, D.J.; Song, M.; Miele, M.M.; Li, Z.; Wang, P.; et al. Targeted delivery of a PD-1-blocking scFv by CAR-T cells enhances anti-tumor efficacy in vivo. *Nat. Biotechnol.* **2018**, *36*, 847–856. [CrossRef] [PubMed]
12. Rupp, L.J.; Schumann, K.; Roybal, K.T.; Gate, R.E.; Ye, C.J.; Lim, W.A.; Marson, A. CRISPR/Cas9-mediated PD-1 disruption enhances anti-tumor efficacy of human chimeric antigen receptor T cells. *Sci. Rep.* **2017**, *7*, 737. [CrossRef] [PubMed]
13. Anagnostou, T.; Ansell, S.M. Immunomodulators in Lymphoma. *Curr. Treat. Options Oncol.* **2020**, *21*, 28. [CrossRef] [PubMed]
14. Chauvin, J.M.; Zarour, H.M. TIGIT in cancer immunotherapy. *J. Immunother. Cancer* **2020**, *8*, e000957. [CrossRef]
15. Longo, V.; Brunetti, O.; Azzariti, A.; Galetta, D.; Nardulli, P.; Leonetti, F.; Silvestris, N. Strategies to Improve Cancer Immune Checkpoint Inhibitors Efficacy, Other Than Abscopal Effect: A Systematic Review. *Cancers* **2019**, *11*, 539. [CrossRef]
16. Kilgour, M.K.; Bastin, D.J.; Lee, S.H.; Ardolino, M.; McComb, S.; Visram, A. Advancements in CAR-NK therapy: Lessons to be learned from CAR-T therapy. *Front. Immunol.* **2023**, *14*, 1166038. [CrossRef]
17. Liu, E.; Marin, D.; Banerjee, P.; Macapinlac, H.A.; Thompson, P.; Basar, R.; Kerbauy, L.N.; Overman, B.; Thall, P.; Kaplan, M.; et al. Use of CAR-Transduced Natural Killer Cells in CD19-Positive Lymphoid Tumors. *N. Engl. J. Med.* **2020**, *382*, 545–553. [CrossRef]
18. Merino, A.; Maakaron, J.; Bachanova, V. Advances in NK cell therapy for hematologic malignancies: NK source, persistence and tumor targeting. *Blood Rev.* **2023**, *60*, 101073. [CrossRef]
19. Nowak, J.; Bentele, M.; Kutle, I.; Zimmermann, K.; Luhmann, J.L.; Steinemann, D.; Kloess, S.; Koehl, U.; Roßberg, W.; Ahmed, A.; et al. CAR-NK Cells Targeting HER1 (EGFR) Show Efficient Anti-Tumor Activity against Head and Neck Squamous Cell Carcinoma (HNSCC). *Cancers* **2023**, *15*, 3169. [CrossRef]
20. Romanski, A.; Uherek, C.; Bug, G.; Seifried, E.; Klingemann, H.; Wels, W.S.; Ottmann, O.G.; Tonn, T. CD19-CAR engineered NK-92 cells are sufficient to overcome NK cell resistance in B-cell malignancies. *J. Cell. Mol. Med.* **2016**, *20*, 1287–1294. [CrossRef]
21. Wlodarczyk, M.; Pyrzynska, B. CAR-NK as a Rapidly Developed and Efficient Immunotherapeutic Strategy against Cancer. *Cancers* **2022**, *15*, 117. [CrossRef] [PubMed]
22. Golubovskaya, V.; Sienkiewicz, J.; Sun, J.; Zhang, S.; Huang, Y.; Zhou, H.; Harto, H.; Xu, S.; Berahovich, R.; Wu, L. CAR-NK Cells Generated with mRNA-LNPs Kill Tumor Target Cells In Vitro and In Vivo. *Int. J. Mol. Sci.* **2023**, *24*, 13364. [CrossRef] [PubMed]
23. Forsberg, E.M.V.; Riise, R.; Saellstrom, S.; Karlsson, J.; Alsen, S.; Bucher, V.; Hemminki, A.E.; Bagge, R.O.; Ny, L.; Nilsson, L.M.; et al. Treatment with Anti-HER2 Chimeric Antigen Receptor Tumor-Infiltrating Lymphocytes (CAR-TILs) Is Safe and Associated with Antitumor Efficacy in Mice and Companion Dogs. *Cancers* **2023**, *15*, 648. [CrossRef] [PubMed]
24. Morandi, F.; Yazdanifar, M.; Cocco, C.; Bertaina, A.; Airoldi, I. Engineering the Bridge between Innate and Adaptive Immunity for Cancer Immunotherapy: Focus on gammadelta T and NK Cells. *Cells* **2020**, *9*, 1757. [CrossRef] [PubMed]
25. Capsomidis, A.; Benthall, G.; Van Acker, H.H.; Fisher, J.; Kramer, A.M.; Abeln, Z.; Majani, Y.; Gileadi, T.; Wallace, R.; Gustafsson, K.; et al. Chimeric Antigen Receptor-Engineered Human Gamma Delta T Cells: Enhanced Cytotoxicity with Retention of Cross Presentation. *Mol. Ther.* **2018**, *26*, 354–365. [CrossRef]
26. Du, S.H.; Li, Z.; Chen, C.; Tan, W.K.; Chi, Z.; Kwang, T.W.; Xu, X.H.; Wang, S. Co-Expansion of Cytokine-Induced Killer Cells and Vgamma9Vdelta2 T Cells for CAR T-Cell Therapy. *PLoS ONE* **2016**, *11*, e0161820. [CrossRef]
27. Fleischer, L.C.; Becker, S.A.; Ryan, R.E.; Fedanov, A.; Doering, C.B.; Spencer, H.T. Non-signaling Chimeric Antigen Receptors Enhance Antigen-Directed Killing by gammadelta T Cells in Contrast to alphabeta T Cells. *Mol. Ther. Oncolytics* **2020**, *18*, 149–160. [CrossRef]
28. Bumma, N.; Papadantonakis, N.; Advani, A.S. Structure, development, preclinical and clinical efficacy of blinatumomab in acute lymphoblastic leukemia. *Future Oncol.* **2015**, *11*, 1729–1739. [CrossRef]
29. Nagorsen, D.; Kufer, P.; Baeuerle, P.A.; Bargou, R. Blinatumomab: A historical perspective. *Pharmacol. Ther.* **2012**, *136*, 334–342. [CrossRef]
30. Nagorsen, D.; Bargou, R.; Ruttinger, D.; Kufer, P.; Baeuerle, P.A.; Zugmaier, G. Immunotherapy of lymphoma and leukemia with T-cell engaging BiTE antibody blinatumomab. *Leuk. Lymphoma* **2009**, *50*, 886–891. [CrossRef]
31. d'Argouges, S.; Wissing, S.; Brandl, C.; Prang, N.; Lutterbuese, R.; Kozhich, A.; Suzich, J.; Locher, M.; Kiener, P.; Kufer, P.; et al. Combination of rituximab with blinatumomab (MT103/MEDI-538), a T cell-engaging CD19-/CD3-bispecific antibody, for highly efficient lysis of human B lymphoma cells. *Leuk. Res.* **2009**, *33*, 465–473. [CrossRef] [PubMed]

32. Rentsch, V.; Seipel, K.; Banz, Y.; Wiedemann, G.; Porret, N.; Bacher, U.; Pabst, T. Glofitamab Treatment in Relapsed or Refractory DLBCL after CAR T-Cell Therapy. *Cancers* **2022**, *14*, 2516. [CrossRef] [PubMed]
33. Klein, C.; Schaefer, W.; Regula, J.T.; Dumontet, C.; Brinkmann, U.; Bacac, M.; Umana, P. Engineering therapeutic bispecific antibodies using CrossMab technology. *Methods* **2019**, *154*, 21–31. [CrossRef]
34. Seckinger, A.; Delgado, J.A.; Moser, S.; Moreno, L.; Neuber, B.; Grab, A.; Lipp, S.; Merino, J.; Prosper, F.; Emde, M.; et al. Target Expression, Generation, Preclinical Activity, and Pharmacokinetics of the BCMA-T Cell Bispecific Antibody EM801 for Multiple Myeloma Treatment. *Cancer Cell* **2017**, *31*, 396–410. [CrossRef]
35. Shanshal, M.; Caimi, P.F.; Adjei, A.A.; Ma, W.W. T-Cell Engagers in Solid Cancers-Current Landscape and Future Directions. *Cancers* **2023**, *15*, 2824. [CrossRef] [PubMed]
36. Buchler, T.; Kovarova, L.; Musilova, R.; Bourkova, L.; Ocadlikova, D.; Bulikova, A.; Hanak, L.; Michalek, J.; Hajek, R. Generation of dendritic cells using cell culture bags—Description of a method and review of literature. *Hematology* **2004**, *9*, 199–205. [CrossRef]
37. Dwivedi, R.; Pandey, R.; Chandra, S.; Mehrotra, D. Dendritic cell-based immunotherapy: A potential player in oral cancer therapeutics. *Immunotherapy* **2023**, *15*, 457–469. [CrossRef]
38. Foley, R.; Tozer, R.; Wan, Y. Genetically modified dendritic cells in cancer therapy: Implications for transfusion medicine. *Transfus. Med. Rev.* **2001**, *15*, 292–304. [CrossRef]
39. Hotchkiss, K.M.; Batich, K.A.; Mohan, A.; Rahman, R.; Piantadosi, S.; Khasraw, M. Dendritic cell vaccine trials in gliomas: Untangling the lines. *Neuro Oncol.* **2023**, *25*, 1752–1762. [CrossRef]
40. Lee, K.W.; Yam, J.W.P.; Mao, X. Dendritic Cell Vaccines: A Shift from Conventional Approach to New Generations. *Cells* **2023**, *12*, 2147. [CrossRef]
41. Ma, X.; Shou, P.; Smith, C.; Chen, Y.; Du, H.; Sun, C.; Kren, N.P.; Michaud, D.; Ahn, S.; Vincent, B.; et al. Interleukin-23 engineering improves CAR T cell function in solid tumors. *Nat. Biotechnol.* **2020**, *38*, 448–459. [CrossRef] [PubMed]
42. Ma, J.; Mo, Y.; Tang, M.; Shen, J.; Qi, Y.; Zhao, W.; Huang, Y.; Yanmin Xu, Y.; Qian, C. Bispecific Antibodies: From Research to Clinical Application. *Front. Immunol.* **2021**, *12*, 626616. [CrossRef] [PubMed]
43. Marple, A.H.; Bonifant, C.L.; Shah, N.N. Improving CAR T-cells: The next generation. *Semin. Hematol.* **2020**, *57*, 115–121. [CrossRef]
44. Beck, J.D.; Reidenbach, D.; Salomon, N.; Sahin, U.; Tureci, O.; Vormehr, M.; Kranz, L.M. mRNA therapeutics in cancer immunotherapy. *Mol. Cancer* **2021**, *20*, 69. [CrossRef] [PubMed]
45. Guevara, M.; Persano, F.; Persano, S. Advances in Lipid Nanoparticles for mRNA-Based Cancer Immunotherapy. *Front. Chem.* **2020**, *8*, 589959. [CrossRef]
46. Ge, C.; Yang, X.; Xin, J.; Gong, X.; Wang, X.; Kong, L. Recent Advances in Antitumor Dendritic Cell Vaccines. *Cancer Biother. Radiopharm.* **2023**, *38*, 450–457. [CrossRef]
47. Goutsouliak, K.; Veeraraghavan, J.; Sethunath, V.; De Angelis, C.; Osborne, C.K.; Rimawi, M.F.; Schiff, R. Towards personalized treatment for early stage HER2-positive breast cancer. *Nat. Rev. Clin. Oncol.* **2020**, *17*, 233–250. [CrossRef]
48. Shin, E.C. Cancer immunotherapy: Special issue of BMB Reports in 2021. *BMB Rep.* **2021**, *54*, 1. [CrossRef]
49. Vilgelm, A.E.; Johnson, D.B.; Richmond, A. Combinatorial approach to cancer immunotherapy: Strength in numbers. *J. Leukoc. Biol.* **2016**, *100*, 275–290. [CrossRef]
50. Korman, A.J.; Peggs, K.S.; Allison, J.P. Checkpoint blockade in cancer immunotherapy. *Adv. Immunol.* **2006**, *90*, 297–339.

Disclaimer/Publisher's Note: The statements, opinions and data contained in all publications are solely those of the individual author(s) and contributor(s) and not of MDPI and/or the editor(s). MDPI and/or the editor(s) disclaim responsibility for any injury to people or property resulting from any ideas, methods, instructions or products referred to in the content.

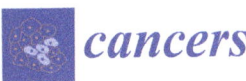

Review

CAR-NK as a Rapidly Developed and Efficient Immunotherapeutic Strategy against Cancer

Marta Włodarczyk [1,2] and Beata Pyrzynska [3,*]

1. Department of Biochemistry and Pharmacogenomics, Faculty of Pharmacy, Medical University of Warsaw, Banacha 1B, 02-097 Warsaw, Poland
2. Centre for Preclinical Research, Medical University of Warsaw, Banacha 1B, 02-097 Warsaw, Poland
3. Department of Biochemistry, Medical University of Warsaw, Banacha 1, 02-097 Warsaw, Poland

* Correspondence: beata.pyrzynska@wum.edu.pl

Simple Summary: New approaches in adoptive immunotherapy using chimeric antigen receptor (CAR)-modified cells have been developing very quickly in recent years, entering into clinical trials and being accepted by health agencies worldwide. Although the classical CAR therapies using genetically engineered T cells (CAR-T) are quite effective in curing resistant and refractory blood disorders, they are less efficient in fighting solid tumors. Therefore, intense research is ongoing to modify the CAR constructs and to use different types of immune cells as platforms for CAR-based therapies in order to make them more efficient and safer. This review summarizes new approaches to CAR therapy, with a particular focus on recent achievements and the benefits of genetic engineering of NK cells.

Abstract: Chimeric antigen receptor (CAR)-modified T cell therapy has been rapidly developing in recent years, ultimately revolutionizing immunotherapeutic strategies and providing significant anti-tumor potency, mainly in treating hematological neoplasms. However, graft-versus-host disease (GVHD) and other adverse effects, such as cytokine release syndromes (CRS) and neurotoxicity associated with CAR-T cell infusion, have raised some concerns about the broad application of this therapy. Natural killer (NK) cells have been identified as promising alternative platforms for CAR-based therapies because of their unique features, such as a lack of human leukocyte antigen (HLA)-matching restriction, superior safety, and better anti-tumor activity when compared with CAR-T cells. The lack of CRS, neurotoxicity, or GVHD, in the case of CAR-NK therapy, in addition to the possibility of using allogeneic NK cells as a CAR platform for "off-the-shelf" therapy, opens new windows for strategic opportunities. This review underlines recent design achievements in CAR constructs and summarizes preclinical studies' results regarding CAR-NK therapies' safety and anti-tumor potency. Additionally, new approaches in CAR-NK technology are briefly described, and currently registered clinical trials are listed.

Keywords: chimeric antigen receptors; CAR-NK; CAR-T

Citation: Włodarczyk, M.; Pyrzynska, B. CAR-NK as a Rapidly Developed and Efficient Immunotherapeutic Strategy against Cancer. *Cancers* **2023**, *15*, 117. https://doi.org/10.3390/cancers15010117

Academic Editor: Vita Golubovskaya

Received: 16 November 2022
Revised: 14 December 2022
Accepted: 20 December 2022
Published: 24 December 2022

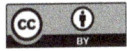

Copyright: © 2022 by the authors. Licensee MDPI, Basel, Switzerland. This article is an open access article distributed under the terms and conditions of the Creative Commons Attribution (CC BY) license (https://creativecommons.org/licenses/by/4.0/).

1. Introduction

NK cells are large granular lymphocytes which are a component of the innate (non-specific) immune defense system. They mature in the bone marrow, lymph nodes, spleen, thymus, and tonsils, and constitute about 5–10% of circulating lymphocytes in the peripheral blood (reviewed in [1]). NK cells are essential components of the anti-tumor, anti-microbial, and anti-parasite defenses of our immune system. Most NK cells recognize antibody-coated tumor cells via their CD16 receptors (also known as FcγRIIIa), the first step that triggers the activation of antibody-dependent cellular cytotoxicity (ADCC). Unlike T lymphocytes, the action of NK cells is less specific, which causes them to respond rapidly to the presence of transformed or infected cells without a prior need for antigen priming or induction of a specific immune response. However, the activation of NK cells is still strictly controlled by the integration of a variety of signals obtained by the activating and inhibitory receptors, as well as cytokine and chemokine receptors on the surface of NK cells (reviewed in [2]). For example, normal cells express MHC class I (MHC-I) molecules, and their proper amount on the cell surface inhibits NK cell activation via interaction with inhibitory killer immunoglobulin receptors (KIR) on their surface. In contrast, cancer cells synthesize a reduced amount of MHC I molecules, leading to reduced signaling from inhibitory receptors and, eventually, activation of NK cells (schema in Figure 1).

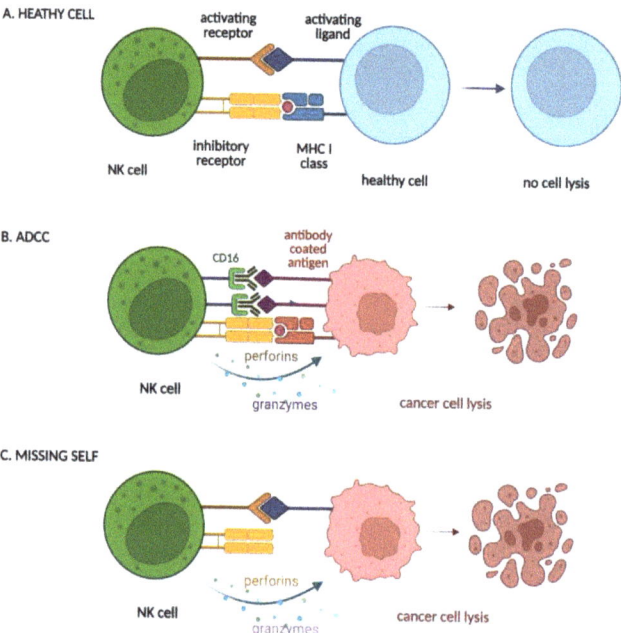

Figure 1. Schematic presenting mechanisms of recognition of healthy cell (**A**), antibody-coated target cell (**B**), or cancer cell missing MHC-I expression (**C**) by NK cell, followed by degranulation of NK cell (**B**,**C**) and cancer cell lysis.

In the case of both cytotoxic T cells and NK cells, similar molecular mechanisms are responsible for their effector function, including (i) degranulation that relies on the directed release of a membrane-disrupting protein (called perforin) and a family of proteases (called granzymes) from the secretory lysosomes; (ii) production of cytokines, such as tumor necrosis factor (TNF-α) and interferon-gamma (INF-γ), as well as production of membrane proteins, such as Fas ligand (FasL) or TNF-related apoptosis-inducing ligand (TRAIL), which are able to activate the death receptor-mediated killing of target cells [3–5].

The efficient cytotoxic activity of T and NK cells makes them the natural choice of cells employed in adoptive cell therapy for cancer, first introduced in the 1980s [6] and later applied in clinical trials to treat metastatic melanoma [7]. Subsequently, AIET therapy (autologous immune enhancement therapy), which uses autologous (patient's own) NK cells and activated T cells to treat various cancers, was developed by Terunuma et al. [8]. In this technique, the NK cells are obtained from the peripheral blood lymphocytes and processed by a selective immune cell expansion kit without needing feeder cells. In the early nineties of the twentieth century, scientists developed the first engineered T cell with a chimeric T-Cell Receptor (TCR) molecule [9] (reviewed in [10]). In recent years, the genetic engineering of cytotoxic lymphocytes to express membrane receptors, called chimeric antigen receptors (CARs), has become one of the most crucial breakthrough approaches in cancer immunotherapy (reviewed in [11,12]). The recognition of antigens on the surface of tumor cells by CAR is independent of the MHC engagement (in contrast to the recognition by the endogenous TCR). The targeting of tumor-associated antigens induces cellular signaling in CAR-bearing lymphocytes, which drives their proliferation, cytokine production, and degranulation, leading to a cytotoxic attack directed toward tumor cells [13]. CAR therapy is referred to as "living therapy," as the genetically modified immune cells multiply in the patient's body and provide long-term anti-cancer memory.

2. CAR Engineering

The term "chimeric" refers to the fact that synthetic CAR molecules are engineered as fusion proteins consisting of at least three essential components; (i) extracellular single chain variable fragment (scFv), classically derived from a murine monoclonal antibody, ensuring specific and efficient recognition of the target antigen on the surface of tumor cell; (ii) extracellular hinge and transmembrane domains; and (iii) intracellular signaling domains ensuring efficient activation of a signaling cascade generating cytotoxic effects toward tumor cells (schema in Figure 2).

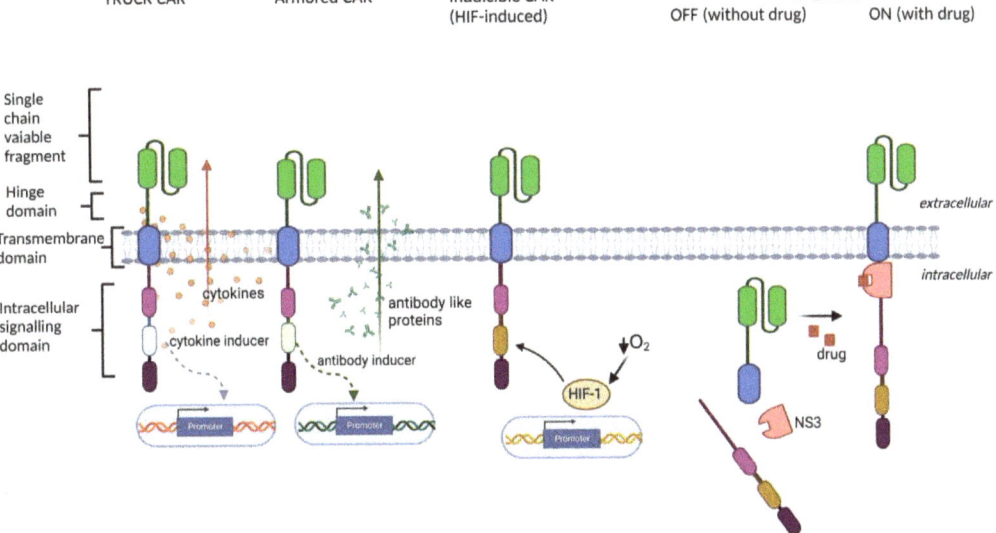

Figure 2. Schema presenting examples of the 4th generation of CAR constructs, including TRUCK CAR, Armored CAR, inducible CAR, and ON/OFF-controllable VIPER CAR.

Most often, CAR technology employs the T cells (called CAR-T cells shortly) since they are relatively easy to expand and genetically modify (reviewed in [14]). Briefly, CAR-Ts are made by harvesting T cells from a patient's blood and reprogramming them in the laboratory to express CAR. Once genetically reprogrammed, grown in large numbers, and administered to the patient's blood, CAR-T cells circulate through the body and end up binding to a specific surface protein which they recognize. This binding event stimulates immune attack, cancer cell destruction, and further CAR-T cell proliferation, leading to long-term fighting of the tumor cells by CAR-T (reviewed in [15]). The first impressive body of evidence supporting the rationale of such an approach came ten years ago, from studies on genetic engineering and adoptive transfer of T cells expressing CAR proteins that targeted CD19-positive relapsed leukemia [16]. This approach continued to develop further until the first approval of CAR therapy by the US Food and Drug Administration (FDA) in 2017 [17]. After the remarkable success of CAR-T cell therapy for acute lymphoblastic leukemia (ALL), non-Hodgkin lymphoma (NHL), and multiple myeloma, this immunotherapy has been called "The 2018 Advance of the Year" by the American Society of Clinical Oncology (ASCO) [18]. Hundreds of CAR-T cell therapy clinical trials are underway [19].

However, it should be emphasized that CAR-T cell therapies are not free from side effects. For example, some tumor antigens, although highly abundant on the surface of tumor cells, are also present in certain normal cell populations, leading to the recognition and killing of these normal cells by CAR-T cells (a phenomenon called the "on-target/off-tumor" effect). Another possible side effect originates from the uncontrolled proliferation of active CAR-T cells, as well as the excessive release of cytokines and other inflammatory signals throughout the body (called cytokine release syndrome; CRS), which leads to neurotoxicity and other adverse events, ranging from mild fever to life-threatening organ failure (reviewed in [20]).

Modifications to CAR engineering strategies are the subject of intense research and investigation, aiming to develop a selective and effective approach, with enhanced potency and CAR expression taking place at the tumor site only (reviewed in [21]).

Recently, the scFv extracellular fragment of CAR constructs has been engineered in various ways by adding the following features:

- Dual or multi-targeting, leading to the recognition of two different epitopes on the same target antigen (to intensify target antigen binding by CAR) or recognition of two or more different antigens (bispecific or multi-specific CARs recognizing antigenic pattern) on the surface of tumor cells (to prevent antigen escape by tumor cells; reviewed in [22]);
- Shorter extracellular fragment, such as single domain variable heavy-chain (VH), derived from camelid antibody (called nanobody; reviewed in [23]) or fully-human heavy-chain-only variable domain (FHVH) instead of conventional scFv fragment (for better expression of smaller CAR constructs on T cells and less immunogenicity induced in the patient's organism toward foreign human protein [24]);
- switchable CAR-T cells (sCAR-T) with CAR molecules that do not directly recognize tumor antigens, but instead recognize the molecule that targets the antigen, such as the Fab fragment of an antigen-specific recombinant antibody [25–28] or the adaptor protein zipFv [29], consisting of scFv and a fragment of the leucine zipper, functioning in this case as a "switch" (for more precise control of CAR-T specificity and activity).

The newest, fourth generation of CAR constructs is devoted to improving the tumor penetration and function of CAR-T cells in the immunosuppressive tumor microenvironment (TME), which usually efficiently blocks the function of both endogenous tumor-resident and adoptively transferred T cells, particularly in solid tumors (reviewed in [21,30,31]). The recent innovative approaches to boost CAR-T cell function in TME are shortly summarized below and in Figure 2:

- TRUCK (T cells Redirected for antigen-Unrestricted Cytokine-initiated Killing) approach, based on engineering CAR-T cells to release particular transgenic cytokine upon CAR engagement, including IL-7 [32,33], IL-12 [34,35], IL-15 [36], IL-18 [37,38], IL-23 [39], and IL-33 [40]. TRUCK CARs stimulate the release of cytokines specifically at the tumor site to provide either an auto-stimulatory effect for CAR-bearing cells or activation of other immune cell types in the TME;
- Armored CAR-T cells engineered to express various proteins alongside the CAR (reviewed in [30], such as antibodies or their fragments, which are able to inhibit immune checkpoints [41,42], or dominant-negative TGF-β receptors [43,44], which are able to overcome TGF-β-induced T cell repression in the TME;
- Inducible CAR expression, regulated by specific cellular signaling and transcription factors, including synthetic Notch signaling [45,46], STAT5, AP-1, NFκB [44] (to improve the control over timing and magnitude of CAR expression), or HIF-1α [47] (to restrict the CAR expression to hypoxic areas of the solid tumors);
- ON- and OFF-controllable CAR signaling, regulated by clinically-approved drugs, including CAR regulated by lenalidomide-induced degradation [48], by dasatinib-

induced downregulation [49] and by proteolytical cleavage [50,51] (to avoid CAR-T exhaustion and to obtain complete control over CAR activity by drug dosing);
- Multiplex CAR circuits [29,51] combining various CAR technologies, including "AND gate," SUPRA CAR, universal ON-OFF, and switchboard VIPER CARs (for expanded control over CAR specificity and activation).

The labor-intensive manufacturing and high costs of classical customized CAR-T therapy are associated with the T cells being isolated, modified, and expanded for each patient individually [52]. Therefore, very intensive studies are currently underway to generate Universal CAR-T (UCAR-T) cell therapy (reviewed in [53]) using healthy donor-derived T cells (allogeneic T cells taken from different individuals, immunologically incompatible), which allows for large-scale batch manufacturing and storage with a significantly reduced cost of production. Although such an "off-the-shelf" product can be ready to use when needed, the manufacturing process of UCAR-T requires additional genetic modification, such as deletion of the gene encoding TCR, to prevent severe immune rejection due to the mismatch of MHC between the donor and the patient.

3. Advantages and Limitations of NK Cells as a CAR Platform

The success of novel immunotherapeutic tools, such as CAR-T cells, has inspired scientists to focus on similar genetic modification of other types of cytotoxic lymphocytes, including NK cells (reviewed in [54–56]). Additionally, there is a constant demand for exploring other lymphocytes as CAR platforms, since many patients treated with CAR-T still experience a progressive disease [57], severe therapy-related toxicities, or other adverse effects. Most importantly, CAR-NK cells are considered an "off-the-shelf" product, as they can be produced from allogeneic sources, such as the blood of healthy donors. Although NK cells have limited persistence in vivo and are more difficult to employ for genetic modification and expansion in vitro than T cells are, they are considered a safer, more powerful, and universal platform for CAR-based therapies due to their unique biological features (Figure 3) (reviewed in [58]).

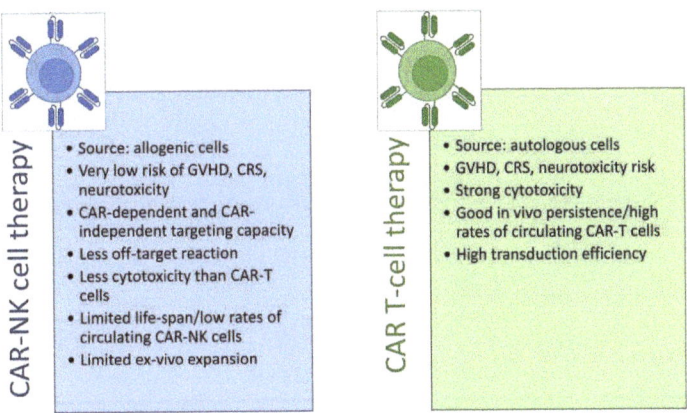

Figure 3. Summary of CAR-NK cell therapy features (list on the left) and CAR-T cell therapy features (list on the right).

NK cells are quick and potent in eliminating abnormal cells without the prior requirement for antigen priming (in contrast to T cells). The CAR-modified NK cells retain their natural ability to recognize abnormal cells by native receptors in a non-antigen-specific manner and efficiently eliminate them, in addition to CAR-mediated antigen-specific killing.

Importantly, CAR-NK therapies have the potential to be used as "off-the-shelf" types of therapy, since it has been documented that the HLA-mismatched NK cells can be employed as a CAR platform [59]. As a matter of safety, CAR-NK therapy is characterized by less toxicity than CAR-T therapies, with no substantial GVHD or CRS effects [59]. While administration of engineered T cells can cause the release of a variety of cytokines, among them IL-6, which is crucial for the occurrence of CRS (reviewed in [60]), the NK cells produce mainly pro-inflammatory cytokines such as IFN-γ, IL-3, and TNF-α [61]. In the case of allogeneic NK cells' dose-limiting toxicities, CRS and GvHD are rarely observed, only after being administered in multiple doses or with other agents. For example, in the NSG mouse model, co-expression of CAR and IL-15 in NK cells, when administered in large amounts, resulted in toxicity, indicating the critical need to control NK cell survival in the body [62]. In a recently published paper, expanded autologous NK cells were transduced with NKG2D-based CAR. Such cells exhibited in vitro cytotoxicity against multiple myeloma cells, with minimal activity against normal cells. Mice injected with these CAR-NK cells did not show any sign of GvHD or treatment-related toxicities during the 150 days of the experiment [63]. Infusions of NK cells expressing IL-2, transduced with a lentiviral construct bearing a third-generation CAR which contained CD28 and 4-1BB co-stimulatory molecules, with an Fc fragment inserted between the CD33 scFv and CD28, have been safely used without significant side effects [64]. Cord blood-derived anti-CD19 CAR-NK cells used to cure B-cell malignancies did not produce CRS or symptoms related to neurotoxicity [59]. Additionally, a clinical study of 11 patients with relapsed or refractory CD19-positive tumors showed that most of them responded to CAR-NK treatment without toxic side effects (NCT03056339). CAR-NK therapy is also undoubtedly safer for the treatment of T cell-derived malignancies. Treatment of these tumor types using CAR-T therapy is limited, as both transformed T cells and CAR-T cells (but not CAR-NK cells) share common antigens. Therefore, a high risk of fratricide attack exists, which may lead to the elimination of CAR-T cells themselves.

The short lifespan of NK cells (typically about two weeks [65]) guarantees the safety of CAR-NK therapy. On the other hand, it compromises the potency and sustained responses to this therapy. Therefore, significant efforts have been made to increase the potency and persistence of CAR-NK treatment without compromising its safety and without reaching NK cell exhaustion. It has been shown that lymphodepletion with fludarabine and cyclophosphamide is crucial to NK cells' expansion [66]. Additionally, interleukins IL-2 and IL-15 seem to play a critical role in extending the life span and persistence of NK cells in vivo. IL-2 needs to be administered in vivo to expand the NK cells upon injection. However, high doses of this cytokine are associated with organ toxicity (heart, lung, kidney, and central nervous system), while low doses activate mobilization of suppressive Treg cells, affecting NK cell function [67]. An alternative to IL-2 is the cytokine IL-15, as it does not induce suppressive Tregs and has been shown to improve NK cell cytolytic function [68]. Therefore, CAR constructs incorporating cytokine transgenes could be used for genetic modification of NK cells, allowing parallel expression of CAR and IL-15. Some studies have already proven that such an approach is efficient for improving the persistence of CAR-NK cells [59].

Numerous approaches to improving CAR technologies and construct designs have been used to genetically modify NK cells (reviewed in [69]). Unfortunately, NK cells are more resistant to genetic engineering than T cells. The lack of an efficient and standardized method for exogenous gene transfer represents one of the most critical limitations in the production of CAR-NK cells. Retroviral transduction is, so far, the most commonly used method for gene delivery into NK cells (reviewed in [70]). However, it typically ranges between 27–52% of NK cells transduced after a single treatment with retroviruses [71]. The low transduction rates can be improved by stimulating NK cells with IL-2 and IL-21 [72,73]. Lentiviral vectors, despite being a safer method for gene transfer due to reduced insertional mutagenic potential [74], Lentiviral vectors are much less efficient in the modification of NK cells. Constant efforts are made to improve the protocols and achieve at least 15% efficiency [75]. Excellent results (70% efficiency) have, however, been reported upon transduction of primary NK cells with lentiviral vectors which have been pseudotyped with modified envelope proteins derived from baboons or gibbons [76–78].

Non-viral methods, such as electroporation or lipofection, provide transient expression from the CAR construct, which drops down in 3–5 days since it is usually not integrated into the NK cell genome (reviewed in [70]). Both virus vectors and transfection methods can also be used to deliver the CRISPR/Cas9 genome editing system [79] for precise gene deletion (knockout) [80], repair, or introduction of a new gene (knock-in) [81,82], and could be used for delivery of CAR constructs to NK cells. Recent studies have confirmed the good efficiency of such approaches, including the adeno-associated virus for delivery of the CAR construct and its precise introduction into primary NK cell genome using CRISPR/Cas9 technology [83].

Interesting technologies combining transfection with stable integration of exogenous genes or large DNA fragments into the genome are transposon systems, such as sleeping beauty or PiggyBac [84]. These systems are considered safe and have already been successfully used for "pasting" CAR constructs into the genome of NK cells [85]. Further optimization of this method is needed, since it is still characterized by low efficiency [86].

For the generation of CAR-NK therapy, different sources of NK cells can be used, including cord blood, peripheral blood, hematopoietic and induced pluripotent stem cells (iPSCs) [87], and NK-like cell lines (reviewed in [54]). NK cells from different sources exhibit different levels of potency and persistence (reviewed in [88]). However, all of them have already reached clinical trial levels.

4. CAR-Engineered NK-92 Cell Line

The NK-92 cell line derives from the lymphoma cells of a 50-year-old male. It exhibits features of activated NK cells in vitro; its growth is interleukin 2 (IL-2)-dependent, and it expresses NK cell markers, such as the CD56 antigen, activating receptors as well as the NK cell's typical adhesion molecule CD2. The potent cytotoxicity toward leukemia, lymphoma, myeloma [89], and some solid tumors, as well as the easy expansion of NK-92 in vitro [90], qualified this cell line as a good target for genetic modification with CAR constructs. The high cytotoxicity of NK-92 results from the expression of activating receptors and adhesion molecules, as well as the lack of most KIR inhibitory receptors [91]. NK-92 cells can be easily modified by non-viral transfection methods (reviewed in [92]), and are well-suited for clinical development, since molecularly- and functionally-characterized single-cell clones can be isolated from the NK-92 cell line for further genetic modification with CAR constructs.

The possibility of continuous expansion in the presence of IL-2, according to the Good Manufacturing Practice (GMP) principles, is the most important advantage of the NK-92 cell line [93]. The safety and clinical activity of NK-92 cells have been initially evaluated in early-phase clinical trials in patients with advanced cancers [94,95]. Positive results encouraged scientists to test the CAR-modified NK-92 in preclinical studies [96–98]. However, as in the case of any other tumor cell line that carries a potential tumorigenicity risk, the preparation of the CAR-NK-92 cell line for clinical injection requires the additional step of cell irradiation [99]. Although irradiated NK-92 cells still retain their cytotoxic activity, they have minimal persistence in vivo, typically reaching only one week [100,101]. However, extremely short persistence of NK-92 has also been reported. In the study conducted by Wiliams et al., NK-92 cells were detected in only one of the three patients by flow cytometry 15 minutes after infusion, suggesting a rapid capture of NK-92 from the circulation [102]. Tonn et al. performed Y-chromosome PCR on two female patients who received an NK-92 infusion from a male donor, and also detected a post-infusion signal at very low levels [95]. The lack of an effective diagnostic tool to assess the presence of cells with the CAR transcript [103] can be partially overcome with the direct or indirect labeling of cells with fluorophores, contrast agents, or radioactive isotopes before infusion [104]. However, leakage of tags from cells and release of tags from dying cells is quite common phenomena. A further disadvantage of these solutions is the dilution of the intracellular tracer as the cells divide. Therefore, imaging after a few weeks is not always feasible [105]. Another option is to use a specific label (e.g., antibody or peptide) capable of binding a particular antigen on the surface of target cells in vivo, and followed by optical imaging (OI), magnetic resonance imaging (MR), and nuclear medicine (NM) [105,106]. A disadvantage of this method is the non-specific uptake by healthy tissues (mainly the liver and/or kidneys) due to the physiological biodistribution of the labeling agent.

Interestingly, in patients with colon carcinomas, autologous NK cells labeled with a radiopharmaceutical ^{111}In-oxine ex vivo were infused and traced, proving NK cell migration to the tumor metastatic regions [107]. ^{111}In-oxine has a 67 h-long half-life; therefore, accumulation of the labeled NK cells can be proven up to 72 h after injection [107]. Recently, Shamalov et al. developed a non-invasive cell tracking technique based on gold nanoparticles to evaluate the kinetics, migration, and biodistribution of NK cells in tumor-bearing mice, which could be applied in the future in human studies [108]. Unfortunately, until now, there has been no precise method for long-term monitoring of CAR-NK therapy persistence in humans.

Compared with the autologous or allogeneic CAR-NK cells and CAR-T therapies, CAR-NK-92 therapy is fairly cheap, since no labor- and cost-intensive cell purification is required in the case of CAR-NK-92 cells. Therefore, even repeated cycles of CAR-modified NK-92 infusions are affordable [109]. The results of clinical trials with NK-92 adoptive therapy have already confirmed the safety of NK-92 cell infusion, even at high doses [93]. A reduced risk of CRS characterizes CAR-engineered NK-92 and NK-92MI (a modified IL-2-independent NK-92 cell line), as they release a small amount of cytokines and exhibit direct killing of tumor cells by releasing toxic granules [110].

NK-92 cells are characterized by the lack of CD16 expression on their surface, which makes them unsuitable for ADCC assays. In contrast, an average population of NK cells in peripheral blood exhibits polymorphisms in CD16 receptors, leading to the expression of CD16 proteins with different affinities to Fc fragments of antibodies [111]. Therefore, for CAR applications, some emphasis is placed on genetic modification of NK-92 cells to obtain cell clones with expression of the high-affinity CD16 receptors [112], in order to increase their anti-tumor activity through ADCC (reviewed in [109]). Additionally, some other approaches have been undertaken to obtain clones of NK-92 cells with particular features. Some inhibitory receptors and checkpoint molecules, such as NKG2A, TIGIT, and CBLB, blocking the NK cell activation, can be knocked out by CRISPR/Cas9 gene-editing technology to increase the anti-tumor cytotoxicity of NK-92 cells clones used for modification with CAR constructs [80].

Series of CAR-NK-92 cell lines have been generated and tested in numerous preclinical in vitro and in vivo models of hematologic and solid tumors, proving the good potency of these therapies against different cancer types, including anti-CD3 [113], anti-CD4 [114], anti-CD5 [115], and anti-CD7 [116] CAR-NK-92 treatment for T cell-derived malignancies; anti-EGFR CAR treatment for metastatic breast cancer [117]; and anti-CS1- and anti-CD138 CAR treatment for multiple myeloma [118,119]. Other CAR-modified NK-92 cells used in the preclinical studies targeted the following antigens: CD33 (Rafiq et al., 2015 Cytotherapy [120]), GPA7 [121], HER2 [100,122,123], CD19 (Romanski et al., 2004 Blood [124]), CD20 [125], and GD2 [126]. Additionally, dual and multi-targeting CAR approaches have also been applied to generate CAR-NK-92 cells targeting CD19 and CD138 antigens [127]. Generally, in syngeneic animal models, the treatment with CAR-expressing NK-92 cells results in the activation of endogenous anti-tumor immunity, leading to tumor destruction and the emergence of a long-term immunological memory against tumor rechallenge (reviewed in [110]).

Following CAR-T cell therapy progress, advanced approaches to designing CAR constructs, such as the TRUCK technology, have also been used to modify NK cells in order to improve their anti-tumor function. The work of Rudek et al. investigated the functionality of inducible promoters responsive to NFAT or NFκB transcription factors for the induction of cytokine release. Such TRUCK anti-GD2-CAR-NK-92 cells and -CAR-primary NK cells exhibited great potency, and also enhanced cytotoxic activity and specific activation [128].

The first clinical trial results regarding CAR-NK-92 targeting the CD33 antigen on human relapsed and refractory acute myeloid leukemia (AML) cells were reported in 2018 [64]. The paragraph "Clinical trials summary" describes the current clinical trials using CAR-NK-92 therapies.

5. CAR-Engineered Primary NK Cells

The improvement of GMP-compliant procedures for efficient isolation, ex vivo expansion of blood-derived NK cells, and generation of CAR-NK cells [129] brings hope for allogeneic CAR-NK cell transfer as a potential "off-the-shelf" product that can significantly improve availability and reduce the cost of such therapies. However, the need to use the NK cell isolation kits and either the feeder cells or a variety of cytokines for expansion makes the procedure more expensive compared to the preparation of CAR-NK-92 cells [130]. Umbilical cord blood (UCB) seems to be a better source of NK cells than peripheral blood, since NK cells constitute as much as 30% of circulating lymphocytes. Additionally, UCB is easy to harvest and cryopreserve, which makes UCB-derived NK cells even more suitable for "off-the-shelf" applications [131]. On the other hand, they represent a less mature phenotype, lower tumor cell-directed cytotoxicity, and higher expression of inhibitory receptors, such as NKG2A, when compared to the peripheral blood-derived NK cells [132]. Unfortunately, a small volume of cord blood available from a single donor, makes it necessary to expand isolated NK cells and get the sufficient number for infusion [131]. In contrast to NK-92, the primary NK cells-derived therapy is also difficult to standardize, since the peripheral blood and UCB sources are not homogenous.

Due to the shorter lifespan of NK cells, adoptively transferred NK cells exhibit almost no side effects associated with their use. On the other hand, the limited life span of primary NK cells is a source of short-duration responses to CAR-NK therapy. To overcome this challenge, Liu et al. [62] engineered cord blood-derived NK cells with expression of both CAR construct and interleukin 15 (IL-15), which significantly improved the persistence in vivo as well as the cytotoxic function of NK cells. Such CAR-NK cells, with expanded persistence and equipped with additional expression of inducible caspase 9 as a safety switch in case of NK overactivation, have been successfully used in a small clinical trial for the therapy of relapsed and refractory blood malignancies, and exhibited an excellent safety profile [59]. The GVHD, CRS, neurotoxicity, and elevated levels of inflammatory factors were not found [59]. Current clinical trials using UCB and peripheral blood-derived CAR-NK cells are mentioned below in the paragraph "Clinical trials summary".

To improve the proliferation and cytotoxic activity of CD33-targeting CAR-NK cells, Albinger et al. [78] demonstrated the possibility of transducing blood-derived primary NK cells with CAR-encoding pseudotyped baboon envelope lentiviral vectors (BaEV-LVs), leading to stable CAR expression in NK cells and their great anti-tumor potency in mouse models of AML [78]. The CD33 antigen is considered an attractive target for therapy to treat myeloid malignancies. Interestingly, Hejazi et al. [133] discovered that the subpopulation of anti-CD33 CAR-NK cells during expansion in vitro undergoes a fratricide-like elimination due to the expression of CD33 antigen on their surface. CD33-positive NK cells exhibit distinctive biological features, such as higher mobilization of cytotoxic granules and higher production of IFNγ and TNFα, while the CD33-negative NK subset shows increased ADCC activity. The expansion of peripheral blood-derived NK cells in NK MACS medium (Miltenyi Biotech), especially, resulted in the most abundant (up to 50%) appearance of the CD33-positive NK cell population [133]. Therefore, depending on the stimulation protocol, it is possible to produce either CD33-positive NK cells that combine effective target cell killing and cytokine production or CD33-negative NK cells that produce fewer cytokines. Still, they are more efficient in antibody-dependent cytotoxicity [133].

Although the CAR constructs optimized for T cell signaling, consisting of CD3ζ and 4-1BB, are often used to modify NK cells, several NK-specific signaling domains, such as DAP10, DAP12 [134], and activating receptor 2B4 [97], have been incorporated in CAR constructs (reviewed in [54]). Some new CAR-related approaches are based on employing NKG2D, one of the NK activating receptors (NKGs) with broad target specificity, which induces NK intracellular signaling through DAP10 phosphorylation and can be incorporated in the CAR construct [135]. Recently, such a CAR construct, based on NKG2D, has been tested on genetically-modified NK and T cells. Although the CAR expression upon transduction was found to be more stable in T cells, more significant cytotoxicity toward multiple myeloma was detected in the case of CAR-NK cells [63].

6. iPSCs-Derived CAR-NK Cells

As the NK cells derived from either UCB or peripheral blood are neither well-characterized nor homogeneous populations, additional sources of NK cells for modification with CAR constructs have been explored. Some protocols allow the generation of mature NK cells from hematopoietic stem cells (HSCs) [87] or iPSCs [85,136]. NK cells differentiated from HSCs exhibit a mature phenotype, with expression of activating receptors and potent cytotoxicity toward tumor cells [137]. The iPSCs, obtained by reversing the developmental program of somatic cells, are currently an excellent, ever-evolving tool of regenerative medicine [138,139]. Notably, only one CAR-engineered iPSC cell is sufficient to differentiate into many highly homogeneous CAR-NK cells for clinical use. In this case, patients can even be administered with multiple doses of CAR-NK to overcome the limitation of the short lifetime of NK cells. The iPSC-derived NK cells are homogeneous, since they are derived from a clonal population and exhibit long-term expansion potential. CAR-NK therapy with iPSC allows for the large-scale production of a standardized product and its administration in multiple doses [140].

Unfortunately, when compared to HSCs, iPSCs are a source of less mature NK cells, with lower expression of CD16 but higher expression of inhibitory receptor NKG2A [141,142]. Nevertheless, in some animal tumor models, the iPSCs-derived CAR-NK cells exhibit similar anti-tumor activity as the peripheral blood-derived CAR-NK cells [141]. Some new improvements in CAR constructs have been tested in iPSCs-derived CAR-NK platforms, such as CAR containing the transmembrane domain of NKG2D and the 2B4 co-stimulatory domain [85], proving their outstanding performance in animal models. In most cases, CAR constructs are introduced into NK cells by retroviral vectors, with their efficiency reaching a maximum of about 50%. Interestingly, Li et al. [85] have proven that iPSCs-derived NK cells can be genetically modified with large DNA fragments by transposon systems, which provide higher biosafety and low immunogenicity compared to viral vectors [143]. Noteworthily, the process of iPSC-NK cell differentiation and maintaining a stable culture of iPSC-NK cells for clinical use remains a challenge, since many factors can influence the iPSC differentiation process: for example, the components of the culture medium [144] and the oxygen supply [145]. The pluripotent stem cells have a propensity for spontaneous differentiation [139]. The development of new protocols allows for the maintenance of a homogenous population of undifferentiated iPSCs characterized by the expression of pluripotent markers, such as stage-specific embryonic antigen 4 (SSEA4) and TRA-1-81. This enables further usage of these cells in a variety of clinical applications [146], including the production of iPSC-derived NK cells. Chen et al. defined Essential 8TM (E8) as a medium designed for the growth and propagation of human PSCs for up to >50 passages [144]. Essential 8TM does not require the presence of BSA (Bovine Serum Albumin) or HSA (Human Serum Albumin), which can cause batch-to-batch variability. The E8 base medium, in the conditions of 5% CO_2 availability, provides a pH of 7.4. iPSC cultures require a stable environment of 37 °C, 5% CO_2, 5% O_2, and around 95% relative humidity. To minimize spontaneous differentiation and chromosomal abnormalities, while inducing cell proliferation, regulation of oxygen concentration to physiological levels (2%–5%) is critical in pluripotent stem cell culture [147,148]. PSCs form colonies, and a suitable material is needed to cover the dish to ensure proper contact between the growing cells, e.g., synthetic extracellular matrix (ECM) [149]. Ni et al. demonstrated that the synthetic peptide-based surface-coating Synthemax II-SC (Corning) could be used in iPSC culture [150]. In addition, vitronectin (VTN), a recombinant ECM xenon-free protein, has been recognized as a component supporting the proliferation rate of human iPSCs under cGMP requirements [151]. Two- and three-dimensional (2D and 3D) culture systems are used to induce hematopoietic differentiation and pass the hematopoietic progenitor cell (HPC) stage to acquire NK cells. Feeder systems assure higher differentiation efficiency, but also increase cost, as more feeder cells are needed for large-scale manufacturing [152].

7. CAR-NK as a Therapy for Solid Tumors

Although quite efficient in curing blood malignancies, CAR therapy faces the following hurdles in curing solid tumors:

- Higher heterogeneity of tumor cells;
- Weak intratumoral penetration and trafficking of CAR-modified immune cells;
- Inhibition of immune cell activation by checkpoint molecules and immunosuppressive TME.

The higher heterogeneity of tumor cells results in a higher probability of target antigen loss on tumor cells during CAR therapy [153]. However, CAR-NK therapy is considered advantageous over CAR-T treatment due to the innate anti-tumor cytolytic capacity of NK cells, which allows the CAR-NK cells to kill tumors using diversified mechanisms, both CAR-dependent and CAR-independent. Additionally, it has been reported that NK cells can eliminate cancer stem cells, usually the most therapy-resistant types of cells residing in solid tumors [154]. The elimination of cancer stem cells is based on decreased MHC-I expression on their surface and the presence of ligands (such as MICA/B proteins) stimulating NKG2D, one of the activating receptors on NK cells [155–157]. Certain cytokines secreted by activated NK cells, such as INF-γ and TNF-α, have been reported to stimulate the differentiation of cancer stem cells, leading to the loss of their self-renewal abilities and chemotherapy resistance (reviewed in [158]).

Several solutions have been implemented to overcome the immunosuppressive TME and enhance the antitumor function of CAR-NK cells. In preclinical studies, some approaches, such as overexpression of chemokine receptors CXCR4 or CXCR1 in CAR-NK cells, have been reported to improve significantly their infiltration into glioblastoma [159] and ovarian cancer [160], respectively. The function of infiltrating immune cells, including NK cells, can, however, be efficiently blocked by tumor cells using the immune checkpoint molecules (reviewed in [161]). Therefore, the blockade of checkpoint receptor TIGIT, associated with the exhaustion of tumor-infiltrating NK cells, has been shown as a promising strategy in the preclinical treatment of colon cancer [162]. An exciting approach to blocking the axis of checkpoint molecules PD1/PD-L1 has been proposed by expression of a chimeric protein PD1-NKG2D-41BB in NK cells, which switches the inhibitory signal from the PD1 receptor to the activating one [163].

The cytotoxic functions of T and NK cells can also be efficiently inhibited by various cytokines and metabolites released by both tumor cells and other cell types present in the solid tumor microenvironment (reviewed in [164]). Expressing a dominant-negative TGFβ receptor II, which blocks TGFβ function, in NK cells has been shown as a strategy to overcome the loss of cytotoxicity by NK cells in the glioblastoma TME [165].

Numerous tumor-type-associated antigens have been used as targets for CAR-NK therapy in preclinical studies, whereas primarily NK-92 cells have been used as CAR platforms. Progression of high-grade glioblastoma is often driven by the expression of EGFRvIII antigen, a constitutively active mutant of the EGF receptor. Interestingly, to prevent EGFRvIII antigen escape, a therapy with dual-specificity CAR-NK cells, recognizing both mutated and wild-type variants of EGFR, has been shown to prolong the survival of glioblastoma-bearing animals [166,167]. Breast cancers have been efficiently treated by CAR-NK therapy targeting a variety of antigens highly expressed on the surface of breast cancer cells, including HER-2 [100,122,123], tissue factor [168], and EpCAM [169]. Ovarian cancer has been treated by CAR-NK targeting mesothelin antigens [170] or CD24 receptors [171], while pancreatic cancer has been targeted by CAR-NK cells via recognition of ROBO1 antigens [172,173] or folate receptors, used as an antigen for therapy of both tumor types [174,175]. Additionally, c-Met receptors [176] and PSMA [177] have been targeted by CAR-NK cells in therapy for liver and prostate cancers, respectively. An interesting approach with switchable CAR (described in more detail in the "CAR engineering" paragraph), recognizing specific target molecules with GD2 antigen-binding moiety, has been proven useful for the treatment of neuroblastoma and melanoma [126].

8. Clinical Trials Summary

In Table 1, we summarize the currently registered clinical studies. According to ClinicalTrials.gov, by November 2022, 42 clinical trials were testing CAR-NK therapy alone or CAR-NK in combination with other drugs. Patient enrollment is ongoing for 27 studies; 4 still need to enter the recruitment phase, and the status of 11 studies is unknown. Most of the presented clinical trials are being conducted in China (n = 28), eight studies are being performed in the United States, one study is located in Germany, and five have an unknown location.

Table 1. The summary of currently registered clinical trials based on CAR-NK therapy.

Title	Trial Number (Number of Participants); Phase	Cancer Type	Treatment; Dosage †	Location
Intracranial Injection of NK-92/5.28.z Cells in Combination With Intravenous Ezabenlimab in Patients With Recurrent HER2-positive Glioblastoma *	NCT03383978 (42); 1	Glioblastoma	CAR-NK-92/5.28.z Doses: 1×10^7–1×10^8 CAR-NK cells Ezabenlimab: 240 mg The standard therapy for glioblastoma (radiotherapy and alkylating chemotherapy) allowed until two weeks and Temozolomide allowed up to 48 h prior to the study	Germany
Clinical Research of Adoptive BCMA CAR-NK Cells on Relapse/Refractory MM +	NCT03940833 (20); 1,2	Multiple Myeloma	BCMA CAR-NK 92 cells	China
CAR-pNK Cell Immunotherapy in CD7 Positive Leukemia and Lymphoma *	NCT02742727 (10); 1,2	Myeloid Leukemia Acute Precursor T-Cell Lymphoblastic Leukemia-Lymphoma T-cell Prolymphocytic Leukemia	anti-CD7 CAR-pNK cells; The allogeneic NK-92 cell line engineered to contain anti-CD7 attached to TCRzeta, CD28 and 4-1BB signaling domains	China
CAR-pNK Cell Immunotherapy for Relapsed/Refractory CD33+ AML+	NCT02944162 (10); 1,2	Myeloid Leukemia Acute	CD33 CAR-NK NK92cells; chimeric antigen receptor NK92 cells transduced with the anti-CD33 vector anti-CD33 CAR-NK (coupled with CD28, CD137 and CD3 zeta signaling domains)	China
NKG2D CAR-NK Cell Therapy in Patients With Relapsed or Refractory Acute Myeloid Leukemia *	NCT05247957 (9); 1	Myeloid Leukemia Relapsed/Refractory Acute	NKG2D ligand-specific umbilical cord blood CAR-NK cells Doses: 2×10^6/kg, 6×10^6/kg, 18×10^6/kg CAR-NK cells, Preconditioning: standard chemotherapy	China
NKG2D-CAR-NK92 Cells Immunotherapy for Solid Tumors *	NCT05528341 (20); 1	Solid Tumors Relapsed/Refractory	NKG2D-CAR-NK92 cells; CAR-NK92 cells targeting NKG2D ligands, Doses: 0.5×10^6, 2×10^6/kg	China
NKG2D CAR-NK Cell Therapy in Patients With Refractory Metastatic Colorectal Cancer *	NCT05213195 (38); 1	Refractory Metastatic Colorectal Cancer	NKG2DL-CAR-NK cells; CAR-NK cells targeting NKG2D ligands,	China

Table 1. *Cont.*

Title	Trial Number (Number of Participants); Phase	Cancer Type	Treatment; Dosage †	Location
Pilot Study of NKG2D-Ligand Targeted CAR-NK Cells in Patients With Metastatic Solid Tumors +	NCT03415100 (30); 1	Solid Tumors	NKG2DL-CAR-NK cells; CAR-NK cells targeting NKG2D ligands	China
NKX101, Intravenous Allogeneic CAR NK Cells, in Adults With AML or MDS *	NCT04623944 (90); 1	AML, AML Relapsed/Refractory, Adult MDS	NKX101 allogeneic CAR NK cells targeting NKG2D ligands NK cells from haplo-matched related or unrelated donor Doses: 1×10^8 CAR-NK cells (2×10^6/kg for weight < 50 kg), 1.5×10^8 CAR-NK cells (3×10^6/kg for weight < 50 kg) Lymphodepletion: fludarabine/cyclophosphamide or fludarabine/cytarabine (ara-C)	United States
NKX019, Intravenous Allogeneic Chimeric Antigen Receptor Natural Killer Cells (CAR NK), in Adults With B-cell Cancers *	NCT05020678 (60); 1	Lymphoma, Non-Hodgkin B-cell Acute Lymphoblastic Leukemia, Large B-cell Lymphoma	NKX019 allogeneic CAR NK product targeting CD19 on cells. Doses: 3×10^8 NK cells (2×10^6/kg for weight < 50 kg). Lymphodepletion: fludarabine/cyclophosphamide	United States
Anti-CD19 Universal CAR-NK Cells Therapy Combined With HSCT for B Cell Hematologic Malignancies	NCT05570188 (30); 1,2 (Withdrawn -the principal investigator decides to stop)	B-cell Lymphoma B-cell Leukemia	anti-CD19 UCAR-NK cells; Preconditioning: Hematopoietic Stem Cell Transplantation(HSCT) Doses: $5-10 \times 10^6$/kg, $1-2 \times 10^7$/kg, $2-5 \times 10^7$/kg	China
Anti-CD19 CAR-Engineered NK Cells in the Treatment of Relapsed/Refractory Acute Lymphoblastic Leukemia	NCT05563545 (Completed, November 28, 2023) (21); 1	recurrent or refractory CD19 positive acute lymphoblastic leukemia	CAR-NK-CD19 Cells; Doses: 1.0×10^7, 2.0×10^7 and 3.0×10^7 cells /kg, Lymphodepletion: Fludarabine (25–30 mg/kg), Cyclophosphamide (250–300 mg/kg)	China
Anti-CD19 CAR-Engineered NK Cells in the Treatment of Relapsed/Refractory Acute Lymphoblastic Leukemia *	NCT05410041 (21); 1	lymphocyte leukemia, B-cell non-Hodgkin's lymphoma and chronic B-lymphocyte leukemia	CAR-NK-CD19 Cells; Doses: 1.0×10^7, 2.0×10^7 and 3.0×10^7 cells /kg, Lymphodepletion: Fludarabine (25–30 mg/kg), Cyclophosphamide (250–300 mg/kg)	China
Natural Killer (NK) Cell Therapy for B-Cell Malignancies *	NCT05379647 (24); 1	B-cell Lymphoma B-cell Acute Lymphoblastic Leukemia	QN-019-a (allogeneic CAR-NK cells targeting CD19) as monotherapy or in combination with Rituximab, Lymphodepletion: Cyclophosphamid, Fludarabine, VP-16	China
Study of Anti-CD19 CAR NK Cells in Relapsed and Refractory B Cell Lymphoma +	NCT03690310 (15); 1	Refractory B-Cell Lymphoma	anti-CD19 CAR NK Cells; Doses: $50-600 \; 10^3$/kg	unknown
Clinical Study of HLA Haploidentical CAR-NK Cells Targeting CD19 in the Treatment of Refractory/Relapsed B-cell NHL *	NCT04887012 (25); 1	B-cell Non-Hodgkin Lymphoma	anti-CD19 CAR-NK; lentiviral vector-transduced HLA haploidentical NK cells express anti-CD19 CAR	China

Table 1. Cont.

Title	Trial Number (Number of Participants); Phase	Cancer Type	Treatment; Dosage †	Location
Anti-CD19 CAR NK Cell Therapy for R/R Non-Hodgkin Lymphoma #	NCT04639739 (9); 1	Non-Hodgkin Lymphoma	anti-CD19 CAR-NK; Doses: 2×10^6 /kg, 6×10^6 /kg, 2×10^7/kg Lymphodepletion: Fludarabine (30 mg/m^2) Cyclophosphamide (500 mg/m^2)	China
Anti-CD19 CAR-Engineered NK Cells in the Treatment of Relapsed/Refractory B-cell Malignancies *	NCT05410041 NCT03690310 (9); 1	Lymphocytic Leukemia Chronic/Acute Non-Hodgkin Lymphoma	CAR-NK-CD19 Cells; Derived from allogenic NK cells Doses: $1–3 \times 10^7$ /KG, Lymphodepletion: Fludarabine (25–30 mg/kg) Cyclophosphamide (250–300 mg/kg)	China
Allogeneic NK T-Cells Expressing CD19 Specific CAR in B-Cell Malignancies (ANCHOR2) *	NCT05487651 (36); 1	Non-Hodgkin Lymphoma, Relapsed, Adult B-cell Lymphoma B-cell Leukemia	KUR-502 - transduced allogeneic natural killer T cells against CD19 (CD19.CAR-aNKT cells) Doses: 1×10^7/m^2, 3×10^7/m^2, 1×10^8/m^2. Body surface area (BSA) capped at 2.4 m^2. Lymphodepletion: cyclophosphamide (500 mg/m^2/day) Fludarabine (30 mg/m^2/day)	United States
Study of Anti-CD19/CD22 CAR NK Cells in Relapsed and Refractory B Cell Lymphoma +	NCT03824964 (10); 1	Relapsed/Refractory B-Cell Lymphoma	Anti-CD19/CD22 CAR NK Cells; Doses: 50–600 10^3 cells/kg	unknown
Study of Anti-CD22 CAR NK Cells in Relapsed and Refractory B Cell Lymphoma +	NCT03692767 (9); 1	Relapsed /Refractory B-Cell Lymphoma	Anti-CD22 CAR NK Cells Derived from allogenic NK cells Doses: 50–600 10^3 cells /kg	unknown
Study of Anti-CD33/CLL1 CAR-NK in Acute Myeloid Leukemia *	NCT05215015 (18); 1	Myeloid Leukemia Acute	Anti-CD33/CLL1 CAR-NK Cells; Doses: 2.0×10^9, 3.0×10^9, 3.0×10^9 cells	China
Anti-CD33 CAR NK Cells in the Treatment of Relapsed/Refractory Acute Myeloid Leukemia *	NCT05008575 (27); 1	Leukemia, Myeloid, Acute	anti-CD33 CAR NK cells; Doses: 6×10^8, 12×10^8, 18×10^8 cells/KG Lymphodepletion: Fludarabine (30 mg/m^2) Cytoxan (300–500 mg/m^2)	China
Study of Anti-5T4 CAR-NK Cell Therapy in Advanced Solid Tumors *	NCT05194709 (40); 1	Solid Tumors Advanced	Anti-5T4 Oncofetal Trophoblast Glycoprotein (5T4) Conjugated Antibody Redirecting Natural Killer (CAR-NK) Cells Doses: 3.0×10^9, 4.0×10^9, 4.0×10^9 cells	China
Allogenic CD123-CAR-NK Cells in the Treatment of Refractory/Relapsed Acute Myeloid Leukemia #	NCT05574608 (12); 1	Acute Myeloid Leukemia Refractory/ Recurrent	Allogenic CD123-CAR-NK cells; Doses: 1×10^6/kg, 5×10^6/kg, 2×10^7/kg Lymphodepletion: Fludarabine, Cyclophosphamide	unknown
Phase I/II Study of CAR.70-Engineered IL15-transduced Cord Blood-derived NK Cells in Conjunction With Lymphodepleting Chemotherapy for the Management of Relapse/Refractory Hematological Malignancies *	NCT05092451 (94); 1,2	Leukemia, Lymphoma, or Multiple Myeloma	CAR.70/IL15-transduced Cord blood NK cells; Lymphodepletion: Cyclophosphamide Fludarabine phosphate	United States

Table 1. Cont.

Title	Trial Number (Number of Participants); Phase	Cancer Type	Treatment; Dosage †	Location
Anti-BCMA CAR-NK Cell Therapy for the Relapsed or Refractory Multiple Myeloma *	NCT05008536 (27); 1	Multiple Myeloma, Refractory	Anti-BCMA CAR-NK, NK Cells from umbilical cord blood, Doses: $1-3 \times 10^6$/KG, $3-6 \times 10^6$/KG, $0.6-1.2 \times 10^7$/KG Lymphodepletion: Fludarabine (30 mg/m^2), Cytoxan (300–500 mg/m^2)	China
Cord Blood Derived Anti-CD19 CAR-Engineered NK Cells for B Lymphoid Malignancies *	NCT04796675 (27); 1	Lymphocytic Leukemia Chronic/Acute Non-Hodgkin's Lymphoma	Cord blood derived NK cells from healthy donor, transduced with a retroviral vector encoding the anti-CD19 CAR and interleukin-15.CAR-NK-CD19 Cells; Doses: $0.01 \times 10^7, 0.1 \times 10^7, 1.0 \times 10^7$/kg Lymphodepletion: fludarabine (30 mg/kg) cyclophosphamide (300 mg/kg)	China
Clinical Study of Cord Blood-derived CAR-NK Cells Targeting CD19 in the Treatment of Refractory/Relapsed B-cell NHL *	NCT05472558 (48); 1	B-cell Non-Hodgkin Lymphoma	anti-CD19 CAR-NK; Doses: 2.5×10^8 cells, 5×10^8 cells, 1×10^9 cells	China
Phase I/II Study of CD5 CAR Engineered IL15-Transduced Cord Blood-Derived NK Cells in Conjunction With Lymphodepleting Chemotherapy for the Management of Relapsed/Refractory Hematological Malignancies #	NCT05110742 (48); 1,2	Hematological Malignancy	CAR.5/IL15-transduced cord blood NK cells; Doses: $1 \times 10^7, 1 \times 10^8, 1 \times 10^9, 1 \times 10^{10}$ cells Lymphodepletion: Cyclophosphamide and Fludarabine or Fludarabine Phosphate	United States
Umbilical & Cord Blood (CB) Derived CAR-Engineered NK Cells for B Lymphoid Malignancies #	NCT03056339 (36); 1,2	B-Lymphoid Malignancies Lymphocytic Leukemia Chronic/Acute Non-Hodgkin Lymphoma	CAR-NK cells CD19-CD28-zeta-2A-iCasp9-IL15-transduced cord blood natural killer (CB-NK) cells Lymphodepletion: Fludarabine Cyclophosphamide (AP1903 in case of graft-versus-host disease (GvHD) or cytokine release syndrome after the NK cell infusion)	United States
Study of Anti-Mesothelin Car NK Cells in Epithelial Ovarian Cancer +	NCT03692637 (30); 1	Epithelial Ovarian Cancer	anti-Mesothelin CAR NK Cells; Doses: $0.5-3 \times 10^6$/kg cells	unknown
Study of Anti-PSMA CAR NK Cell (TABP EIC) in Metastatic Castration-Resistant Prostate Cancer *	NCT03692663 (9); 1	Metastatic Castration-resistant Prostate Cancer	TABP EIC (anti-PSMA CAR NK cells) Doses: 0.5, 10, and 30×10^6 CAR NK cells Lymphodepletion: Cyclophosphamide 250 mg/m^2, fludarabine 25 mg/m^2	China
CLDN6-CAR-NK Cell Therapy for Advanced Solid Tumors *	NCT05410717 (40); 1,2	Stage IV Ovarian Cancer Testis Cancer, Refractory Endometrial Cancer Recurrent	CAR-NK cells from patients PMBC; (some CAR-NK cells are genetically engineered to express and secret IL7/CCL19 and/or SCFVs against PD1/CTLA4/Lag3)	China
Study of DLL3-CAR-NK Cells in the Treatment of Extensive Stage Small Cell Lung Cancer *	NCT05507593 (18); 1	SCLC, Extensive Stage	DLL3-CAR-NK cells; Doses: $1 \times 10^7, 1 \times 10^8, 1 \times 10^9$ DLL3-CAR-NK cells	China

Table 1. Cont.

Title	Trial Number (Number of Participants); Phase	Cancer Type	Treatment; Dosage †	Location
Irradiated PD-L1 CAR-NK Cells Plus Pembrolizumab Plus N-803 for Subjects With Recurrent/Metastatic Gastric or Head and Neck Cancer *	NCT04847466 (55); 2	Gastroesophageal Junction (GEJ) Cancers Advanced HNSCC	Irradiated PD-L1 CAR-NK Cells Plus Pembrolizumab Plus N-803 Doses: 2×10^9 cells Pembrolizumab 400 mg N-803 (15 mcg/kg)	United States
FT576 in Subjects With Multiple Myeloma * (Allogenic CAR NK cells with BCMA expression)	NCT05182073 (168);1	Multiple Myeloma Myeloma	FT576 as monotherapy and in combination with the monoclonal antibody daratumumab FT576: allogeneic natural killer (NK) cells, derived from a clonal, CD38-knockout, iPSC that expresses BCMA, CAR, high-affinity, non-cleavable CD16 (hnCD16), and IL-15/IL-15 receptor fusion protein (IL-15RF). Lymphodepletion: Cyclophosphamide Fludarabine	United States
Induced-T Cell Like NK Cellular Immunotherapy for Cancer Lack of MHC-I +	NCT03882840 (30); 1,2	Anti-cancer Cell Immunotherapy T Cell and NK Cell	Induced-T cell-like NK cells; T-like NK cells (ITNK) from patient's T cells,	China
Induced-T Cell Like NK Cells for B Cell Malignancies *	NCT04747093 (12); 1,2	B Cell Leukemia B Cell Lymphoma B-cell Acute Lymphoblastic	CAR-ITNK cells; Induced-T cell-like NK cells with chimeric antigen receptor	China
Clinical Research of ROBO1 Specific BiCAR-NK Cells on Patients With Pancreatic Cancer +	NCT03941457 (9); 1,2	Pancreatic Cancer	BiCAR-NK cells- (ROBO1 CAR-NK cells) Derived from allogenic NK cells	China
Clinical Research of ROBO1 Specific BiCAR-NK/T Cells on Patients With Malignant Tumor +	NCT03931720 (20); 1,2	Malignant Tumor	BiCAR-NK/T cells (ROBO1 CAR-NK/T cells) Derived from allogenic NK cells	China
Clinical Research of ROBO1 Specific CAR-NK Cells on Patients With Solid Tumors +	NCT03940820 (20); 1,2	Solid Tumor	ROBO1 CAR-NK cells; Derived from allogenic NK cells	China

* recruiting; # not yet recruiting; + unknown status; † information about pre-condition treatment, type of cells used, and the dosage of CAR-NK cells, if available.

Almost all trials are open-label, single-group assignment studies. Some of them have parallel assignment (NCT05379647 and NCT05487651) or sequential assignment (NCT03692767, NCT05574608, NCT05110742, and NCT05507593). Only one study is characterized as a randomized trial: Phase I/II Study of CAR.70-Engineered IL15-transduced Cord Blood-derived NK Cells in Conjunction With Lymphodepleting Chemotherapy for the Management of Relapse/Refractory Hematological Malignances (NCT05092451).

The clinical trials conducted using CAR-NK have mainly focused on the neoplastic diseases of hematopoietic organs, such as lymphoma and leukemia, NHL, multiple myeloma, and myelodysplastic syndromes (MDS). Some trials concern reproductive tract tumors: prostate cancer, ovarian cancer, testis cancer, endometrial cancer, and epithelial ovarian cancer. Therapy with CAR-NK is also being tested for other solid tumors, such as small cell lung cancer (SCLC), head and neck squamous cell carcinoma (HNSCC), pancreatic cancer, colorectal cancer, and gastroesophageal junction (GEJ) cancer.

The results from a few clinical trials testing CAR-NK therapy's potential for solid tumors have been published (reviewed in [178]). The Phase I / II clinical trials of allogeneic cellular immunotherapy with CAR-NK-92 indicate the possibility of treating non-hematological neoplasms with ROBO-1-CAR-NK cells [179,180]. The combination of CAR-NK cells and anti-cancer drugs is a promising type of therapy to alter the immunosuppressive TME and the metastatic capacity of refractory tumors (reviewed in [178]).

NKG2D is an activated receptor expressed on the surface of human NK cells and some T cells. However, it is absent in healthy tissue. It plays a vital role in innate immunity, as it is involved in recognizing virus-infected cells and killing cancer cells with NK. Five clinical studies developed NKG2D-based CAR-NK therapies to treat myeloid leukemia and solid tumors. The in vitro studies have already demonstrated the anti-tumor action of NKG2D-DAP10-CD3ζ-CAR-NK cells against osteosarcoma cell lines, pancreatic cancer, and breast cancer. A few NKG2D-based CAR therapies are described, with anti-mesothelin-NKG2D-2B4 CARs showing the best results regarding anti-tumor response, proving the potential of 2B4 as the co-stimulatory domain in CAR constructs (reviewed in [181]).

Table 1 presents clinical trial schemas, including CAR-NK cell infusions combined with chemotherapeutics such as cyclophosphamide, fludarabine, and Cytoxan. Phase II trial of PD-L1-CAR-NK cell immunotherapy, in combination with an IL-15 agonist (N-803) and pembrolizumab (NCT04847466), is currently underway among patients with head and neck cancers and gastric cancers in the United States. A German clinical trial is testing the combination therapy of CAR-NK-92 with the anti-PD-1 antibody Ezabenlimab in Patients With Recurrent HER2-positive Glioblastoma (NCT03383978).

A clinical trial with the CAR NK cells targeting the prostate-specific membrane antigen (PSMA) is being carried out in a group of patients with metastatic castration-resistant prostate cancer (NCT03692663). Published results of combined treatment with CAR NK-92 and anti-PD-L1 monoclonal antibody have confirmed its anti-tumor efficacy against prostate cancer in a mouse model [182].

Another phase I/IIa study (NCT05410717) is being carried out in 40 patients with Claudin 6-positive advanced solid tumors. Engineered Claudin 6-targeting CAR is introduced into NK cells isolated from the peripheral blood of patients with advanced ovarian cancer or other cancers expressing Claudin 6. To enhance the killing capability, the CAR-NK cells are genetically engineered to express and secrete IL7/CCL19 and/or scFvs against PD1/CTLA4/Lag3.

Table 1 also summarizes the target antigens used in current clinical trials employing CAR-NK cells. The CD19 antigen is the most prevalent in engineering CAR-NK and CAR-T cells [92]. Treatments of B cell tumors based on the anti-CD19 CAR-T cell products axicabtagene ciloleucel and tisagenlecleucel were the first to be approved by FDA (reviewed in [183]). The phase 1 and 2 trial results of 11 patients with relapsed or refractory CD19-positive cancers showed a favorable response to CD19-targeting CAR-NK therapy without developing significant toxic effects (NCT03056339 [59]).

Few CAR-NK therapies target AML with anti-CD33, anti-CLL1, and anti-CD123 CARs. The interest in CD33 is based on the fact that about 85–90% of AML cases express the CD33 antigen, whereas, on normal pluripotent hematopoietic stem cells, CD33 expression is absent [184,185]. The clinical trial results using CD33-CAR NK-92 cell infusion indicated that this therapy is safe, but exhibits low anti-leukemia efficacy [64]. Two clinical trials based on anti-CD33 CAR-NK (NCT05215015 and NCT05008575) are currently recruiting AML patients.

Another molecule, highly expressed in AML blasts but not on normal HSC cells, is the family of 12 C lectin domains (CLL1, also known as CLEC12A and MICL) [186]. The in vitro study confirmed that CLL1 CAR-NK cells efficiently eliminate the primary AML cells (Gurney et al., 2021 Blood [187]). Previously, CLL1 and CD33 were successfully used as targets for AML CAR-T cell therapy (Liu et al., 2018 Blood [188]). Please cite the two in number.

The highly expressed molecule in most AML cases is CD123 (Interleukin-3 receptor alpha; IL-3RA) [189]. NK cells expressing CARs targeting CD123 show antigen-specific anti-AML activity in vitro [190]. NK cells expressing a second-generation CAR directed against CD123 exhibit significantly higher cytotoxicity in AML cell lines [191]. In a planned, but not yet underway, clinical trial (NCT05574608), 12 patients with relapsed/refractory AML will receive fludarabine and cyclophosphamide chemotherapy followed by infusion of CD123-CAR-NK cells.

We found two registered clinical trials based on NK cells engineered with anti-CD22 CARs. Several studies have been performed previously with anti-CD22-CAR T-cells, since the expression of CD22, a sialic acid-binding adhesion molecule, is specific to most B-lineage malignancies [57]. Current clinical trial studies of anti-CD22 CAR-NK cells (NCT03692767) and dual anti-CD19/CD22 CAR-NK cells (NCT03824964) are planned against relapsed and refractory B Cell lymphoma. To prevent antigen escape, the CAR-NK cells simultaneously express the CD22-targeting CAR and CD19-specific T cell receptors. Previous in vitro studies have demonstrated that dual CD19/CD22 CAR-NK cells have anti-tumor activity against the ALL cell line [192]. In the murine xenograft model, CD22-CAR/CD19-engager NK cells recognized tumor cells in an antigen-dependent manner, redirected T cells to tumor cells, and caused significant leukemia regression (Szoor et al., 2017 J Immunol [193]).

For the treatment of relapsed or refractory multiple myeloma, clinical trials with CAR-NK cells that express an anti-BCMA (B-cell maturation antigen highly expressed on myeloma cells) construct, together with chemotherapy, are underway (NCT03940833, NCT05008536). The sources of allogeneic NK cells for these therapies are iPSCs and UCB. In a xenograft mouse model, anti-BCMA CAR-NK cells revealed anti-tumor efficiency against multiple myeloma [194]. Roex et al. developed a dual-CAR NK-92 cell line simultaneously targeting CD19 and BCMA, which efficiently recognize and eliminate single- and double-positive target cells, including primary tumor cells [195].

In three clinical trials, CAR-NK cells will target ROBO1 antigen on solid tumors. Bi- and tri-specific antibodies, as well as BiCARs, are novel immunotherapy strategies that can engage the immune effector cells so that they eliminate tumor cells by binding simultaneously to both cell types (NK and tumor cells). The forced proximity between these cells causes the release of cytotoxic molecules by effector cells, followed by apoptosis of tumor cells. This method previously showed good anti-cancer activity against several types of non-Hodgkin lymphomas [196,197].

T-cell-like NK cells are cytotoxic T-cells that co-express NK receptors such as CD56, CD16, and/or CD57. They are involved in cytotoxic killing, and, like NK cells, are not restricted by MHC recognition [198]. Two studies (NCT04747093 and NCT03882840) are already recruiting patients with B-cell leukemia/lymphoma/acute lymphoblastic leukemia for therapy based on induced T cell-like NK cells.

9. Conclusions

Almost a decade has passed since the *Science* magazine named cancer immunotherapy the "Breakthrough of the Year 2013." Indeed, today, immunology is the most promising field of cancer research, raising great hopes for finding cures for cancer. Clinical approaches, such as CAR therapy or immune checkpoints blockade with antibodies, have revolutionized medicine. In recent years, more attention has been paid to NK cells and their potential usage in adoptive therapy, including CAR therapy, by administering these genetically modified effector cells to patients in order to fight cancer. There has already been significant evidence collected from the results of in vitro studies and animal models for the effective anti-tumor activity of CAR-NK therapies. In parallel, the engineering of CAR constructs is developing rapidly to create "smart" tools to support and improve existing CAR therapies. Numerous clinical trials using blood- or iPSCs-derived NK cells and NK-like cell lines are currently ongoing. However, further large-scale clinical trials are still required to improve the potency of CAR-NK therapy, not only against the most commonly targeted hematological tumor, but also to tackle solid tumors more efficiently.

Author Contributions: M.W. and B.P. wrote and approved the manuscript. All authors have read and agreed to the published version of the manuscript.

Funding: This work was funded by the National Science Centre (NCN, Poland), grant no: 2016/23/B/NZ5/02622.

Acknowledgments: The publication costs were partially covered by the Medical University of Warsaw internal funds. The figures were prepared using BioRender icons and templates.

Conflicts of Interest: The authors declare no conflict of interest.

References

1. Abel, A.M.; Yang, C.; Thakar, M.S.; Malarkannan, S. Natural Killer Cells: Development, Maturation, and Clinical Utilization. *Front. Immunol.* **2018**, *9*, 1869. [CrossRef] [PubMed]
2. Sivori, S.; Vacca, P.; Del Zotto, G.; Munari, E.; Mingari, M.C.; Moretta, L. Human NK cells: Surface receptors, inhibitory checkpoints, and translational applications. *Cell Mol. Immunol.* **2019**, *16*, 430–441. [CrossRef] [PubMed]
3. Prager, I.; Watzl, C. Mechanisms of natural killer cell-mediated cellular cytotoxicity. *J. Leukoc. Biol.* **2019**, *105*, 1319–1329. [CrossRef]
4. Prager, I.; Liesche, C.; van Ooijen, H.; Urlaub, D.; Verron, Q.; Sandstrom, N.; Fasbender, F.; Claus, M.; Eils, R.; Beaudouin, J.; et al. NK cells switch from granzyme B to death receptor-mediated cytotoxicity during serial killing. *J. Exp. Med.* **2019**, *216*, 2113–2127. [CrossRef] [PubMed]
5. Verron, Q.; Forslund, E.; Brandt, L.; Leino, M.; Frisk, T.W.; Olofsson, P.E.; Onfelt, B. NK cells integrate signals over large areas when building immune synapses but require local stimuli for degranulation. *Sci. Signal.* **2021**, *14*. [CrossRef] [PubMed]
6. Grimm, E.A.; Mazumder, A.; Zhang, H.Z.; Rosenberg, S.A. Lymphokine-activated killer cell phenomenon: Lysis of natural killer-resistant fresh solid tumor cells by interleukin 2-activated autologous human peripheral blood lymphocytes. *J. Exp. Med.* **1982**, *155*, 1823–1841. [CrossRef]
7. Rosenberg, S.A.; Yang, J.C.; Sherry, R.M.; Kammula, U.S.; Hughes, M.S.; Phan, G.Q.; Citrin, D.E.; Restifo, N.P.; Robbins, P.F.; Wunderlich, J.R.; et al. Durable complete responses in heavily pretreated patients with metastatic melanoma using T-cell transfer immunotherapy. *Clin. Cancer. Res.* **2011**, *17*, 4550–4557. [CrossRef]
8. Terunuma, H.; Deng, X.; Nishino, N.; Watanabe, K. NK cell-based autologous immune enhancement therapy (AIET) for cancer. *J. Stem. Cells. Regen. Med.* **2013**, *9*, 9–13.
9. Gross, G.; Gorochov, G.; Waks, T.; Eshhar, Z. Generation of effector T cells expressing chimeric T cell receptor with antibody type-specificity. *Transplant. Proc.* **1989**, *21*, 127–130.
10. Decker, W.K.; da Silva, R.F.; Sanabria, M.H.; Angelo, L.S.; Guimaraes, F.; Burt, B.M.; Kheradmand, F.; Paust, S. Cancer Immunotherapy: Historical Perspective of a Clinical Revolution and Emerging Preclinical Animal Models. *Front. Immunol.* **2017**, *8*, 829. [CrossRef]
11. Graham, C.; Hewitson, R.; Pagliuca, A.; Benjamin, R. Cancer immunotherapy with CAR-T cells—Behold the future. *Clin. Med.* **2018**, *18*, 324–328. [CrossRef] [PubMed]
12. June, C.H.; O'Connor, R.S.; Kawalekar, O.U.; Ghassemi, S.; Milone, M.C. CAR T cell immunotherapy for human cancer. *Science* **2018**, *359*, 1361–1365. [CrossRef] [PubMed]
13. Dirar, Q.; Russell, T.; Liu, L.; Ahn, S.; Dotti, G.; Aravamudhan, S.; Conforti, L.; Yun, Y. Activation and degranulation of CAR-T cells using engineered antigen-presenting cell surfaces. *PLoS One* **2020**, *15*, e0238819. [CrossRef]
14. Sterner, R.C.; Sterner, R.M. CAR-T cell therapy: Current limitations and potential strategies. *Blood Cancer J.* **2021**, *11*, 69. [CrossRef]
15. Wang, X.; Riviere, I. Clinical manufacturing of CAR T cells: Foundation of a promising therapy. *Mol. Ther. Oncolytics* **2016**, *3*, 16015. [CrossRef] [PubMed]
16. Grupp, S.A.; Kalos, M.; Barrett, D.; Aplenc, R.; Porter, D.L.; Rheingold, S.R.; Teachey, D.T.; Chew, A.; Hauck, B.; Wright, J.F.; et al. Chimeric antigen receptor-modified T cells for acute lymphoid leukemia. *N. Engl. J. Med.* **2013**, *368*, 1509–1518. [CrossRef]
17. First-Ever CAR T-cell Therapy Approved in U.S. *Cancer Discov.* **2017**, *7*, OF1. [CrossRef]
18. Heymach, J.; Krilov, L.; Alberg, A.; Baxter, N.; Chang, S.M.; Corcoran, R.B.; Dale, W.; DeMichele, A.; Magid Diefenbach, C.S.; Dreicer, R.; et al. Clinical Cancer Advances 2018: Annual Report on Progress Against Cancer from the American Society of Clinical Oncology. *J. Clin. Oncol.* **2018**, *36*, 1020–1044. [CrossRef]
19. Seo, B.; Kim, S.; Kim, J. The 100 Most Influential Studies in Chimeric Antigen Receptor T-Cell: A Bibliometric Analysis. *Front. Med. Technol.* **2020**, *2*, 3. [CrossRef]
20. Lundh, S.; Maji, S.; Melenhorst, J.J. Next-generation CAR T cells to overcome current drawbacks. *Int. J. Hematol.* **2021**, *114*, 532–543. [CrossRef]
21. Rodriguez-Garcia, A.; Palazon, A.; Noguera-Ortega, E.; Powell, D.J., Jr.; Guedan, S. CAR-T Cells Hit the Tumor Microenvironment: Strategies to Overcome Tumor Escape. *Front. Immunol.* **2020**, *11*, 1109. [CrossRef] [PubMed]
22. Tahmasebi, S.; Elahi, R.; Khosh, E.; Esmaeilzadeh, A. Programmable and multi-targeted CARs: A new breakthrough in cancer CAR-T cell therapy. *Clin. Transl. Oncol.* **2021**, *23*, 1003–1019. [CrossRef] [PubMed]
23. Safarzadeh Kozani, P.; Naseri, A.; Mirarefin, S.M.J.; Salem, F.; Nikbakht, M.; Evazi Bakhshi, S.; Safarzadeh Kozani, P. Nanobody-based CAR-T cells for cancer immunotherapy. *Biomark. Res.* **2022**, *10*, 24. [CrossRef]
24. Lam, N.; Trinklein, N.D.; Buelow, B.; Patterson, G.H.; Ojha, N.; Kochenderfer, J.N. Anti-BCMA chimeric antigen receptors with fully human heavy-chain-only antigen recognition domains. *Nat. Commun.* **2020**, *11*, 283. [CrossRef] [PubMed]
25. Raj, D.; Yang, M.H.; Rodgers, D.; Hampton, E.N.; Begum, J.; Mustafa, A.; Lorizio, D.; Garces, I.; Propper, D.; Kench, J.G.; et al. Switchable CAR-T cells mediate remission in metastatic pancreatic ductal adenocarcinoma. *Gut* **2019**, *68*, 1052–1064. [CrossRef]
26. Cao, Y.J.; Wang, X.; Wang, Z.; Zhao, L.; Li, S.; Zhang, Z.; Wei, X.; Yun, H.; Choi, S.H.; Liu, Z.; et al. Switchable CAR-T Cells Outperformed Traditional Antibody-Redirected Therapeutics Targeting Breast Cancers. *ACS Synth. Biol.* **2021**, *10*, 1176–1183. [CrossRef]

27. Qi, J.; Tsuji, K.; Hymel, D.; Burke, T.R., Jr.; Hudecek, M.; Rader, C.; Peng, H. Chemically Programmable and Switchable CAR-T Therapy. *Angew. Chem. Int. Ed. Engl.* **2020**, *59*, 12178–12185. [CrossRef]
28. Kuo, Y.C.; Kuo, C.F.; Jenkins, K.; Hung, A.F.; Chang, W.C.; Park, M.; Aguilar, B.; Starr, R.; Hibbard, J.; Brown, C.; et al. Antibody-based redirection of universal Fabrack-CAR T cells selectively kill antigen bearing tumor cells. *J. Immunother. Cancer* **2022**, *10*, e003752. [CrossRef]
29. Cho, J.H.; Collins, J.J.; Wong, W.W. Universal Chimeric Antigen Receptors for Multiplexed and Logical Control of T Cell Responses. *Cell* **2018**, *173*, 1426–1438.e1411. [CrossRef]
30. Hawkins, E.R.; D'Souza, R.R.; Klampatsa, A. Armored CAR T-Cells: The Next Chapter in T-Cell Cancer Immunotherapy. *Biologics* **2021**, *15*, 95–105. [CrossRef]
31. Nguyen, A.; Johanning, G.; Shi, Y. Emerging Novel Combined CAR-T Cell Therapies. *Cancers* **2022**, *14*, 1403. [CrossRef] [PubMed]
32. Adachi, K.; Kano, Y.; Nagai, T.; Okuyama, N.; Sakoda, Y.; Tamada, K. IL-7 and CCL19 expression in CAR-T cells improves immune cell infiltration and CAR-T cell survival in the tumor. *Nat. Biotechnol.* **2018**, *36*, 346–351. [CrossRef] [PubMed]
33. Golumba-Nagy, V.; Kuehle, J.; Hombach, A.A.; Abken, H. CD28-zeta CAR T Cells Resist TGF-beta Repression through IL-2 Signaling, Which Can Be Mimicked by an Engineered IL-7 Autocrine Loop. *Mol. Ther.* **2018**, *26*, 2218–2230. [CrossRef] [PubMed]
34. Koneru, M.; O'Cearbhaill, R.; Pendharkar, S.; Spriggs, D.R.; Brentjens, R.J. A phase I clinical trial of adoptive T cell therapy using IL-12 secreting MUC-16(ecto) directed chimeric antigen receptors for recurrent ovarian cancer. *J. Transl. Med.* **2015**, *13*, 102. [CrossRef]
35. Yeku, O.O.; Purdon, T.J.; Koneru, M.; Spriggs, D.; Brentjens, R.J. Armored CAR T cells enhance antitumor efficacy and overcome the tumor microenvironment. *Sci. Rep.* **2017**, *7*, 10541. [CrossRef]
36. Chen, Y.; Sun, C.; Landoni, E.; Metelitsa, L.; Dotti, G.; Savoldo, B. Eradication of Neuroblastoma by T Cells Redirected with an Optimized GD2-Specific Chimeric Antigen Receptor and Interleukin-15. *Clin. Cancer Res.* **2019**, *25*, 2915–2924. [CrossRef]
37. Chmielewski, M.; Abken, H. CAR T Cells Releasing IL-18 Convert to T-Bet(high) FoxO1(low) Effectors that Exhibit Augmented Activity against Advanced Solid Tumors. *Cell Rep.* **2017**, *21*, 3205–3219. [CrossRef]
38. Hu, B.; Ren, J.; Luo, Y.; Keith, B.; Young, R.M.; Scholler, J.; Zhao, Y.; June, C.H. Augmentation of Antitumor Immunity by Human and Mouse CAR T Cells Secreting IL-18. *Cell Rep.* **2017**, *20*, 3025–3033. [CrossRef]
39. Ma, X.; Shou, P.; Smith, C.; Chen, Y.; Du, H.; Sun, C.; Porterfield Kren, N.; Michaud, D.; Ahn, S.; Vincent, B.; et al. Interleukin-23 engineering improves CAR T cell function in solid tumors. *Nat. Biotechnol.* **2020**, *38*, 448–459. [CrossRef]
40. Brog, R.A.; Ferry, S.L.; Schiebout, C.T.; Messier, C.M.; Cook, W.J.; Abdullah, L.; Zou, J.; Kumar, P.; Sentman, C.L.; Frost, H.R.; et al. Superkine IL-2 and IL-33 Armored CAR T Cells Reshape the Tumor Microenvironment and Reduce Growth of Multiple Solid Tumors. *Cancer. Immunol. Res.* **2022**, *10*, 962–977. [CrossRef]
41. Suarez, E.R.; Chang de, K.; Sun, J.; Sui, J.; Freeman, G.J.; Signoretti, S.; Zhu, Q.; Marasco, W.A. Chimeric antigen receptor T cells secreting anti-PD-L1 antibodies more effectively regress renal cell carcinoma in a humanized mouse model. *Oncotarget* **2016**, *7*, 34341–34355. [CrossRef] [PubMed]
42. Rafiq, S.; Yeku, O.O.; Jackson, H.J.; Purdon, T.J.; van Leeuwen, D.G.; Drakes, D.J.; Song, M.; Miele, M.M.; Li, Z.; Wang, P.; et al. Targeted delivery of a PD-1-blocking scFv by CAR-T cells enhances anti-tumor efficacy in vivo. *Nat. Biotechnol.* **2018**, *36*, 847–856. [CrossRef] [PubMed]
43. Narayan, V.; Barber-Rotenberg, J.S.; Jung, I.Y.; Lacey, S.F.; Rech, A.J.; Davis, M.M.; Hwang, W.T.; Lal, P.; Carpenter, E.L.; Maude, S.L.; et al. PSMA-targeting TGFbeta-insensitive armored CAR T cells in metastatic castration-resistant prostate cancer: A phase 1 trial. *Nat. Med.* **2022**, *28*, 724–734. [CrossRef] [PubMed]
44. Webster, B.; Xiong, Y.; Hu, P.; Wu, D.; Alabanza, L.; Orentas, R.J.; Dropulic, B.; Schneider, D. Self-driving armored CAR-T cells overcome a suppressive milieu and eradicate CD19(+) Raji lymphoma in preclinical models. *Mol. Ther.* **2021**, *29*, 2691–2706. [CrossRef] [PubMed]
45. Srivastava, S.; Salter, A.I.; Liggitt, D.; Yechan-Gunja, S.; Sarvothama, M.; Cooper, K.; Smythe, K.S.; Dudakov, J.A.; Pierce, R.H.; Rader, C.; et al. Logic-Gated ROR1 Chimeric Antigen Receptor Expression Rescues T Cell-Mediated Toxicity to Normal Tissues and Enables Selective Tumor Targeting. *Cancer Cell* **2019**, *35*, 489–503.e488. [CrossRef]
46. Roybal, K.T.; Rupp, L.J.; Morsut, L.; Walker, W.J.; McNally, K.A.; Park, J.S.; Lim, W.A. Precision Tumor Recognition by T Cells With Combinatorial Antigen-Sensing Circuits. *Cell* **2016**, *164*, 770–779. [CrossRef]
47. Kosti, P.; Opzoomer, J.W.; Larios-Martinez, K.I.; Henley-Smith, R.; Scudamore, C.L.; Okesola, M.; Taher, M.Y.M.; Davies, D.M.; Muliaditan, T.; Larcombe-Young, D.; et al. Hypoxia-sensing CAR T cells provide safety and efficacy in treating solid tumors. *Cell Rep. Med.* **2021**, *2*, 100227. [CrossRef]
48. Jan, M.; Scarfo, I.; Larson, R.C.; Walker, A.; Schmidts, A.; Guirguis, A.A.; Gasser, J.A.; Slabicki, M.; Bouffard, A.A.; Castano, A.P.; et al. Reversible ON- and OFF-switch chimeric antigen receptors controlled by lenalidomide. *Sci. Transl. Med.* **2021**, *13*, eabb629. [CrossRef]
49. Weber, E.W.; Parker, K.R.; Sotillo, E.; Lynn, R.C.; Anbunathan, H.; Lattin, J.; Good, Z.; Belk, J.A.; Daniel, B.; Klysz, D.; et al. Transient rest restores functionality in exhausted CAR-T cells through epigenetic remodeling. *Science* **2021**, *372*, 239. [CrossRef]
50. Labanieh, L.; Majzner, R.G.; Klysz, D.; Sotillo, E.; Fisher, C.J.; Vilches-Moure, J.G.; Pacheco, K.Z.B.; Malipatlolla, M.; Xu, P.; Hui, J.H.; et al. Enhanced safety and efficacy of protease-regulated CAR-T cell receptors. *Cell* **2022**, *185*, 1745–1763.e1722. [CrossRef]
51. Li, H.S.; Wong, N.M.; Tague, E.; Ngo, J.T.; Khalil, A.S.; Wong, W.W. High-performance multiplex drug-gated CAR circuits. *Cancer Cell* **2022**, *40*, 1294–1305.e4. [CrossRef] [PubMed]

52. Lin, J.K.; Lerman, B.J.; Barnes, J.I.; Boursiquot, B.C.; Tan, Y.J.; Robinson, A.Q.L.; Davis, K.L.; Owens, D.K.; Goldhaber-Fiebert, J.D. Cost Effectiveness of Chimeric Antigen Receptor T-Cell Therapy in Relapsed or Refractory Pediatric B-Cell Acute Lymphoblastic Leukemia. *J. Clin. Oncol.* **2018**, *36*, 3192–3202. [CrossRef] [PubMed]
53. Lin, H.; Cheng, J.; Mu, W.; Zhou, J.; Zhu, L. Advances in Universal CAR-T Cell Therapy. *Front. Immunol.* **2021**, *12*, 744823. [CrossRef] [PubMed]
54. Daher, M.; Rezvani, K. Outlook for New CAR-Based Therapies with a Focus on CAR NK Cells: What Lies Beyond CAR-Engineered T Cells in the Race against Cancer. *Cancer Discov.* **2021**, *11*, 45–58. [CrossRef]
55. Goldenson, B.H.; Hor, P.; Kaufman, D.S. iPSC-Derived Natural Killer Cell Therapies—Expansion and Targeting. *Front. Immunol.* **2022**, *13*, 841107. [CrossRef]
56. Xie, G.; Dong, H.; Liang, Y.; Ham, J.D.; Rizwan, R.; Chen, J. CAR-NK cells: A promising cellular immunotherapy for cancer. *EBioMedicine* **2020**, *59*, 102975. [CrossRef]
57. Spiegel, J.Y.; Patel, S.; Muffly, L.; Hossain, N.M.; Oak, J.; Baird, J.H.; Frank, M.J.; Shiraz, P.; Sahaf, B.; Craig, J.; et al. CAR T cells with dual targeting of CD19 and CD22 in adult patients with recurrent or refractory B cell malignancies: A phase 1 trial. *Nat. Med.* **2021**, *27*, 1419–1431. [CrossRef]
58. Myers, J.A.; Miller, J.S. Exploring the NK cell platform for cancer immunotherapy. *Nat. Rev. Clin. Oncol.* **2021**, *18*, 85–100. [CrossRef]
59. Liu, E.; Marin, D.; Banerjee, P.; Macapinlac, H.A.; Thompson, P.; Basar, R.; Nassif Kerbauy, L.; Overman, B.; Thall, P.; Kaplan, M.; et al. Use of CAR-Transduced Natural Killer Cells in CD19-Positive Lymphoid Tumors. *N. Engl. J. Med.* **2020**, *382*, 545–553. [CrossRef]
60. Morris, E.C.; Neelapu, S.S.; Giavridis, T.; Sadelain, M. Cytokine release syndrome and associated neurotoxicity in cancer immunotherapy. *Nat. Rev. Immunol.* **2022**, *22*, 85–96. [CrossRef]
61. Habib, S.; Tariq, S.M.; Tariq, M. Chimeric Antigen Receptor-Natural Killer Cells: The Future of Cancer Immunotherapy. *Ochsner. J.* **2019**, *19*, 186–187. [CrossRef] [PubMed]
62. Liu, E.; Tong, Y.; Dotti, G.; Shaim, H.; Savoldo, B.; Mukherjee, M.; Orange, J.; Wan, X.; Lu, X.; Reynolds, A.; et al. Cord blood NK cells engineered to express IL-15 and a CD19-targeted CAR show long-term persistence and potent antitumor activity. *Leukemia* **2018**, *32*, 520–531. [CrossRef] [PubMed]
63. Leivas, A.; Valeri, A.; Cordoba, L.; Garcia-Ortiz, A.; Ortiz, A.; Sanchez-Vega, L.; Grana-Castro, O.; Fernandez, L.; Carreno-Tarragona, G.; Perez, M.; et al. NKG2D-CAR-transduced natural killer cells efficiently target multiple myeloma. *Blood Cancer J.* **2021**, *11*, 146. [CrossRef] [PubMed]
64. Tang, X.; Yang, L.; Li, Z.; Nalin, A.P.; Dai, H.; Xu, T.; Yin, J.; You, F.; Zhu, M.; Shen, W.; et al. First-in-man clinical trial of CAR NK-92 cells: Safety test of CD33-CAR NK-92 cells in patients with relapsed and refractory acute myeloid leukemia. *Am. J. Cancer Res.* **2018**, *8*, 1083–1089.
65. Vivier, E.; Tomasello, E.; Baratin, M.; Walzer, T.; Ugolini, S. Functions of natural killer cells. *Nat. Immunol.* **2008**, *9*, 503–510. [CrossRef]
66. Geller, M.A.; Miller, J.S. Use of allogeneic NK cells for cancer immunotherapy. *Immunotherapy* **2011**, *3*, 1445–1459. [CrossRef]
67. West, W.H.; Tauer, K.W.; Yannelli, J.R.; Marshall, G.D.; Orr, D.W.; Thurman, G.B.; Oldham, R.K. Constant-infusion recombinant interleukin-2 in adoptive immunotherapy of advanced cancer. *N. Engl. J. Med.* **1987**, *316*, 898–905. [CrossRef]
68. Tornroos, H.; Hagerstrand, H.; Lindqvist, C. Culturing the Human Natural Killer Cell Line NK-92 in Interleukin-2 and Interleukin-15—Implications for Clinical Trials. *Anticancer Res.* **2019**, *39*, 107–112. [CrossRef]
69. Morgan, M.A.; Buning, H.; Sauer, M.; Schambach, A. Use of Cell and Genome Modification Technologies to Generate Improved "Off-the-Shelf"CAR T and CAR NK Cells. *Front. Immunol.* **2020**, *11*, 1965. [CrossRef]
70. Carlsten, M.; Childs, R.W. Genetic Manipulation of NK Cells for Cancer Immunotherapy: Techniques and Clinical Implications. *Front. Immunol.* **2015**, *6*, 266. [CrossRef]
71. Guven, H.; Konstantinidis, K.V.; Alici, E.; Aints, A.; Abedi-Valugerdi, M.; Christensson, B.; Ljunggren, H.G.; Dilber, M.S. Efficient gene transfer into primary human natural killer cells by retroviral transduction. *Exp. Hematol.* **2005**, *33*, 1320–1328. [CrossRef] [PubMed]
72. Streltsova, M.A.; Barsov, E.; Erokhina, S.A.; Kovalenko, E.I. Retroviral gene transfer into primary human NK cells activated by IL-2 and K562 feeder cells expressing membrane-bound IL-21. *J. Immunol. Methods* **2017**, *450*, 90–94. [CrossRef] [PubMed]
73. Ma, M.; Badeti, S.; Kim, J.K.; Liu, D. Natural Killer (NK) and CAR-NK Cell Expansion Method using Membrane Bound-IL-21-Modified B Cell Line. *J. Vis. Exp.* **2022**. [CrossRef]
74. Papayannakos, C.; Daniel, R. Understanding lentiviral vector chromatin targeting: Working to reduce insertional mutagenic potential for gene therapy. *Gene Ther.* **2013**, *20*, 581–588. [CrossRef]
75. Portillo, A.L.; Hogg, R.; Ashkar, A.A. Production of human CAR-NK cells with lentiviral vectors and functional assessment in vitro. *STAR Protoc.* **2021**, *2*, 100956. [CrossRef]
76. Bari, R.; Granzin, M.; Tsang, K.S.; Roy, A.; Krueger, W.; Orentas, R.; Schneider, D.; Pfeifer, R.; Moeker, N.; Verhoeyen, E.; et al. A Distinct Subset of Highly Proliferative and Lentiviral Vector (LV)-Transducible NK Cells Define a Readily Engineered Subset for Adoptive Cellular Therapy. *Front. Immunol.* **2019**, *10*, 2001. [CrossRef]

77. Tomas, H.A.; Mestre, D.A.; Rodrigues, A.F.; Guerreiro, M.R.; Carrondo, M.J.T.; Coroadinha, A.S. Improved GaLV-TR Glycoproteins to Pseudotype Lentiviral Vectors: Impact of Viral Protease Activity in the Production of LV Pseudotypes. *Mol. Ther. Methods Clin. Dev.* **2019**, *15*, 1–8. [CrossRef]
78. Albinger, N.; Pfeifer, R.; Nitsche, M.; Mertlitz, S.; Campe, J.; Stein, K.; Kreyenberg, H.; Schubert, R.; Quadflieg, M.; Schneider, D.; et al. Primary CD33-targeting CAR-NK cells for the treatment of acute myeloid leukemia. *Blood Cancer J.* **2022**, *12*, 61. [CrossRef]
79. Ran, F.A.; Hsu, P.D.; Wright, J.; Agarwala, V.; Scott, D.A.; Zhang, F. Genome engineering using the CRISPR-Cas9 system. *Nat. Protoc.* **2013**, *8*, 2281–2308. [CrossRef]
80. Urena-Bailen, G.; Dobrowolski, J.M.; Hou, Y.; Dirlam, A.; Roig-Merino, A.; Schleicher, S.; Atar, D.; Seitz, C.; Feucht, J.; Antony, J.S.; et al. Preclinical Evaluation of CRISPR-Edited CAR-NK-92 Cells for Off-the-Shelf Treatment of AML and B-ALL. *Int. J. Mol. Sci.* **2022**, *23*, 12828. [CrossRef]
81. Huang, R.S.; Shih, H.A.; Lai, M.C.; Chang, Y.J.; Lin, S. Enhanced NK-92 Cytotoxicity by CRISPR Genome Engineering Using Cas9 Ribonucleoproteins. *Front. Immunol.* **2020**, *11*, 1008. [CrossRef] [PubMed]
82. Elmas, E.; Saljoughian, N.; de Souza Fernandes Pereira, M.; Tullius, B.P.; Sorathia, K.; Nakkula, R.J.; Lee, D.A.; Naeimi Kararoudi, M. CRISPR Gene Editing of Human Primary NK and T Cells for Cancer Immunotherapy. *Front. Oncol.* **2022**, *12*, 834002. [CrossRef] [PubMed]
83. Naeimi Kararoudi, M.; Likhite, S.; Elmas, E.; Yamamoto, K.; Schwartz, M.; Sorathia, K.; de Souza Fernandes Pereira, M.; Sezgin, Y.; Devine, R.D.; Lyberger, J.M.; et al. Optimization and validation of CAR transduction into human primary NK cells using CRISPR and AAV. *Cell Rep. Methods* **2022**, *2*, 100236. [CrossRef] [PubMed]
84. Kim, A.; Pyykko, I. Size matters: Versatile use of PiggyBac transposons as a genetic manipulation tool. *Mol. Cell Biochem.* **2011**, *354*, 301–309. [CrossRef] [PubMed]
85. Li, Y.; Hermanson, D.L.; Moriarity, B.S.; Kaufman, D.S. Human iPSC-Derived Natural Killer Cells Engineered with Chimeric Antigen Receptors Enhance Anti-tumor Activity. *Cell Stem Cell* **2018**, *23*, 181–192 e185. [CrossRef]
86. Monjezi, R.; Miskey, C.; Gogishvili, T.; Schleef, M.; Schmeer, M.; Einsele, H.; Ivics, Z.; Hudecek, M. Enhanced CAR T-cell engineering using non-viral Sleeping Beauty transposition from minicircle vectors. *Leukemia* **2017**, *31*, 186–194. [CrossRef]
87. Lowe, E.; Truscott, L.C.; De Oliveira, S.N. In Vitro Generation of Human NK Cells Expressing Chimeric Antigen Receptor Through Differentiation of Gene-Modified Hematopoietic Stem Cells. *Methods Mol. Biol.* **2016**, *1441*, 241–251.
88. Sabbah, M.; Jondreville, L.; Lacan, C.; Norol, F.; Vieillard, V.; Roos-Weil, D.; Nguyen, S. CAR-NK Cells: A Chimeric Hope or a Promising Therapy? *Cancers* **2022**, *14*, 3839. [CrossRef]
89. Yan, Y.; Steinherz, P.; Klingemann, H.G.; Dennig, D.; Childs, B.H.; McGuirk, J.; O'Reilly, R.J. Antileukemia activity of a natural killer cell line against human leukemias. *Clin. Cancer Res.* **1998**, *4*, 2859–2868.
90. Gong, J.H.; Maki, G.; Klingemann, H.G. Characterization of a human cell line (NK-92) with phenotypical and functional characteristics of activated natural killer cells. *Leukemia* **1994**, *8*, 652–658.
91. Maki, G.; Klingemann, H.G.; Martinson, J.A.; Tam, Y.K. Factors regulating the cytotoxic activity of the human natural killer cell line, NK-92. *J. Hematother. Stem Cell Res.* **2001**, *10*, 369–383. [CrossRef] [PubMed]
92. Gong, Y.; Klein Wolterink, R.G.J.; Wang, J.; Bos, G.M.J.; Germeraad, W.T.V. Chimeric antigen receptor natural killer (CAR-NK) cell design and engineering for cancer therapy. *J. Hematol. Oncol.* **2021**, *14*, 73. [CrossRef] [PubMed]
93. Suck, G.; Odendahl, M.; Nowakowska, P.; Seidl, C.; Wels, W.S.; Klingemann, H.G.; Tonn, T. NK-92: An 'off-the-shelf therapeutic' for adoptive natural killer cell-based cancer immunotherapy. *Cancer Immunol. Immunother.* **2016**, *65*, 485–492. [CrossRef] [PubMed]
94. Arai, S.; Meagher, R.; Swearingen, M.; Myint, H.; Rich, E.; Martinson, J.; Klingemann, H. Infusion of the allogeneic cell line NK-92 in patients with advanced renal cell cancer or melanoma: A phase I trial. *Cytotherapy* **2008**, *10*, 625–632. [CrossRef] [PubMed]
95. Tonn, T.; Schwabe, D.; Klingemann, H.G.; Becker, S.; Esser, R.; Koehl, U.; Suttorp, M.; Seifried, E.; Ottmann, O.G.; Bug, G. Treatment of patients with advanced cancer with the natural killer cell line NK-92. *Cytotherapy* **2013**, *15*, 1563–1570. [CrossRef]
96. Boissel, L.; Betancur, M.; Wels, W.S.; Tuncer, H.; Klingemann, H. Transfection with mRNA for CD19 specific chimeric antigen receptor restores NK cell mediated killing of CLL cells. *Leuk. Res.* **2009**, *33*, 1255–1259. [CrossRef]
97. Altvater, B.; Landmeier, S.; Pscherer, S.; Temme, J.; Schweer, K.; Kailayangiri, S.; Campana, D.; Juergens, H.; Pule, M.; Rossig, C. 2B4 (CD244) signaling by recombinant antigen-specific chimeric receptors costimulates natural killer cell activation to leukemia and neuroblastoma cells. *Clin. Cancer Res.* **2009**, *15*, 4857–4866. [CrossRef]
98. Oelsner, S.; Friede, M.E.; Zhang, C.; Wagner, J.; Badura, S.; Bader, P.; Ullrich, E.; Ottmann, O.G.; Klingemann, H.; Tonn, T.; et al. Continuously expanding CAR NK-92 cells display selective cytotoxicity against B-cell leukemia and lymphoma. *Cytotherapy* **2017**, *19*, 235–249. [CrossRef]
99. Liu, Q.; Xu, Y.; Mou, J.; Tang, K.; Fu, X.; Li, Y.; Xing, Y.; Rao, Q.; Xing, H.; Tian, Z.; et al. Irradiated chimeric antigen receptor engineered NK-92MI cells show effective cytotoxicity against CD19(+) malignancy in a mouse model. *Cytotherapy* **2020**, *22*, 552–562. [CrossRef]
100. Schonfeld, K.; Sahm, C.; Zhang, C.; Naundorf, S.; Brendel, C.; Odendahl, M.; Nowakowska, P.; Bonig, H.; Kohl, U.; Kloess, S.; et al. Selective inhibition of tumor growth by clonal NK cells expressing an ErbB2/HER2-specific chimeric antigen receptor. *Mol. Ther.* **2015**, *23*, 330–338. [CrossRef]
101. Zhang, C.; Burger, M.C.; Jennewein, L.; Genssler, S.; Schonfeld, K.; Zeiner, P.; Hattingen, E.; Harter, P.N.; Mittelbronn, M.; Tonn, T.; et al. ErbB2/HER2-Specific NK Cells for Targeted Therapy of Glioblastoma. *J. Natl. Cancer Inst.* **2016**, *108*. [CrossRef] [PubMed]

102. Williams, B.A.; Law, A.D.; Routy, B.; denHollander, N.; Gupta, V.; Wang, X.H.; Chaboureau, A.; Viswanathan, S.; Keating, A. A phase I trial of NK-92 cells for refractory hematological malignancies relapsing after autologous hematopoietic cell transplantation shows safety and evidence of efficacy. *Oncotarget* **2017**, *8*, 89256–89268. [CrossRef] [PubMed]
103. Varani, M.; Auletta, S.; Signore, A.; Galli, F. State of the Art of Natural Killer Cell Imaging: A Systematic Review. *Cancers* **2019**, *11*, 967. [CrossRef]
104. Zhu, L.; Li, X.J.; Kalimuthu, S.; Gangadaran, P.; Lee, H.W.; Oh, J.M.; Baek, S.H.; Jeong, S.Y.; Lee, S.W.; Lee, J.; et al. Natural Killer Cell (NK-92MI)-Based Therapy for Pulmonary Metastasis of Anaplastic Thyroid Cancer in a Nude Mouse Model. *Front. Immunol.* **2017**, *8*, 816. [CrossRef] [PubMed]
105. Gangadaran, P.; Ahn, B.C. Molecular Imaging: A Useful Tool for the Development of Natural Killer Cell-Based Immunotherapies. *Front. Immunol.* **2017**, *8*, 1090. [CrossRef] [PubMed]
106. Ottobrini, L.; Martelli, C.; Trabattoni, D.L.; Clerici, M.; Lucignani, G. In vivo imaging of immune cell trafficking in cancer. *Eur. J. Nucl. Med. Mol. Imaging* **2011**, *38*, 949–968. [CrossRef]
107. Matera, L.; Galetto, A.; Bello, M.; Baiocco, C.; Chiappino, I.; Castellano, G.; Stacchini, A.; Satolli, M.A.; Mele, M.; Sandrucci, S.; et al. In vivo migration of labeled autologous natural killer cells to liver metastases in patients with colon carcinoma. *J. Transl. Med.* **2006**, *4*, 49. [CrossRef]
108. Shamalov, K.; Meir, R.; Motiei, M.; Popovtzer, R.; Cohen, C.J. Noninvasive Tracking of Natural Killer Cells Using Gold Nanoparticles. *ACS Omega* **2021**, *6*, 28507–28514. [CrossRef]
109. Klingemann, H.; Boissel, L.; Toneguzzo, F. Natural Killer Cells for Immunotherapy—Advantages of the NK-92 Cell Line over Blood NK Cells. *Front. Immunol.* **2016**, *7*, 91. [CrossRef]
110. Zhang, C.; Oberoi, P.; Oelsner, S.; Waldmann, A.; Lindner, A.; Tonn, T.; Wels, W.S. Chimeric Antigen Receptor-Engineered NK-92 Cells: An Off-the-Shelf Cellular Therapeutic for Targeted Elimination of Cancer Cells and Induction of Protective Antitumor Immunity. *Front. Immunol.* **2017**, *8*, 533. [CrossRef]
111. Paul, P.; Pedini, P.; Lyonnet, L.; Di Cristofaro, J.; Loundou, A.; Pelardy, M.; Basire, A.; Dignat-George, F.; Chiaroni, J.; Thomas, P.; et al. FCGR3A and FCGR2A Genotypes Differentially Impact Allograft Rejection and Patients' Survival After Lung Transplant. *Front. Immunol.* **2019**, *10*, 1208. [CrossRef] [PubMed]
112. Jochems, C.; Hodge, J.W.; Fantini, M.; Fujii, R.; Morillon, Y.M., 2nd; Greiner, J.W.; Padget, M.R.; Tritsch, S.R.; Tsang, K.Y.; Campbell, K.S.; et al. An NK cell line (haNK) expressing high levels of granzyme and engineered to express the high affinity CD16 allele. *Oncotarget* **2016**, *7*, 86359–86373. [CrossRef] [PubMed]
113. Chen, K.H.; Wada, M.; Firor, A.E.; Pinz, K.G.; Jares, A.; Liu, H.; Salman, H.; Golightly, M.; Lan, F.; Jiang, X.; et al. Novel anti-CD3 chimeric antigen receptor targeting of aggressive T cell malignancies. *Oncotarget* **2016**, *7*, 56219–56232. [CrossRef]
114. Pinz, K.G.; Yakaboski, E.; Jares, A.; Liu, H.; Firor, A.E.; Chen, K.H.; Wada, M.; Salman, H.; Tse, W.; Hagag, N.; et al. Targeting T-cell malignancies using anti-CD4 CAR NK-92 cells. *Oncotarget* **2017**, *8*, 112783–112796. [CrossRef] [PubMed]
115. Xu, Y.; Liu, Q.; Zhong, M.; Wang, Z.; Chen, Z.; Zhang, Y.; Xing, H.; Tian, Z.; Tang, K.; Liao, X.; et al. 2B4 costimulatory domain enhancing cytotoxic ability of anti-CD5 chimeric antigen receptor engineered natural killer cells against T cell malignancies. *J. Hematol. Oncol.* **2019**, *12*, 49. [CrossRef]
116. You, F.; Wang, Y.; Jiang, L.; Zhu, X.; Chen, D.; Yuan, L.; An, G.; Meng, H.; Yang, L. A novel CD7 chimeric antigen receptor-modified NK-92MI cell line targeting T-cell acute lymphoblastic leukemia. *Am. J. Cancer Res.* **2019**, *9*, 64–78.
117. Chen, X.; Han, J.; Chu, J.; Zhang, L.; Zhang, J.; Chen, C.; Chen, L.; Wang, Y.; Wang, H.; Yi, L.; et al. A combinational therapy of EGFR-CAR NK cells and oncolytic herpes simplex virus 1 for breast cancer brain metastases. *Oncotarget* **2016**, *7*, 27764–27777. [CrossRef]
118. Chu, J.; Deng, Y.; Benson, D.M.; He, S.; Hughes, T.; Zhang, J.; Peng, Y.; Mao, H.; Yi, L.; Ghoshal, K.; et al. CS1-specific chimeric antigen receptor (CAR)-engineered natural killer cells enhance in vitro and in vivo antitumor activity against human multiple myeloma. *Leukemia* **2014**, *28*, 917–927. [CrossRef]
119. Jiang, H.; Zhang, W.; Shang, P.; Zhang, H.; Fu, W.; Ye, F.; Zeng, T.; Huang, H.; Zhang, X.; Sun, W.; et al. Transfection of chimeric anti-CD138 gene enhances natural killer cell activation and killing of multiple myeloma cells. *Mol. Oncol.* **2014**, *8*, 297–310. [CrossRef]
120. Rafiq, S.; Purdon, T.; Schultz, L.; Klingemann, H.; Brentjens, R. NK-92 cells engineered with anti-CD33 chimeric antigen receptors (CAR) for the treatment of Acute Myeloid Leukemia (AML). *Cytotherapy* **2015**, *17*, S23. [CrossRef]
121. Zhang, G.; Liu, R.; Zhu, X.; Wang, L.; Ma, J.; Han, H.; Wang, X.; Zhang, G.; He, W.; Wang, W.; et al. Retargeting NK-92 for anti-melanoma activity by a TCR-like single-domain antibody. *Immunol. Cell Biol.* **2013**, *91*, 615–624. [CrossRef] [PubMed]
122. Daldrup-Link, H.E.; Meier, R.; Rudelius, M.; Piontek, G.; Piert, M.; Metz, S.; Settles, M.; Uherek, C.; Wels, W.; Schlegel, J.; et al. In vivo tracking of genetically engineered, anti-HER2/neu directed natural killer cells to HER2/neu positive mammary tumors with magnetic resonance imaging. *Eur. Radiol.* **2005**, *15*, 4–13. [CrossRef] [PubMed]
123. Kruschinski, A.; Moosmann, A.; Poschke, I.; Norell, H.; Chmielewski, M.; Seliger, B.; Kiessling, R.; Blankenstein, T.; Abken, H.; Charo, J. Engineering antigen-specific primary human NK cells against HER-2 positive carcinomas. *Proc. Natl. Acad. Sci. USA* **2008**, *105*, 17481–17486. [CrossRef] [PubMed]
124. Romanski, A.; Uherek, C.; Bug, G.; Muller, T.; Rossig, C.; Kampfmann, M.; Krossok, N.; Hoelzer, D.; Seifried, E.; Wels, W.; et al. Re-Targeting of an NK Cell Line (NK92) with Specificity for CD19 Efficiently Kills Human B-Precursor Leukemia Cells. *Blood* **2004**, *104*, 2747. [CrossRef]

125. Muller, T.; Uherek, C.; Maki, G.; Chow, K.U.; Schimpf, A.; Klingemann, H.G.; Tonn, T.; Wels, W.S. Expression of a CD20-specific chimeric antigen receptor enhances cytotoxic activity of NK cells and overcomes NK-resistance of lymphoma and leukemia cells. *Cancer Immunol. Immunother.* **2008**, *57*, 411–423. [CrossRef]
126. Mitwasi, N.; Feldmann, A.; Arndt, C.; Koristka, S.; Berndt, N.; Jureczek, J.; Loureiro, L.R.; Bergmann, R.; Mathe, D.; Hegedus, N.; et al. "UniCAR"-modified off-the-shelf NK-92 cells for targeting of GD2-expressing tumour cells. *Sci. Rep.* **2020**, *10*, 2141. [CrossRef]
127. Luanpitpong, S.; Poohadsuan, J.; Klaihmon, P.; Issaragrisil, S. Selective Cytotoxicity of Single and Dual Anti-CD19 and Anti-CD138 Chimeric Antigen Receptor-Natural Killer Cells against Hematologic Malignancies. *J. Immunol. Res.* **2021**, *2021*, 5562630. [CrossRef]
128. Rudek, L.S.; Zimmermann, K.; Galla, M.; Meyer, J.; Kuehle, J.; Stamopoulou, A.; Brand, D.; Sandalcioglu, I.E.; Neyazi, B.; Moritz, T.; et al. Generation of an NFkappaB-Driven Alpharetroviral "All-in-One" Vector Construct as a Potent Tool for CAR NK Cell Therapy. *Front. Immunol.* **2021**, *12*, 751138. [CrossRef]
129. Kloss, S.; Oberschmidt, O.; Morgan, M.; Dahlke, J.; Arseniev, L.; Huppert, V.; Granzin, M.; Gardlowski, T.; Matthies, N.; Soltenborn, S.; et al. Optimization of Human NK Cell Manufacturing: Fully Automated Separation, Improved Ex Vivo Expansion Using IL-21 with Autologous Feeder Cells, and Generation of Anti-CD123-CAR-Expressing Effector Cells. *Hum. Gene Ther.* **2017**, *28*, 897–913. [CrossRef]
130. Shimasaki, N.; Jain, A.; Campana, D. NK cells for cancer immunotherapy. *Nat. Rev. Drug Discov.* **2020**, *19*, 200–218. [CrossRef]
131. Luevano, M.; Daryouzeh, M.; Alnabhan, R.; Querol, S.; Khakoo, S.; Madrigal, A.; Saudemont, A. The unique profile of cord blood natural killer cells balances incomplete maturation and effective killing function upon activation. *Hum. Immunol.* **2012**, *73*, 248–257. [CrossRef] [PubMed]
132. Sarvaria, A.; Jawdat, D.; Madrigal, J.A.; Saudemont, A. Umbilical Cord Blood Natural Killer Cells, Their Characteristics, and Potential Clinical Applications. *Front. Immunol.* **2017**, *8*, 329. [CrossRef] [PubMed]
133. Hejazi, M.; Zhang, C.; Bennstein, S.B.; Balz, V.; Reusing, S.B.; Quadflieg, M.; Hoerster, K.; Heinrichs, S.; Hanenberg, H.; Oberbeck, S.; et al. CD33 Delineates Two Functionally Distinct NK Cell Populations Divergent in Cytokine Production and Antibody-Mediated Cellular Cytotoxicity. *Front. Immunol.* **2021**, *12*, 798087. [CrossRef] [PubMed]
134. Topfer, K.; Cartellieri, M.; Michen, S.; Wiedemuth, R.; Muller, N.; Lindemann, D.; Bachmann, M.; Fussel, M.; Schackert, G.; Temme, A. DAP12-based activating chimeric antigen receptor for NK cell tumor immunotherapy. *J. Immunol.* **2015**, *194*, 3201–3212. [CrossRef] [PubMed]
135. Rezvani, K.; Rouce, R.; Liu, E.; Shpall, E. Engineering Natural Killer Cells for Cancer Immunotherapy. *Mol. Ther.* **2017**, *25*, 1769–1781. [CrossRef]
136. Passweg, J.R.; Tichelli, A.; Meyer-Monard, S.; Heim, D.; Stern, M.; Kuhne, T.; Favre, G.; Gratwohl, A. Purified donor NK-lymphocyte infusion to consolidate engraftment after haploidentical stem cell transplantation. *Leukemia* **2004**, *18*, 1835–1838. [CrossRef]
137. Cany, J.; van der Waart, A.B.; Spanholtz, J.; Tordoir, M.; Jansen, J.H.; van der Voort, R.; Schaap, N.M.; Dolstra, H. Combined IL-15 and IL-12 drives the generation of CD34(+)-derived natural killer cells with superior maturation and alloreactivity potential following adoptive transfer. *Oncoimmunology* **2015**, *4*, e1017701. [CrossRef]
138. Takahashi, K.; Yamanaka, S. Induction of pluripotent stem cells from mouse embryonic and adult fibroblast cultures by defined factors. *Cell* **2006**, *126*, 663–676. [CrossRef]
139. Valamehr, B.; Tsutsui, H.; Ho, C.M.; Wu, H. Developing defined culture systems for human pluripotent stem cells. *Regen. Med.* **2011**, *6*, 623–634. [CrossRef]
140. Knorr, D.A.; Ni, Z.; Hermanson, D.; Hexum, M.K.; Bendzick, L.; Cooper, L.J.; Lee, D.A.; Kaufman, D.S. Clinical-scale derivation of natural killer cells from human pluripotent stem cells for cancer therapy. *Stem Cells Transl. Med.* **2013**, *2*, 274–283. [CrossRef]
141. Hermanson, D.L.; Bendzick, L.; Pribyl, L.; McCullar, V.; Vogel, R.I.; Miller, J.S.; Geller, M.A.; Kaufman, D.S. Induced Pluripotent Stem Cell-Derived Natural Killer Cells for Treatment of Ovarian Cancer. *Stem Cells* **2016**, *34*, 93–101. [CrossRef] [PubMed]
142. Saetersmoen, M.L.; Hammer, Q.; Valamehr, B.; Kaufman, D.S.; Malmberg, K.J. Off-the-shelf cell therapy with induced pluripotent stem cell-derived natural killer cells. *Semin. Immunopathol.* **2019**, *41*, 59–68. [CrossRef] [PubMed]
143. Vargas, J.E.; Chicaybam, L.; Stein, R.T.; Tanuri, A.; Delgado-Canedo, A.; Bonamino, M.H. Retroviral vectors and transposons for stable gene therapy: Advances, current challenges and perspectives. *J. Transl. Med.* **2016**, *14*, 288. [CrossRef] [PubMed]
144. Chen, G.; Gulbranson, D.R.; Hou, Z.; Bolin, J.M.; Ruotti, V.; Probasco, M.D.; Smuga-Otto, K.; Howden, S.E.; Diol, N.R.; Propson, N.E.; et al. Chemically defined conditions for human iPSC derivation and culture. *Nat. Methods* **2011**, *8*, 424–429. [CrossRef] [PubMed]
145. Dashtban, M.; Panchalingam, K.M.; Shafa, M.; Ahmadian Baghbaderani, B. Addressing Manufacturing Challenges for Commercialization of iPSC-Based Therapies. *Methods Mol. Biol.* **2021**, *2286*, 179–198. [PubMed]
146. Valamehr, B.; Robinson, M.; Abujarour, R.; Rezner, B.; Vranceanu, F.; Le, T.; Medcalf, A.; Lee, T.T.; Fitch, M.; Robbins, D.; et al. Platform for induction and maintenance of transgene-free hiPSCs resembling ground state pluripotent stem cells. *Stem Cell Reports* **2014**, *2*, 366–381. [CrossRef] [PubMed]
147. Nit, K.; Tyszka-Czochara, M.; Bobis-Wozowicz, S. Oxygen as a Master Regulator of Human Pluripotent Stem Cell Function and Metabolism. *J. Pers. Med.* **2021**, *11*, 905. [CrossRef]

148. Dakhore, S.; Nayer, B.; Hasegawa, K. Human Pluripotent Stem Cell Culture: Current Status, Challenges, and Advancement. *Stem Cells Int.* **2018**, *2018*, 7396905. [CrossRef]
149. Yamamoto, T.; Arita, M.; Kuroda, H.; Suzuki, T.; Kawamata, S. Improving the differentiation potential of pluripotent stem cells by optimizing culture conditions. *Sci. Rep.* **2022**, *12*, 14147. [CrossRef]
150. Ni, Y.; Zhao, Y.; Warren, L.; Higginbotham, J.; Wang, J. cGMP Generation of Human Induced Pluripotent Stem Cells with Messenger RNA. *Curr. Protoc. Stem. Cell Biol.* **2016**, *39*, 4A.6.1–4A.6.25. [CrossRef]
151. Rivera, T.; Zhao, Y.; Ni, Y.; Wang, J. Human-Induced Pluripotent Stem Cell Culture Methods Under cGMP Conditions. *Curr. Protoc. Stem. Cell Biol.* **2020**, *54*, e117. [CrossRef] [PubMed]
152. Karagiannis, P.; Kim, S.I. iPSC-Derived Natural Killer Cells for Cancer Immunotherapy. *Mol. Cells* **2021**, *44*, 541–548. [CrossRef] [PubMed]
153. Kailayangiri, S.; Altvater, B.; Wiebel, M.; Jamitzky, S.; Rossig, C. Overcoming Heterogeneity of Antigen Expression for Effective CAR T Cell Targeting of Cancers. *Cancers* **2020**, *12*, 1075. [CrossRef] [PubMed]
154. Luna, J.I.; Grossenbacher, S.K.; Murphy, W.J.; Canter, R.J. Targeting Cancer Stem Cells with Natural Killer Cell Immunotherapy. *Expert Opin. Biol. Ther.* **2017**, *17*, 313–324. [CrossRef] [PubMed]
155. Yin, T.; Wang, G.; He, S.; Liu, Q.; Sun, J.; Wang, Y. Human cancer cells with stem cell-like phenotype exhibit enhanced sensitivity to the cytotoxicity of IL-2 and IL-15 activated natural killer cells. *Cell Immunol.* **2016**, *300*, 41–45. [CrossRef]
156. Ferrari de Andrade, L.; Tay, R.E.; Pan, D.; Luoma, A.M.; Ito, Y.; Badrinath, S.; Tsoucas, D.; Franz, B.; May, K.F., Jr.; Harvey, C.J.; et al. Antibody-mediated inhibition of MICA and MICB shedding promotes NK cell-driven tumor immunity. *Science* **2018**, *359*, 1537–1542. [CrossRef]
157. Ferrari de Andrade, L.; Kumar, S.; Luoma, A.M.; Ito, Y.; Alves da Silva, P.H.; Pan, D.; Pyrdol, J.W.; Yoon, C.H.; Wucherpfennig, K.W. Inhibition of MICA and MICB Shedding Elicits NK-Cell-Mediated Immunity against Tumors Resistant to Cytotoxic T Cells. *Cancer Immunol. Res.* **2020**, *8*, 769–780. [CrossRef]
158. Atashzar, M.R.; Baharlou, R.; Karami, J.; Abdollahi, H.; Rezaei, R.; Pourramezan, F.; Zoljalali Moghaddam, S.H. Cancer stem cells: A review from origin to therapeutic implications. *J. Cell Physiol.* **2020**, *235*, 790–803. [CrossRef]
159. Muller, N.; Michen, S.; Tietze, S.; Topfer, K.; Schulte, A.; Lamszus, K.; Schmitz, M.; Schackert, G.; Pastan, I.; Temme, A. Engineering NK Cells Modified with an EGFRvIII-specific Chimeric Antigen Receptor to Overexpress CXCR4 Improves Immunotherapy of CXCL12/SDF-1alpha-secreting Glioblastoma. *J. Immunother.* **2015**, *38*, 197–210. [CrossRef]
160. Ng, Y.Y.; Tay, J.C.K.; Wang, S. CXCR1 Expression to Improve Anti-Cancer Efficacy of Intravenously Injected CAR-NK Cells in Mice with Peritoneal Xenografts. *Mol. Ther. Oncolytics* **2020**, *16*, 75–85. [CrossRef]
161. Cao, Y.; Wang, X.; Jin, T.; Tian, Y.; Dai, C.; Widarma, C.; Song, R.; Xu, F. Immune checkpoint molecules in natural killer cells as potential targets for cancer immunotherapy. *Signal Transduct. Target. Ther.* **2020**, *5*, 250. [CrossRef] [PubMed]
162. Zhang, Q.; Bi, J.; Zheng, X.; Chen, Y.; Wang, H.; Wu, W.; Wang, Z.; Wu, Q.; Peng, H.; Wei, H.; et al. Blockade of the checkpoint receptor TIGIT prevents NK cell exhaustion and elicits potent anti-tumor immunity. *Nat. Immunol.* **2018**, *19*, 723–732. [CrossRef]
163. Lu, C.; Guo, C.; Chen, H.; Zhang, H.; Zhi, L.; Lv, T.; Li, M.; Niu, Z.; Lu, P.; Zhu, W. A novel chimeric PD1-NKG2D-41BB receptor enhances antitumor activity of NK92 cells against human lung cancer H1299 cells by triggering pyroptosis. *Mol. Immunol.* **2020**, *122*, 200–206. [CrossRef] [PubMed]
164. Tong, L.; Jimenez-Cortegana, C.; Tay, A.H.M.; Wickstrom, S.; Galluzzi, L.; Lundqvist, A. NK cells and solid tumors: Therapeutic potential and persisting obstacles. *Mol. Cancer* **2022**, *21*, 206. [CrossRef] [PubMed]
165. Yvon, E.S.; Burga, R.; Powell, A.; Cruz, C.R.; Fernandes, R.; Barese, C.; Nguyen, T.; Abdel-Baki, M.S.; Bollard, C.M. Cord blood natural killer cells expressing a dominant negative TGF-beta receptor: Implications for adoptive immunotherapy for glioblastoma. *Cytotherapy* **2017**, *19*, 408–418. [CrossRef]
166. Han, J.; Chu, J.; Keung Chan, W.; Zhang, J.; Wang, Y.; Cohen, J.B.; Victor, A.; Meisen, W.H.; Kim, S.H.; Grandi, P.; et al. CAR-Engineered NK Cells Targeting Wild-Type EGFR and EGFRvIII Enhance Killing of Glioblastoma and Patient-Derived Glioblastoma Stem Cells. *Sci. Rep.* **2015**, *5*, 11483. [CrossRef] [PubMed]
167. Genssler, S.; Burger, M.C.; Zhang, C.; Oelsner, S.; Mildenberger, I.; Wagner, M.; Steinbach, J.P.; Wels, W.S. Dual targeting of glioblastoma with chimeric antigen receptor-engineered natural killer cells overcomes heterogeneity of target antigen expression and enhances antitumor activity and survival. *Oncoimmunology* **2016**, *5*, e1119354. [CrossRef]
168. Hu, Z. Tissue factor as a new target for CAR-NK cell immunotherapy of triple-negative breast cancer. *Sci. Rep.* **2020**, *10*, 2815. [CrossRef]
169. Sahm, C.; Schonfeld, K.; Wels, W.S. Expression of IL-15 in NK cells results in rapid enrichment and selective cytotoxicity of gene-modified effectors that carry a tumor-specific antigen receptor. *Cancer Immunol. Immunother.* **2012**, *61*, 1451–1461. [CrossRef]
170. Cao, B.; Liu, M.; Wang, L.; Liang, B.; Feng, Y.; Chen, X.; Shi, Y.; Zhang, J.; Ye, X.; Tian, Y.; et al. Use of chimeric antigen receptor NK-92 cells to target mesothelin in ovarian cancer. *Biochem. Biophys. Res. Commun.* **2020**, *524*, 96–102. [CrossRef]
171. Klapdor, R.; Wang, S.; Morgan, M.; Dork, T.; Hacker, U.; Hillemanns, P.; Buning, H.; Schambach, A. Characterization of a Novel Third-Generation Anti-CD24-CAR against Ovarian Cancer. *Int. J. Mol. Sci.* **2019**, *20*, 660. [CrossRef] [PubMed]
172. Xia, N.; Haopeng, P.; Gong, J.U.; Lu, J.; Chen, Z.; Zheng, Y.; Wang, Z.; Sun, Y.U.; Yang, Z.; Hoffman, R.M.; et al. Robo1-specific CAR-NK Immunotherapy Enhances Efficacy of (125)I Seed Brachytherapy in an Orthotopic Mouse Model of Human Pancreatic Carcinoma. *Anticancer. Res.* **2019**, *39*, 5919–5925. [CrossRef] [PubMed]

173. Li, C.; Yang, N.; Li, H.; Wang, Z. Robo1-specific chimeric antigen receptor natural killer cell therapy for pancreatic ductal adenocarcinoma with liver metastasis. *J. Cancer Res. Ther.* **2020**, *16*, 393–396.
174. Ao, X.; Yang, Y.; Li, W.; Tan, Y.; Guo, W.; Ao, L.; He, X.; Wu, X.; Xia, J.; Xu, X.; et al. Anti-alphaFR CAR-engineered NK-92 Cells Display Potent Cytotoxicity Against alphaFR-positive Ovarian Cancer. *J. Immunother.* **2019**, *42*, 284–296. [CrossRef] [PubMed]
175. Lee, Y.E.; Ju, A.; Choi, H.W.; Kim, J.C.; Kim, E.E.; Kim, T.S.; Kang, H.J.; Kim, S.Y.; Jang, J.Y.; Ku, J.L.; et al. Rationally designed redirection of natural killer cells anchoring a cytotoxic ligand for pancreatic cancer treatment. *J. Control Release* **2020**, *326*, 310–323. [CrossRef] [PubMed]
176. Liu, B.; Liu, Z.Z.; Zhou, M.L.; Lin, J.W.; Chen, X.M.; Li, Z.; Gao, W.B.; Yu, Z.D.; Liu, T. Development of c-MET-specific chimeric antigen receptor-engineered natural killer cells with cytotoxic effects on human liver cancer HepG2 cells. *Mol. Med. Rep.* **2019**, *20*, 2823–2831. [CrossRef]
177. Subrakova, V.G.; Kulemzin, S.V.; Belovezhets, T.N.; Chikaev, A.N.; Chikaev, N.A.; Koval, O.A.; Gorchakov, A.A.; Taranin, A.V. shp-2 gene knockout upregulates CAR-driven cytotoxicity of YT NK cells. *Vavilovskii Zhurnal Genet. Sel.* **2020**, *24*, 80–86. [CrossRef]
178. Wrona, E.; Borowiec, M.; Potemski, P. CAR-NK Cells in the Treatment of Solid Tumors. *Int. J. Mol. Sci.* **2021**, *22*, 5899. [CrossRef]
179. Geller, M.A.; Cooley, S.; Judson, P.L.; Ghebre, R.; Carson, L.F.; Argenta, P.A.; Jonson, A.L.; Panoskaltsis-Mortari, A.; Curtsinger, J.; McKenna, D.; et al. A phase II study of allogeneic natural killer cell therapy to treat patients with recurrent ovarian and breast cancer. *Cytotherapy* **2011**, *13*, 98–107. [CrossRef]
180. Yang, Y.; Lim, O.; Kim, T.M.; Ahn, Y.O.; Choi, H.; Chung, H.; Min, B.; Her, J.H.; Cho, S.Y.; Keam, B.; et al. Phase I Study of Random Healthy Donor-Derived Allogeneic Natural Killer Cell Therapy in Patients with Malignant Lymphoma or Advanced Solid Tumors. *Cancer Immunol. Res.* **2016**, *4*, 215–224. [CrossRef]
181. Lin, C.; Zhang, J. Reformation in chimeric antigen receptor based cancer immunotherapy: Redirecting natural killer cell. *Biochim. Biophys. Acta Rev. Cancer* **2018**, *1869*, 200–215. [CrossRef] [PubMed]
182. Wang, F.; Wu, L.; Yin, L.; Shi, H.; Gu, Y.; Xing, N. Combined treatment with anti-PSMA CAR NK-92 cell and anti-PD-L1 monoclonal antibody enhances the antitumour efficacy against castration-resistant prostate cancer. *Clin. Transl. Med.* **2022**, *12*, e901. [CrossRef] [PubMed]
183. Sengsayadeth, S.; Savani, B.N.; Oluwole, O.; Dholaria, B. Overview of approved CAR-T therapies, ongoing clinical trials, and its impact on clinical practice. *EJHaem* **2022**, *3*, 6–10. [CrossRef] [PubMed]
184. Hauswirth, A.W.; Florian, S.; Printz, D.; Sotlar, K.; Krauth, M.T.; Fritsch, G.; Schernthaner, G.H.; Wacheck, V.; Selzer, E.; Sperr, W.R.; et al. Expression of the target receptor CD33 in CD34+/CD38-/CD123+ AML stem cells. *Eur. J. Clin. Investig.* **2007**, *37*, 73–82. [CrossRef]
185. Walter, R.B. The role of CD33 as therapeutic target in acute myeloid leukemia. *Expert Opin. Ther. Targets* **2014**, *18*, 715–718. [CrossRef]
186. Jiang, Y.P.; Liu, B.Y.; Zheng, Q.; Panuganti, S.; Chen, R.; Zhu, J.; Mishra, M.; Huang, J.; Dao-Pick, T.; Roy, S.; et al. CLT030, a leukemic stem cell-targeting CLL1 antibody-drug conjugate for treatment of acute myeloid leukemia. *Blood Adv.* **2018**, *2*, 1738–1749. [CrossRef]
187. Gurney, M.; O'Reilly, E.; Corcoran, S.; Brophy, S.; Hardwicke, D.; Krawczyk, J.; Hermanson, D.; Childs, R.; Szegezdi, E.; O'Dwyer, M.E. Tc Buster Transposon Engineered CLL-1 CAR-NK Cells Efficiently Target Acute Myeloid Leukemia. *Blood* **2021**, *138*, 1725. [CrossRef]
188. Liu, F.; Cao, Y.; Pinz, K.; Ma, Y.; Wada, M.; Chen, K.; Ma, G.; Shen, J.; Tse, C.; Su, Y.; et al. First-in-Human CLL1-CD33 Compound CAR T Cell Therapy Induces Complete Remission in Patients with Refractory Acute Myeloid Leukemia: Update on Phase 1 Clinical Trial. *Blood* **2018**, *132*, 901. [CrossRef]
189. Bras, A.E.; de Haas, V.; van Stigt, A.; Jongen-Lavrencic, M.; Beverloo, H.B.; Te Marvelde, J.G.; Zwaan, C.M.; van Dongen, J.J.M.; Leusen, J.H.W.; van der Velden, V.H.J. CD123 expression levels in 846 acute leukemia patients based on standardized immunophenotyping. *Cytom. B Clin. Cytom.* **2019**, *96*, 134–142. [CrossRef]
190. Christodoulou, I.; Ho, W.J.; Marple, A.; Ravich, J.W.; Tam, A.; Rahnama, R.; Fearnow, A.; Rietberg, C.; Yanik, S.; Solomou, E.E.; et al. Engineering CAR-NK cells to secrete IL-15 sustains their anti-AML functionality but is associated with systemic toxicities. *J. Immunother. Cancer* **2021**, *9*, e003894. [CrossRef]
191. Caruso, S.; De Angelis, B.; Del Bufalo, F.; Ciccone, R.; Donsante, S.; Volpe, G.; Manni, S.; Guercio, M.; Pezzella, M.; Iaffaldano, L.; et al. Safe and effective off-the-shelf immunotherapy based on CAR.CD123-NK cells for the treatment of acute myeloid leukaemia. *J. Hematol. Oncol.* **2022**, *15*, 163. [CrossRef] [PubMed]
192. Colamartino, A.B.L.; Lemieux, W.; Bifsha, P.; Nicoletti, S.; Chakravarti, N.; Sanz, J.; Romero, H.; Selleri, S.; Beland, K.; Guiot, M.; et al. Efficient and Robust NK-Cell Transduction With Baboon Envelope Pseudotyped Lentivector. *Front. Immunol.* **2019**, *10*, 2873. [CrossRef] [PubMed]
193. Szoor, A.; Velasquez, M.; Bonifant, C.; Vaidya, A.; Brunetti, L.; Gundry, M.; Parihar, R.; Goodell, M.; Gottschalk, S. Two-pronged Cell Therapy: Engineering NK cells to target CD22 and redirect bystander T cells to CD19 for the adoptive immunotherapy of B-cell malignancies. *J. Immunol.* **2017**, *198*, 6. [CrossRef]
194. Ng, Y.Y.; Du, Z.; Zhang, X.; Chng, W.J.; Wang, S. CXCR4 and anti-BCMA CAR co-modified natural killer cells suppress multiple myeloma progression in a xenograft mouse model. *Cancer Gene Ther.* **2022**, *29*, 475–483. [CrossRef] [PubMed]

195. Roex, G.; Campillo-Davo, D.; Flumens, D.; Shaw, P.A.G.; Krekelbergh, L.; De Reu, H.; Berneman, Z.N.; Lion, E.; Anguille, S. Two for one: Targeting BCMA and CD19 in B-cell malignancies with off-the-shelf dual-CAR NK-92 cells. *J. Transl. Med.* **2022**, *20*, 124. [CrossRef]
196. Goebeler, M.E.; Knop, S.; Viardot, A.; Kufer, P.; Topp, M.S.; Einsele, H.; Noppeney, R.; Hess, G.; Kallert, S.; Mackensen, A.; et al. Bispecific T-Cell Engager (BiTE) Antibody Construct Blinatumomab for the Treatment of Patients With Relapsed/Refractory Non-Hodgkin Lymphoma: Final Results From a Phase I Study. *J. Clin. Oncol.* **2016**, *34*, 1104–1111. [CrossRef]
197. Spiess, C.; Zhai, Q.; Carter, P.J. Alternative molecular formats and therapeutic applications for bispecific antibodies. *Mol. Immunol.* **2015**, *67*, 95–106. [CrossRef]
198. Jiang, Z.; Qin, L.; Tang, Y.; Liao, R.; Shi, J.; He, B.; Li, S.; Zheng, D.; Cui, Y.; Wu, Q.; et al. Human induced-T-to-natural killer cells have potent anti-tumour activities. *Biomark. Res.* **2022**, *10*, 13. [CrossRef]

Disclaimer/Publisher's Note: The statements, opinions and data contained in all publications are solely those of the individual author(s) and contributor(s) and not of MDPI and/or the editor(s). MDPI and/or the editor(s) disclaim responsibility for any injury to people or property resulting from any ideas, methods, instructions or products referred to in the content.

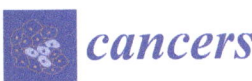

Article

TIGIT Expression on Activated NK Cells Correlates with Greater Anti-Tumor Activity but Promotes Functional Decline upon Lung Cancer Exposure: Implications for Adoptive Cell Therapy and TIGIT-Targeted Therapies

Md Faqrul Hasan, Tayler J. Croom-Perez, Jeremiah L. Oyer, Thomas A. Dieffenthaller, Liza D. Robles-Carrillo, Jonathan E. Eloriaga, Sanjana Kumar, Brendan W. Andersen and Alicja J. Copik *

Burnett School of Biomedical Science, College of Medicine, University of Central Florida, Orlando, FL 32827, USA; sanjanakumar@knights.ucf.edu (S.K.); brendanandersen@knights.ucf.edu (B.W.A.)
* Correspondence: alicja.copik@ucf.edu

Simple Summary: Therapies targeting TIGIT have garnered tremendous interest, but have so far failed to reach primary endpoints in PhIII trials in lung cancer settings. This study examined the function of TIGIT on NK cells and how NK cells may impact the success of TIGIT therapeutics. This study demonstrated that TIGIT expression is increased on activated NK cells, including those expanded with clinical protocols for cell therapy. Activated TIGIT$^+$ NK cells have a better anti-tumor response as compared to TIGIT$^-$ NK cells. More importantly, higher tumor infiltration of activated NK cells correlates with better patient outcomes in lung adenocarcinoma. However, chronic TIGIT engagement with its ligands in the tumor microenvironment leads to the functional decline of NK cells, which can be prevented with anti-TIGIT. This demonstrates that TIGIT-expressing cells are not inherently exhausted but can represent NK cells with the highest anti-tumor activity. These findings support the joint application of NK cells with blocking, non-depleting anti-TIGIT for improved treatment outcomes.

Abstract: Treatments targeting TIGIT have gained a lot of attention due to strong preclinical and early clinical results, particularly with anti-PD-(L)1 therapeutics. However, this combination has failed to meet progression-free survival endpoints in phase III trials. Most of our understanding of TIGIT comes from studies of T cell function. Yet, this inhibitory receptor is often upregulated to the same, or higher, extent on NK cells in cancers. Studies in murine models have demonstrated that TIGIT inhibits NK cells and promotes exhaustion, with its effects on tumor control also being dependent on NK cells. However, there are limited studies assessing the role of TIGIT on the function of human NK cells (hNK), particularly in lung cancer. Most studies used NK cell lines or tested TIGIT blockade to reactivate exhausted cells obtained from cancer patients. For therapeutic advancement, a better understanding of TIGIT in the context of activated hNK cells is crucial, which is different than exhausted NK cells, and critical in the context of adoptive NK cell therapeutics that may be combined with TIGIT blockade. In this study, the effect of TIGIT blockade on the anti-tumor activities of human ex vivo-expanded NK cells was evaluated in vitro in the context of lung cancer. TIGIT expression was higher on activated and/or expanded NK cells compared to resting NK cells. More TIGIT$^+$ NK cells expressed major activating receptors and exerted anti-tumor response as compared to TIGIT$^-$ cells, indicating that NK cells with greater anti-tumor function express more TIGIT. However, long-term TIGIT engagement upon exposure to PVR$^+$ tumors downregulated the cytotoxic function of expanded NK cells while the inclusion of TIGIT blockade increased cytotoxicity, restored effector functions against PVR-positive targets, and upregulated immune inflammation-related gene sets. These combined results indicate that TIGIT blockade can preserve the activation state of NK cells during exposure to PVR$^+$ tumors. These results support the notion that a functional NK cell compartment is critical for anti-tumor response and anti-TIGIT/adoptive NK cell combinations have the potential to improve outcomes.

Citation: Hasan, M.F.; Croom-Perez, T.J.; Oyer, J.L.; Dieffenthaller, T.A.; Robles-Carrillo, L.D.; Eloriaga, J.E.; Kumar, S.; Andersen, B.W.; Copik, A.J. TIGIT Expression on Activated NK Cells Correlates with Greater Anti-Tumor Activity but Promotes Functional Decline upon Lung Cancer Exposure: Implications for Adoptive Cell Therapy and TIGIT-Targeted Therapies. *Cancers* 2023, 15, 2712. https://doi.org/10.3390/cancers15102712

Academic Editor: Vita Golubovskaya

Received: 24 March 2023
Revised: 2 May 2023
Accepted: 7 May 2023
Published: 11 May 2023

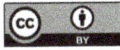

Copyright: © 2023 by the authors. Licensee MDPI, Basel, Switzerland. This article is an open access article distributed under the terms and conditions of the Creative Commons Attribution (CC BY) license (https://creativecommons.org/licenses/by/4.0/).

Keywords: NK cell; cancer immune cell therapy; checkpoint blockade immunotherapy; lung cancer; TIGIT blockade

1. Introduction

T cell immunoreceptor with immunoglobulin and ITIM domain (TIGIT) is a major inhibitory receptor of both T cells and natural killer (NK) cells (reviewed in [1–3]) and is an emerging target for immune checkpoint blockade for the treatment of cancer. TIGIT competes with inhibitory receptors KIR2DL5A [4,5] and PVRIG and activating receptor CD226 (DNAM-1) to bind ligands CD155 (PVR) and CD112 (Nectin-2 or PVRL2) which are commonly expressed on cancer cells and antigen-presenting cells (APCs) (reviewed in [6]). CD96 (TACTILE) also competes for binding to PVR and has been proposed to have a function in human NK-cell-target adhesion [7], but its role as an inhibitory or activating receptor is unclear (reviewed in [8]). Additionally, PVRL3 interacts with PVR and downregulates its surface expression and availability for receptor binding [9]. TIGIT also binds PVRL4 (Nectin-4), a TIGIT-specific ligand almost exclusively expressed on tumor cells [10]. TIGIT signaling regulates the tumor immunity cycle in multiple steps [3]. It prevents T cell proliferation, cytotoxicity, and the production of proinflammatory cytokine IFNγ by these cells (reviewed in [1]). Early clinical testing of anti-TIGIT therapies has shown success. To date, 20 anti-TIGIT antibody therapies are in clinical trials for over two dozen indications, with just over a dozen more anti-TIGIT modalities in preclinical development (reviewed in [11–13]). However, recent phase III trials in NSCLC and ES-SCLC did not show enhancement in PFS or OS at the time of this publication [14,15]. With the mixed clinical results, there is a critical need to further understand the mechanism of function of TIGIT on immune cells to support its clinical use.

Most of the current understanding of TIGIT regulation of immune cell function has been based on T cells and/or comes from murine models, while only limited mechanistic in vitro studies of TIGIT in human NK cells exist, and these predominantly rely on NK cell lines [16–22], despite the same or higher TIGIT expression on NK cells compared to T cells [23–25]. The limited studies that examined the role of TIGIT on primary human NK cells were mostly performed with cells derived from patients with cancer or chronic infection and showed that patient NK cells express TIGIT, and, dependent on the conditions, TIGIT levels were found to be similar to those in healthy cells [22,23,26], downregulated in the case of some metastatic cancer patients [21] or upregulated in patients with chronic infection [27]. In these studies, patient's cells were found to be dysfunctional and TIGIT blockade alone or with cytokines was shown to increase NK cell function, including IFNγ response and degranulation. While TIGIT and PD-1 combined blockade had a synergistic effect in improving tumor control and survival in mouse models and early clinical trials [12,28], in a B16 mouse model the therapeutic efficacy of PD-1 and TIGIT blockade depended on the presence of NK cells, as NK cell depletion abolished the effect [29]. These data show NK cells are an important immune population to consider in the efficacy of TIGIT blockade treatments.

Natural killer (NK) cells are first responders as part of the innate immune system, with an inherent ability to recognize and directly kill cancerous cells, and have emerged as a promising platform for next-generation of cell-based immunotherapies (reviewed in [30–35]). NK cells express a set of activating and inhibitory receptors that bind with their ligands and the balance of these inhibitory and activating receptors' signaling determines NK cell activity [30]. NK cells not only directly kill tumor cells but also "jump-start" the anti-tumor response, as they recruit, coordinate, and activate other immune cells, including cells of the adaptive immune system through the secretion of pro-inflammatory cytokines (e.g., IFNγ and TNFα) and chemokines ([36–38], reviewed in [39]). Recent studies have highlighted NK cells' critical role in the efficacy of immunotherapies where low NK cell numbers correlated with a lack of response to treatment (reviewed in [34]). The addition of adoptive NK cell treatments has the potential to improve the outcomes of current therapeutic strategies. NK cells can be efficiently expanded, viably cryopreserved without loss of efficacy [40–44], and are not associated with graft vs. host disease (GVHD) [45–47], supporting the potential safe use of cryopreserved donor-derived material as an off-the-shelf cell therapy ([48,49], reviewed in [50]). There are now large numbers of clinical trials assessing the efficacy of NK cells, including CAR-NK cells, in various cancer settings (reviewed in [51,52]).

Adoptive NK cell therapy in combination with anti-TIGIT treatment could provide an enhanced treatment option for cancer patients. In mouse models, blockade of TIGIT restored NK cell cytotoxicity, increased IFNγ and TNFα expression, and promoted tumor-specific T cell immunity [29,53–55]. However, there are no studies examining the effect of TIGIT expression on the cytotoxicity and function of highly activated and expanded NK cells used for adoptive cell therapy. Here, a novel exhaustion model was utilized in combination with kinetic live-cell imaging assays and sequencing to assess the impact of long-term exposure to lung cancer spheroids on the function of NK cells expanded with PM21 particles (PM21-NK cells) [48,49,56]. PM21-NK cells are clinically utilized in currently ongoing trials for cancer treatment (NCT04220684 and NCT05115630). Ex vivo expansion and/or activation upregulated TIGIT on NK cells. TIGIT-expressing cells expressed more activating receptors and had a higher frequency of cells producing effector cytokines and degranulating in response to target cell engagement. LUAD-TCGA database analysis demonstrated that TIGIT expression in the tumor tissue positively correlated with activating NK cells, while the presence of activating NK cells correlated with better outcomes. Expanded NK cells were found to be more resistant to TIGIT inhibition, where TIGIT blockade did not increase the anti-tumor activities of PM21-NK cells against K562 cells or lung cancer cells in monolayers, or within the first 24–32 h of spheroid exposure. However long-term spheroid exposure resulted in decreased cytotoxicity and function that could be preserved by the inclusion of TIGIT blockade. TIGIT blockade increased PM21-NK cell cytotoxicity against 3D lung cancer spheroids and prevented PVR-mediated dysfunction after exposure to tumor spheroids. TIGIT blockade upregulated multiple gene sets related to NK cell anti-tumor responses, including inflammatory response-related genes, TNFα signaling via NFκB, and IFNγ response-related gene sets. The implications of these findings on understanding TIGIT-targeted therapies and the use of adoptive NK cell/anti-TIGIT combinations are discussed.

2. Materials and Methods

2.1. Cell Culture

Buffy coats (leukocyte source) from de-identified healthy donors were used as a source of NK cells and were purchased from a local blood bank (OneBlood). Peripheral blood mononuclear cells (PBMC) were separated by density gradient (Ficoll-Paque Plus solution; GE Healthcare, Chicago, IL, USA) and cryopreserved for further use. NK cells were expanded with PM21 particles as described previously [48,49,56]. Briefly, T-cell-depleted PBMCs (EasySep CD3-positive selection kit; StemCell Technologies, Vancouver, Canada) were stimulated with 200 µg/mL PM21 particles and cultured for 2–3 weeks in SCGM media (CellGenix GmbH, Freiburg im Breisgau, Germany) and RPMI media with 100 U/mL IL-2 (PeproTech, Cranbury, NJ, USA). For activated NK cells, T-cell-depleted PBMCs were stimulated overnight with IL-2 (1000 U/mL) or IL-12 (10 µg/mL) + IL-15 (100 µg/mL) + IL-18 (50 µg/mL). Cancer cell line K562, A549, NCI-H358, and NCI-H1975 cells (ATCC) and NCI-H1299 (a generous gift from Dr. Griffith Parks, UCF) were maintained in RPMI media with 10% FBS, 1% antibiotic/antimycotic, and 2 mM Glutamax. A549-NLR, NCI-H358-NLR, NCI-H1975-NLR, and NCI-H1299-NLR cells were generated through stable transduction using commercial Nuclight Red Lentivirus (Sartorius). All cell lines were positively selected via puromycin selection followed by sorting on uniform positive populations (BD FACS Aria II). All cells were maintained in a humidified atmosphere at 37 °C supplemented with 5% (vol/vol) CO_2 in air. Cell lines were routinely assessed for mycoplasma (E-Myco Plus Mycoplasma PCR Detection Kit, Bulldog-Bio, Inc., Portsmouth, NH, USA) and authenticated via human STR profiling (serviced by ATCC).

2.2. Stable Cell Line Generation

PVR-expressing K562-GFPLuc cells were generated via stable transduction using lentiviral particles generated in-house (VectorBuilder Inc., Chicago, IL, USA) containing PVR coding gene sequences and sorted for positive and negative populations with a BD FACSAria II Cell Sorter (BD Biosciences, Franklin Lakes, NJ, USA). PVR$^+$ and PVR$^-$-K562-GFPLuc cell lines were cryopreserved until needed.

2.3. qRT-PCR

NK cells were selected (EasySep CD56-positive selection kit StemCell Technologies, Vancouver, BC, Canada) before and after expansion, and total RNA was isolated (Direct-zol RNA Microprep kit; Zymo Research, Irvine, CA, USA). cDNA was synthesized (High-Capacity cDNA Reverse Transcription Kit; Applied Biosystems, Waltham, MA, USA) and a gene expression primer set for TIGIT (QuantiTect Primer Assay; Qiagen, Hilden, Germany) was used to determine RNA expression levels by qRT-PCR (Quantstudio 7 PCR system, Applied Biosystems, USA). EIF3D and RPL13A were used as control genes. The $2^{-\Delta\Delta CT}$ method [57] was used to determine the relative RNA expression of the target gene.

2.4. Flow Cytometry

The following antibodies were used for flow cytometry analysis: CD56-PE (clone:5.1H11), CD56-APC/Fire™750 (clone:NCAM), CD56-AF®647 (clone:5.1H11), CD3-FITC (Clone:UCHT1), TIGIT-PE/Cy7 (Clone:A15153G), CD96-PE (Clone:NK92.39), DNAM-1-FITC (Clone:TX25), PVRIG-APC (Clone:W16216D), PVR-PE (Clone:SKIL2), PVRL2-APC (Clone:TX31), PVRL4-AF488 (Clone:337516), NKp30-PE (Clone:P30-15), NKp46-PE/Dazzle™594 (Clone:9E2), CD16-PeCy5 (Clone:3G8), NKG2D-APC (Clone:1D11), NKp44-PE-Cy7 (Clone:P44-8), LAG-3-FITC (Clone:11C3C65), PD-1-PE-Dazzle™594 (Clone:EH12.2H7), TIM-3-PE (Clone:F38-2F2), TNFα-PE/Dazzle™594 (Clone:MAB11), IFNγ-PerCP5.5 (Clone:B27), CD107a-PE (Clone:H4A3), CD3-PerCP-eF710 (Clone:OKT3), and NKG2A-APC (Clone:Z199). NK cells were stained with pre-conjugated protein-specific or the corresponding isotype control antibodies. All samples were acquired on a Cytoflex (Beckman Coulter, Brea, CA, USA) or Northern Lights 2000 Full Spectrum (Cytek, Fremont, CA, USA) flow cytometer and analyzed with FlowJo software (v10.6.2). An example gating strategy for NK cells is shown in Supplementary Materials Figure S1.

2.5. Kinetic Live-Cell Imaging Cytotoxicity Assays

Kinetic live-cell imaging cytotoxicity assays were performed as previously described [58]. Lung cancer cell lines A549-NLR, NCI-H358-NLR, NCI-H1975-NLR, and NCI-H1299-NLR, stably expressing nuclear red fluorescent protein (Nuclight Red; NLR) for tracking were used as target cells. For monolayer cytotoxicity assays, 6000 cancer cells were seeded per well in a flat-bottom 96-well plate the day prior to adding NK cells. For spheroid cytotoxicity assays, 5000 cancer cells were seeded in a 96-well clear round-bottom ultra-low attachment microplate (Corning, Corning, NY, USA), centrifuged at $130 \times g$ for 10 min, and incubated for 3 days to form spheroids. Cancer cell monolayers or spheroids were then co-cultured with NK cells at the indicated effector-to-target (E:T) ratios in the presence of Ultra-LEAF isotype or anti-TIGIT antibodies (Biolegend, San Diego, CA, USA). Monolayers were imaged for 72 h, while spheroid experiments were conducted for 7 days with an IncuCyte® S3 Live-Cell Analysis System (Sartorius, Göttingen, Germany). Target tumor cell growth was tracked over time by red object count per well (ROC) in 2D assays and total red object integrated intensity (ROII) (RCU × µm^2/Image) in 3D assays. Relative growth of the target cells alone or in the presence of NK cells with or without TIGIT blockade was determined by normalizing ROC or ROII to the value at time 0 (ROC$_t$/ROC$_{t=0}$ or ROII$_t$/ROII$_{t=0}$) when NK cells were initially added to determine normalized ROC (nROC) or normalized ROII (nROII) [59]. Cytotoxicity (%) was then determined based on the following equations:

$$2D\ Cytotoxicity^{E:T}(\%) = \left(1 - \left(\frac{nROC^{E:T}}{nROC^T}\right)\right) \times 100$$

$$3D\ Cytotoxicity^{E:T}(\%) = \left(1 - \left(\frac{nROII^{E:T}}{nROII^T}\right)\right) \times 100$$

2.6. In Vitro Exhaustion Model

A549-NLR cells (5000/well) were seeded in a 96-well clear round-bottom ultra-low attachment microplate (Corning, Corning, NY, USA), centrifuged at 130× g for 10 min, and incubated for 3–4 days to form spheroids. NK cells were then added in the presence of Ultra-LEAF isotype or anti-TIGIT antibodies (Biolegend, San Diego, CA, USA). After 7 days of incubation, NK cells were stimulated with PVR$^-$ or PVR$^+$-K562-GFPLuc cells for 4–6 h in the presence of Brefeldin A (eBioscience, San Diego, CA, USA) and Golgi Stop™ (BD Biosciences, Franklin Lakes, NJ, USA). Samples were harvested and stained with CD56, CD3, and CD107a antibodies, fixed and permeabilized (eBioscience IC Fixation and Permeabilization buffers), and probed with antibodies for IFNγ and TNFα, followed by analysis using flow cytometry.

2.7. RNA-Seq

NK cells were set up as described in the exhaustion model. After 7 days of coincubation, NK cells were isolated with an NK cell selection kit (EasySep CD56+ selection kit; StemCell technologies, Vancouver, BC, Canada) and analyzed by flow cytometry (Northern Lights 2000 Full Spectrum, Cytek, Fremont, CA, USA) to determine NK cell purity. Total RNA was extracted from the NK cells (Direct-zol Microprep kit, Zymo research, Irvine, CA, USA). RNA quality (RIN value) was determined by TapeStation and used for polyA selection, library preparation, and RNA sequencing (Genewiz, Inc., South Plainfield, NJ, USA). Raw RNA-seq data (Fastq) were analyzed with FastQC for quality control [60]. Trimmomatic was used for trimming adaptor and low-quality reads [61], HISAT2 for mapping genes with the hg38 human genome, and Stringtie for assembly and quantification of read counts [62]. Combat-seq was used to remove batch effects among samples [63] and EdgeR to normalize gene expression and determine differentially expressed genes [64]. A ranked gene list was generated by multiplying $\log_2$-fold change and $-\log_{10}$ (p-value) of individual genes obtained from EdgeR and used for pre-ranked gene set enrichment (GSEA) analysis to determine enriched hallmark-gene sets [65].

2.8. TIMER2.0-Based Analyses

The TIMER2.0 webserver [66–68] was used to report NK cell immune infiltration, gene expression, and patient survival correlations from the lung adenocarcinoma patient cohort of The Cancer Genome Atlas Program (TCGA) (n = 515). Correlation between TIGIT and NK cell infiltration was analyzed after tumor purity adjustment (partial Spearman's correlation) using the CIBERSORT immune deconvolution method in absolute mode. The statistical significance of differential expression between tumor and adjacent normal tissues was analyzed by the Wilcoxon test. The Cox proportional hazard model was used to determine the survival of lung adenocarcinoma patients using the upper and lower 25% of patients. The hazard ratio (HR) and p-value for Kaplan–Meier curves were determined to understand clinical relevance.

2.9. Statistics

Statistical analysis was performed by GraphPad Prism 9.3.1. Paired or unpaired two-tailed Student's t-tests were used unless noted in the figure legend. All experiments were performed for at least 3 biological replicates. p-values less than 0.05 were considered statistically significant. *p*-values are shown as * if $p < 0.05$, ** if $p < 0.01$, *** if $p < 0.001$, and **** if $p < 0.0001$.

3. Results

3.1. PM21-Particle-Expanded or Cytokine-Activated NK Cells Have Increased TIGIT Expression

NK cells obtained from healthy donors were expanded using PM21 particles [48,49]. This feeder cell-free expansion technology utilizes plasma membrane particles derived from K562-mbIL21-41BBL cells (PM21 particles) to stimulate NK cell proliferation, resulting in an average 1700-fold expansion of NK cells in 2 weeks (N = 113 from 18 donors, Supplementary Materials Figure S2). Resting NK cells isolated from PBMCs, and NK cells expanded from matching donors using PM21 particles (PM21-NK cells) were analyzed for TIGIT expression by qRT-PCR and flow cytometry. TIGIT was upregulated on the RNA level in PM21-NK cells compared to resting NK cells, ranging from 2.3-fold to 9.3-fold (average 5.6 ± 2.6-fold; N = 8, $p < 0.002$) (Figure 1A). Furthermore, the percentage of TIGIT$^+$ NK cells was increased in PM21-NK cells compared to resting NK cells (Figure 1B), with the expression ranging from 9% to 54% in resting NK cells and 54% to 90% in PM21-NK cells (N = 9, $p < 0.0001$) (Figure 1C). To determine if other NK cell activation methods also increase TIGIT expression, T-cell-depleted PBMCs were stimulated overnight with either IL-2 (1000 U/mL) or the combination of IL-12 (10 μg/mL), IL-15 (100 μg/mL), and IL-18 (50 μg/mL), and the percentage of NK cells expressing TIGIT was compared to resting NK cells (Figure 1D). TIGIT expression was upregulated on IL-2-activated NK cells (86 ± 7%, $p < 0.0001$) and IL-12/15/18-activated NK cells (79 ± 18%, $p < 0.0001$) compared to resting NK cells (29 ± 13%), and was comparable to the level of expression on PM21-NK cells (74 ± 13%) (Figure 1E). Altogether, these findings demonstrated that NK cells, activated with either PM21 particles or cytokines, upregulated TIGIT on both the RNA and surface protein levels.

3.2. More TIGIT$^+$ PM21-NK Cells Expressed Activating and Inhibitory Receptors Compared to TIGIT$^-$ PM21-NK Cells, and upon Stimulation with K562 Cells, More TIGIT$^+$ NK Cells Produced Effector Cytokines and Had Surface CD107a

To determine if the expression of TIGIT is associated with any changes to the phenotype and/or activation state of NK cells, the level of expression of major activating and inhibitory receptors was compared between TIGIT$^+$ and TIGIT$^-$ PM21-NK cells, determined by flow cytometry gating (Figure 2A, Supplementary Figure S1). Differences were evaluated on cells prior to day 14 of expansion when the expression is not at the maximal level and differential expression can still be assessed. In general, expression of activating and other inhibitory receptors was increased on TIGIT$^+$ PM21-NK cells compared to TIGIT$^-$ PM21-NK cells, as summarized in Figure 2B,C. The percentage of NK cells expressing activating receptors CD16, NKp30, NKp46, DNAM-1, and NKG2D varied between donors but was increased ($p = 0.02$ or less) for TIGIT$^+$ vs. TIGIT$^-$ NK cells in donor-matched pairs for all activating receptors, except for DNAM-1. DNAM-1 was ubiquitously and highly expressed on all PM21-NK cells, averaging more than 98% of both TIGIT$^-$ and TIGIT$^+$ NK cells (Figure 2B). The inhibitory receptors CD96, TIM-3, NKG2A, and LAG-3 were also expressed on PM21-NK cells, while PD-1 was detected on fewer than 2% of PM21-NK cells (Figure 2C). A significantly higher percentage of TIGIT$^+$ NK cells expressed CD96 ($p = 0.01$) and TIM-3 ($p = 0.008$) compared to donor-matched TIGIT$^-$ NK cells, while expression of NKG2A and LAG-3 were not significantly different. These findings showed that TIGIT$^+$ NK cells expressed higher levels of important activating and some inhibitory receptors typically induced upon activation.

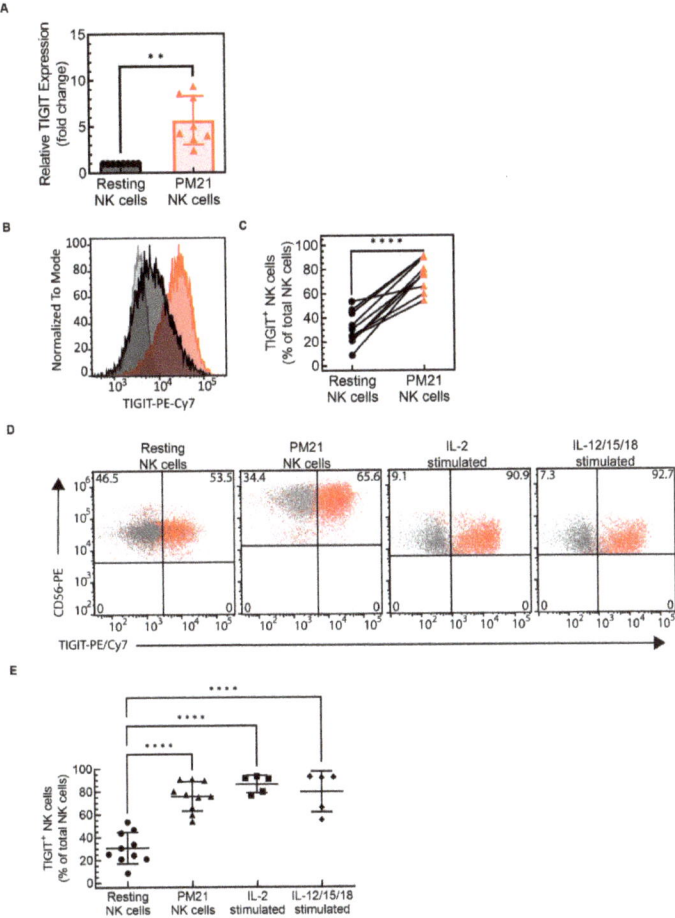

Figure 1. Cytokine-activated or PM21-particle-expanded NK cells highly expressed TIGIT. NK cells were either expanded with PM21 particles from T-cell-depleted PBMCs (PM21-NK cells) or were isolated from PBMCs by negative selection and analyzed for TIGIT expression directly (resting NK cells) or after overnight stimulation with cytokines. TIGIT expression was analyzed on the mRNA level by qPCR and on the protein level by flow cytometry. (**A**) TIGIT RNA level was on average 5.6 ± 2.6-fold greater in PM21-particle-expanded NK cells compared to resting NK cells ($N = 8$ donors). TIGIT expression was measured on the protein level by flow cytometry. (**B**) A representative histogram overlay is shown comparing PM21-NK cells (red) and resting NK cells (black) to isotype control (gray). (**C**) Summary data from 10 donors showed TIGIT protein expression significantly increased in PM21-NK cells (red triangles) compared to donor-matched resting NK cells (black circles). (**D**) Flow cytometry was also used to analyze TIGIT expression on NK cells activated by other methods, with dot plots showing examples of TIGIT expression on resting and activated cells as indicated above the graphs (red—anti-TIGIT vs. black—isotype ctrl.). (**E**) Consistent with PM21-NK cells (triangles), TIGIT expression is also increased in NK cells activated overnight with 1000 U/mL of IL-2 (squares) or 10 μg/mL IL-12, 100 μg/mL IL-15, and 50 μg/mL IL-18 (diamonds) compared to resting NK cells (circles) ($N = 5$–10 donors). Data are presented as a mean with error bars representing standard deviation (SD), scatter plots with donor-pair lines, or scatter plots with mean and SD. Paired two-tailed Student's t-tests were used to compare TIGIT expression in PM21-NK cells to that in resting cells and one-way ANOVA corrected for multiple comparisons using a Turkey post hoc test was used to compare TIGIT expression across different NK cell activation methods using GraphPad Prism software v. 9.3.1. *p*-values are shown as ** if $p < 0.01$, and **** if $p < 0.0001$.

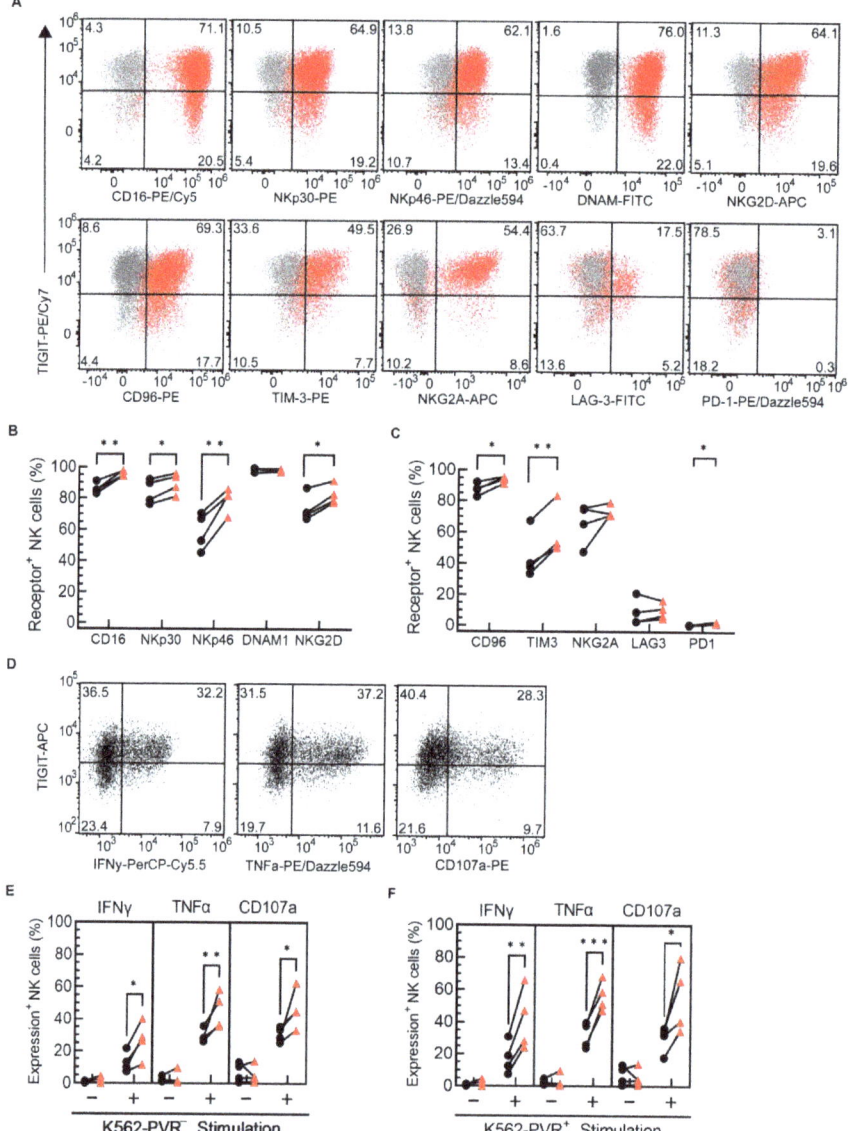

Figure 2. TIGIT⁺ NK cells have increased expression of NK cell receptors compared to TIGIT⁻ NK cells and have enhanced anti-tumor function. NK cells from four donors were expanded with PM21 particles from T-cell-depleted PBMCs for 12 days. Expression of NK cell activating and inhibitory receptors was determined by flow cytometry and gated on TIGIT⁻ or TIGIT⁺ NK cells. (**A**) Representative flow cytometry dot plots with gating are shown comparing NK cells with isotype control (gray) or the indicated receptor-specific antibody (red). The percentages of NK cells expressing (**B**) activating receptors CD16, NKp30, NKp46, DNAM1, and NKG2D and (**C**) inhibitory receptors CD96, TIM3, NKG2A, LAG3, and PD1 were determined for TIGIT⁺ NK cells (red triangles) and TIGIT⁻ NK cells (black circles) (N = 4 donors, avg. of duplicates). PM21-NK cells were stimulated with either PVR⁻ or PVR⁺-K562 cells and the percentage of TIGIT⁻ or TIGIT⁺ NK cells expressing IFNγ, TNFα, or CD107a was determined by flow cytometry with (**D**) representative dot plots shown for stimulation with PVR⁻ for each effector function measured. Significantly more TIGIT⁺-PM21-NK

cells (red triangles) produced IFNγ and TNFα, and expressed CD107a after stimulation with either PVR⁻ (**E**) or PVR⁺ (**F**) K562 cells compared to TIGIT⁻-PM21-NK cells (black circles) ($N = 4$ donors, avg. of 2–3 replicates). Data are presented as scatter plots with donor-pair lines. Statistical significance was determined by multiple paired t-tests. p-values are shown as * if $p < 0.05$, ** if $p < 0.01$ and *** if $p < 0.001$.

Next, the functional status of TIGIT⁺ vs. TIGIT⁻ PM21-NK cells was assessed to determine if TIGIT expression on NK cells also corresponds to higher function. For this, the production of effector cytokines and degranulation in unstimulated PM21-NK cells or cells stimulated with either PVR⁻ or PVR⁺-K562 cells was measured and compared based on TIGIT expression (Figure 2D). Significantly more TIGIT⁺ PM21-NK cells than TIGIT⁻ cells produced IFNγ ($27 \pm 12\%$ vs. $13 \pm 6\%$, $p = 0.014$) and TNFα ($45 \pm 11\%$ vs. $30 \pm 4\%$, $p = 0.005$) and stained for more surface CD107a ($46 \pm 12\%$ vs. $31 \pm 5\%$, $p = 0.013$) in response to PVR⁻-K562 cells (Figure 2E). Similarly, PVR⁺-K562 cell stimulation resulted in more TIGIT⁺ PM21-NK cells than TIGIT⁻ cells producing IFNγ ($41 \pm 19\%$ vs. $17 \pm 10\%$, $p = 0.009$) and TNFα ($56 \pm 9\%$ vs. $32 \pm 8\%$, $p < 0.001$) and with surface CD107a ($55 \pm 21\%$ vs. $30 \pm 8\%$, $p = 0.013$) (Figure 2F). There was no inhibition of TIGIT⁺ PM21-NK cells stimulated with PVR⁺-K562 cells compared to PVR⁻; in fact, the percentage of IFNγ⁺ and TNFα⁺ NK cells trended higher for PVR⁺-K562 stimulation (IFNγ $41 \pm 19\%$ vs. $27 \pm 12\%$, $p = 0.06$; TNFα $56 \pm 9\%$ vs. $45 \pm 11\%$, $p = 0.07$). This suggests that the response to PVR is overpowered by signaling through activating receptors DNAM-1 and/or NKG2D which are highly expressed on PM21-NK cells, while TIGIT inhibition is less evident. Consistent with the observations made with regard to PM21-NK cells, when NK cells were activated with IL-2 or IL-12/15/18, more TIGIT⁺ NK cells than TIGIT⁻ cells produced TNFα and had more cells with surface CD107a in response to both PVR⁻ and PVR⁺ K562 cell stimulation (Supplementary Materials Figure S3). However, no significant difference was observed between TIGIT⁺ and TIGIT⁻ NK cells in IFNγ, with overall low levels of IFNγ-expressing cells with O/N IL-2 activation (less than 14%) and overall high levels of IFNγ-expressing cells even without any stimulation with O/N IL-12/15/18 (more than 40%). The high basal level of IFNγ secretion with O/N IL-12/15/18 could be overpowering the response, not allowing for the detection of induction by target cell stimulation. No significant difference in effector cytokine production or degranulation between TIGIT⁺ and TIGIT⁻ PM21-NK cells was observed in response to cytokine stimulation with IL-12/15/18 (Supplementary Materials Figure S4), indicating this greater function is specific to anti-tumor response. Taken together, these data suggest that TIGIT⁺ NK cells represent a more activated cell subpopulation of NK cells with greater anti-tumor response capacity, and those cells are not inherently exhausted.

3.3. TIGIT Blockade Enhanced PM21-NK Cell Cytotoxicity against 3D Lung Tumor Spheroids

To access the effect of TIGIT blockade on PM21-NK cell anti-tumor functions, PM21-NK cell cytotoxicity against A549 lung tumor cells was examined. This cell line expresses TIGIT ligands PVR and PVRL2 but not PVRL3 or PVRL4 (Table 1, Supplementary Figure S5). PM21-NK cells were co-cultured with 2D A549 lung cancer cell monolayers at a 0.33:1 NK:A549 cell ratio in the presence of anti-TIGIT antibodies or isotype controls and cytotoxicity was measured with a live-cell imaging assay. No significant enhancement of PM21-NK cell killing occurred with TIGIT blockade over 72 h (cytotoxicity in the presence of isotype control vs. anti-TIGIT antibodies was $14 \pm 10\%$ vs. $15 \pm 9\%$ at 24 h, $27 \pm 11\%$ vs. $31 \pm 7\%$ at 48 h, and $44 \pm 9\%$ vs. $50 \pm 4\%$ at 72 h, $N = 3$ donors) (Figure 3A,B). Concentration-dependent cytotoxicity curves were determined for each timepoint for one donor and no difference in killing was observed with or without TIGIT blockade (area under the curve was $559 \pm 18\% \times$ cell ratio vs. $525 \pm 24\% \times$ cell ratio at 24 h, $689 \pm 17\% \times$ cell ratio vs. $629 \pm 37\% \times$ cell ratio at 48 h, and $751 \pm 14\% \times$ cell ratio vs. $697 \pm 25\% \times$ cell ratio at 72 h) (Figure 3C–E).

To determine if blockade of TIGIT affects PM21-NK cell cytotoxicity against lung cancer spheroids that better mimic the cancer environment, PM21-NK cells were co-cultured with A549 cell spheroids, and their killing over time as well as NK cell phenotype at the end of the co-culture were assessed. PM21-NK cells were exposed to tumor spheroid for 7 days in the presence of anti-TIGIT or isotype control antibodies. Representative videos and images at several time points show the increased killing of A549 spheroids in the presence of anti-TIGIT after 48 h (Supplementary Figure S6A, Figure 4A), apparent by the smaller size of resulting spheroids (Figure 4A) and reduced relative spheroid growth (Supplementary Figure S6B). Cytotoxicity curves over time were determined and representative curves from one donor and summary cytotoxicity data from multiple donors are shown in Figure 4B–D. The cytotoxicity was increasing over time with a comparable rate of killing observed between the control and anti-TIGIT samples during the first 48 h (Supplementary Figure S6A). Killing slowed down after 28 h in the absence of anti-TIGIT, while the killing rate remained unchanged when NK cells were with anti-TIGIT until 72 h, resulting in greater killing observed in the presence of anti-TIGIT over time. TIGIT blockade enhanced PM21-NK cell cytotoxicity against A549 spheroids at 72 h by an average of 20% across donors ($p < 0.0001$, 1:1 PM21-NK cells:A549 cells, $N = 6$) (Figure 4C,D). Expression of multiple activating and inhibitory receptors was evaluated on unexposed control PM21-NK cells and PM21-NK cells from three donors after exposure to A549 spheroid in the presence of isotype control or anti-TIGIT antibodies. Tumor exposure alone or with TIGIT blockade did not change the frequency of NK cells expressing inhibitory receptors TIM-3, NKG2A, LAG-3, PD-1, or CD96 compared to isotype control or unexposed NK cells (Supplementary Figure S7). Similarly, there was no difference in the expression of activating receptors CD16, NKG2D, NKp30, NKp46, and DNAM-1 after tumor exposure with or without TIGIT blockade, although there was a trend toward a decreased expression of NKG2D upon spheroid exposure, particularly with isotype control (Supplementary Figure S7).

Table 1. TIGIT ligand expression in lung cancer cell lines. Lung cancer cell lines were stained with TIGIT-ligand-specific antibodies and compared to isotype controls to determine ligand expression by flow cytometry. Data are presented as percentage of cancer cells that are ligand-positive (%) averaged from 2–3 different passages, in duplicate.

Lung Cancer Cell Line	PVR (%)	PVRL2 (%)	PVRL3 (%)	PVRL4 (%)
A549	100 ± 1	100 ± 1	2 ± 1	1 ± 1
NCI-H358	100 ± 1	100 ± 1	0 ± 1	82 ± 18
NCI-H1299	100 ± 1	100 ± 1	2 ± 1	1 ± 1
NCI-H1975	100 ± 1	100 ± 1	2 ± 2	16 ± 13

To confirm that the enhancement in NK cell cytotoxicity against lung cancer spheroids upon TIGIT blockade is not limited to a single cell line, testing of the anti-TIGIT antibody was also performed in the NCI-H1299, NCI-H358, and NCI-1975 lung cancer cell lines. These cell lines also highly express PVR and PVRL2 while H358 additionally expresses PVRL4 among the TIGIT ligands assessed (Table 1).

PM21-NK cell cytotoxicity against spheroids of these cell lines was determined using the live-cell imaging assay. Each cell line was killed at different rates, but all demonstrated enhanced cytotoxicity upon TIGIT blockade after the 24 h time point, with the effect increasing over time (Figure 5A–C). While there was donor-dependent variability in the extent of killing, TIGIT blockade increased cytotoxicity in donor-matched comparisons against all cell lines tested (NCI-H1299 $p = 0.02$, NCI-H358 $p = 0.01$, and NCI-1975; $p = 0.005$) and modestly enhanced the killing of H1299 (on average by 12%) and H358 (by 18%), while strongly enhancing killing of H1975 (by 88%) (Figure 5D,E). Collectively, these findings indicate that in 3D spheroid models, TIGIT blockade enhanced the cytotoxicity of PM21-NK cells over time against lung cancer cells without a change in the phenotype of the NK cells. The enhancement difference was not observed during the first 24–36 h but increased over time, with the largest differential observed after 72 h.

3.4. TIGIT Blockade Preserved PM21-NK Cell Effector Function against PVR-Positive Cancer Cells after Co-Culture with Cancer Cell Spheroids

NK cell exhaustion can occur in the context of the tumor microenvironment whereby long-term exposure to tumors leads to decreased effector function, altered phenotype, or decreased killing. The mechanisms leading to NK cell exhaustion are not well defined, although recent studies have shown that exacerbated inhibitory receptor signaling plays a role (reviewed in [69]). Previous studies have reported that chronic inhibitory signaling promotes the exhaustion of cytotoxic immune cells [69] and TIGIT has been associated with NK cell exhaustion in tumor-bearing mouse models and cancer patients [28]. In the experiments testing cytotoxicity of PM21-NK cells against lung cancer spheroids (Figures 3A and 4A–C), TIGIT blockade resulted in the enhancement of cytotoxicity that was increasing as a function of the time in co-culture with tumor, indicating that the rate of killing was decreasing in the absence of TIGIT blockade potentially as a result of progressive decline in function. To determine if TIGIT blockade could alleviate signs of exhaustion in PM21-NK cells upon exposure to tumor spheroids, an in vitro exhaustion model was developed. PM21-NK cells were first co-cultured with A549 spheroids for 7 days either in the presence of anti-TIGIT or isotype control antibodies. NK cells were then stimulated with either PVR^- or PVR^+-K562 cells and the production of effector cytokines and degranulation was assessed. Unexposed, unstimulated PM21-NK cells were used as a negative control while unexposed PM21-NK cells, stimulated with either PVR^+-K562 or PVR^--K562 cells, were used as positive controls. A schematic of the in vitro exhaustion model is shown in Figure 6A, and examples of flow cytometry histograms for one donor are shown in Figure 6B. Notably, the cytotoxicity, cytokine production, and degranulation of unexposed PM21-NK cells stimulated with either PVR^+-K562 or PVR^--K562 cells were comparable and were not affected by TIGIT blockade (Supplementary Figure S8).

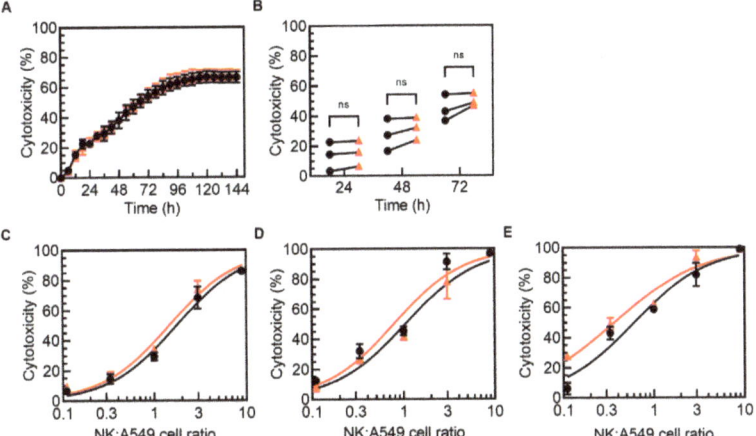

Figure 3. TIGIT blockade did not enhance PM21-NK cell cytotoxicity against A549 lung tumor monolayers. NK cells were expanded with PM21 particles from T-cell-depleted PBMCs obtained from multiple donors for 14–16 days. Cytotoxicity against A549-NLR lung cancer cells in a monolayer, measured by kinetic live-cell imaging, was not significantly improved in the presence of anti-TIGIT antibodies compared to isotype control. (**A**) Representative cytotoxicity time courses from one donor are shown in the presence of 0.3:1 NK cells:A549 cells either with isotype control (black circles) or in the presence of anti-TIGIT antibodies (red triangles). (**B**) Summary plot comparing cytotoxicity at 24, 48, and 72 h for NK cells from multiple donors at 0.3:1 of NK:A549 cells is shown ($N = 3$). Concentration-dependent cytotoxicity curves are shown for one donor at multiple NK cells:A549 cell ratios at 24 h (**C**), 48 h (**D**), and 72 h (**E**). Statistical significance was determined by multiple paired t-tests and represented as ns if $p > 0.05$.

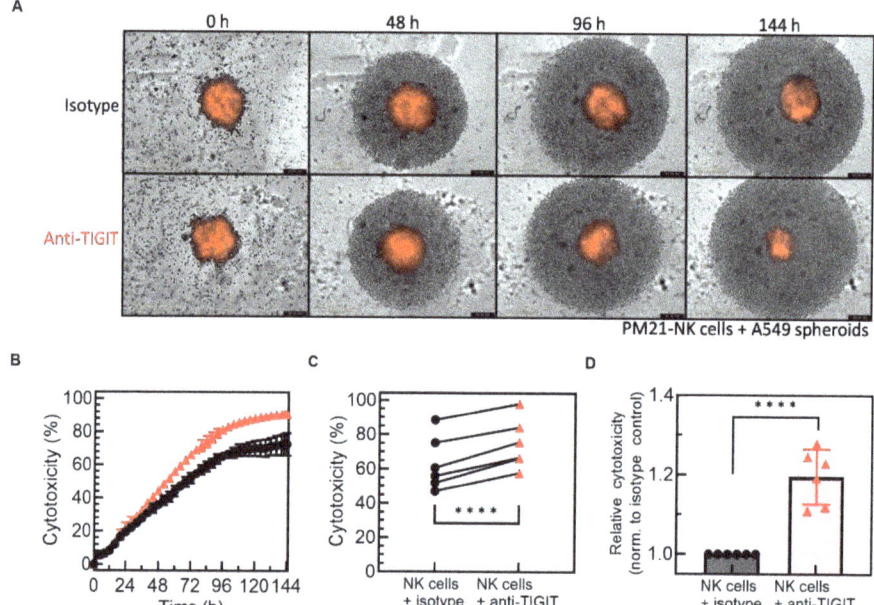

Figure 4. TIGIT blockade enhanced PM21-NK cell cytotoxicity against A549 lung tumor spheroids. Expanded NK cells were co-cultured with A549 tumor spheroids for 7 days. NK cell cytotoxicity was determined by kinetic live-cell imaging. Representative images at 10× magnification from the live-cell imaging cytotoxicity assay of NLR-expressing A549 cancer cell spheroids incubated with 10,000 NK cells in the presence of anti-TIGIT or isotype control after 0, 48, 96, and 144 h showed increased NK cell cytotoxicity in the presence of anti-TIGIT antibodies against A549 spheroids (**A**). Representative cytotoxicity time courses from one donor are shown with isotype control (black circles) or anti-TIGIT (red triangles) antibodies present (**B**). Summary plot comparing NK cell cytotoxicity from multiple donors at 72 h at 1:1 NK:A549 ratio shows that TIGIT blockade significantly increased cytotoxicity ($N = 6$ donors, avg. of 2–3 replicates) (**C**), and relative cytotoxicity increased for each donor when normalized to isotype control (**D**). Data are presented as scatter plots with donor-pair lines or as mean with error bars representing standard deviation. Statistical significance was determined by multiple paired *t*-tests. For concentration-dependent cytotoxicity curves, the area under the curve (AUC) was determined and compared by unpaired *t*-tests. *p*-values are shown as **** if $p < 0.0001$.

When unexposed PM21-NK cells were stimulated with K562 cells, the percentage of NK cells expressing IFNγ increased from less than 1% to 15 ± 5% ($p = 0.0002$) when stimulated with PVR$^-$-K562 cells and to 14 ± 7% ($p < 0.0001$) with PVR$^+$-K562 cells (Figure 6C). Restimulation with K562 cells after A549 spheroid co-culture resulted in a lower percentage of PM21-NK cells expressing IFNγ (8 ± 5% for PVR$^-$ ($p = 0.03$) and 4 ± 3% with PVR$^+$ cells ($p = 0.0002$)) (Figure 6C) and the decrease was greater when PVR$^+$ cells were used ($p = 0.04$). TIGIT blockade during co-culture with A549 spheroids did not mitigate the tumor-induced decrease in IFNγ expression after restimulation with PVR$^-$ cells with still only 9 ± 7% of cells expressing IFNγ. By contrast, restimulation with PVR$^+$-K562 cells increased IFNγ expression in NK cells from 3 ± 2% with isotype control to 7 ± 4% with anti-TIGIT, although without reaching significance ($p = 0.1$) (Figure 6C). Additionally, there was no longer a significant difference in IFNγ expression between PVR$^-$ or PVR$^+$-K562 cell restimulation when anti-TIGIT antibodies were present in the initial tumor co-culture, indicating that the initial difference was TIGIT-dependent. Thus, tumor exposure resulted in close to 80% loss in the IFNγ generation capacity with about 30% of this loss being dependent on TIGIT/PVR engagement.

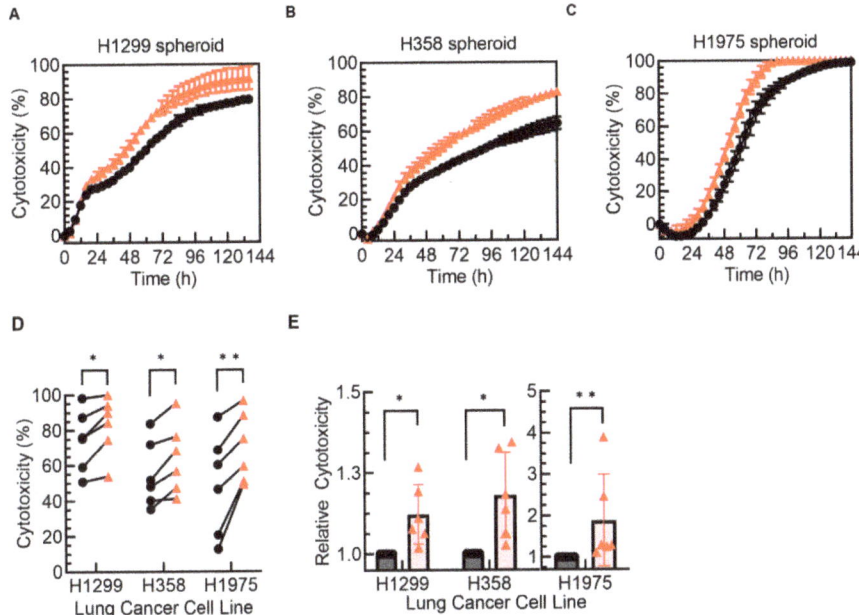

Figure 5. TIGIT blockade enhanced NK-cell-mediated killing in multiple 3D lung tumor spheroid models. NK cells were expanded with PM21 particles from T-cell-depleted PBMCs obtained from multiple donors for 14–16 days. Expanded NK cells were co-cultured with NCI-H1299-NLR, NCI-H358-NLR, or NCI-1975-NLR lung tumor spheroids for 7 days. NK cell cytotoxicity time courses were determined by kinetic live-cell imaging. Representative cytotoxicity curves from one donor are shown against H1299 (**A**), H358 (**B**), and H1975 (**C**) spheroids either with isotype control (black circles) or TIGIT (red triangles) antibodies present. Summary plot comparing NK cell cytotoxicity from multiple donors at 72 h shows that TIGIT blockade significantly increased cytotoxicity (**D**) and enhanced relative cytotoxicity when cytotoxicity with anti-TIGIT for each donor was normalized to isotype control (**E**) (E:T ratios used were 3:1 for NCI-H1299, 1:1 for NCI-H358, and 1:3 for NCI-H1975; N = 6 donors, avg. of 3 replicates). Data are presented as scatter plots with donor-pair lines or as mean with error bars representing standard deviation. Statistical significance was determined by multiple paired t-tests. p-values are shown as * if $p < 0.05$ and ** if $p < 0.01$.

TNFα generation was also negatively impacted by tumor exposure, with most of the decrease being driven by the TIGIT/PVR axis. Stimulation of unexposed PM21-NK cells with K562 cells resulted in an increased frequency of TNFα$^+$ NK cells compared to unstimulated cells (4 ± 1% vs. 29 ± 5% upon PVR$^-$ cell stimulation ($p < 0.0001$) and 4% vs. 28 ± 3% with PVR$^+$ cells ($p < 0.0001$)) (Figure 6D). Compared to unexposed cells, A549 tumor exposure either in the presence of isotype control or anti-TIGIT antibodies did not result in a change in the frequency of TNFα$^+$ NK cells induced in response to PVR$^-$-K562 cell restimulation (27 ± 6% in the presence of isotype control and 30 ± 8% with anti-TIGIT antibodies) (Figure 6D). However, restimulation with PVR$^+$-K562 cells resulted in a lower frequency of TNFα$^+$ NK cells after co-cultures with isotype control antibodies compared to PVR$^-$-K562 cell restimulation (27 ± 6% with PVR$^-$ vs. 15 ± 5% with PVR$^+$ cells; $p = 0.008$) or compared to unexposed NK cells stimulated with PVR$^+$-K562 cells (28 ± 3% in unexposed vs. 15 ± 5% for spheroid exposed; $p = 0.0001$) (Figure 6D). Blocking of TIGIT during spheroid co-culture prevented the decrease in the frequency of TNFα$^+$ NK cells, with 28 ± 7% of NK cells expressing TNFα after restimulation with PVR$^+$-K562 cells, frequencies comparable to unexposed stimulated NK cells (28 ± 3%) and to exposed NK cells stimulated with PVR$^-$-K562 cells (27 ± 6%) (Figure 6D). Thus, blocking TIGIT fully restored the TNFα production capacity of NK cells in response to PVR$^+$ targets.

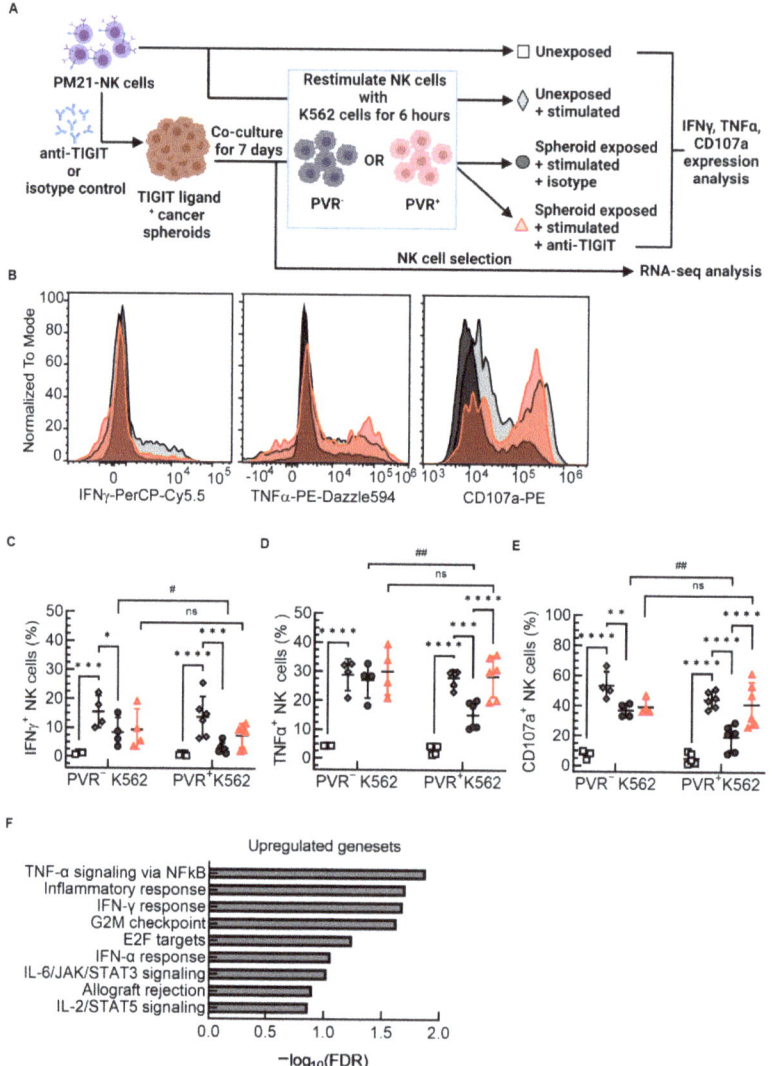

Figure 6. TIGIT blockade prevents PVR-mediated NK cell exhaustion during spheroid exposure. NK cells were expanded from T-cell-depleted PBMCs for 14–16 days. Expanded NK cells were co-cultured with A549 spheroids for 7 days in the presence of anti-TIGIT or isotype control. After 7 days of co-culture, NK cells were stimulated with K562 cancer cells with or without PVR expression for 4–6 h in the presence of Brefeldin A and Golgi Stop, and NK cell expression of surface CD107a, IFNγ, and TNFα was analyzed with flow cytometry. Unexposed PM21-NK cells, either unstimulated or stimulated, were used as controls. Additionally, NK cells were selected after co-culture with A549 spheroids and used for RNA extraction and transcriptomic analysis. A schematic of the experiment is shown in (**A**). IFNγ, TNFα, and CD107a expression on NK cells was determined by flow cytometry, and representative histograms are shown overlaying unexposed stimulated PM21-NK cells (light gray fill with black outline) with PM21-NK cells that were tumor exposed in the presence of a blocking antibody isotype control (dark gray fill with black outline) or anti-TIGIT (red fill and outline) and stimulated with PVR+ K652 cells for all shown conditions (**B**). Unstimulated, unexposed NK cells (open squares), unexposed stimulated NK cells (gray filled diamonds), NK cells that were tumor-exposed in the presence of isotype (dark gray filled circles) or anti-TIGIT antibodies (red filled triangles) are shown for either re-stimulation with PVR−-K562 cells or PVR+-K562 cells. TIGIT blockade

preserved IFNγ (**C**), TNFα (**D**), and CD107a (**E**) expression to levels of unexposed NK cells, when re-challenged with PVR$^+$-K562 cells (N = 4–6 donors, avg. of 2 replicates). GSEA analysis of RNA-seq data from 3 donors shows that TIGIT blockade upregulated IFNγ, TNFα, and other related inflammation response gene sets. Summary graphs show upregulated gene sets upon TIGIT blockade based on their $-\log_{10}$(FDR) (**F**). Data are presented as scatter plots or bar graphs with error bars representing standard deviation. Statistical significance was determined by 2-way ANOVA with p-values shown as * if $p < 0.05$, ** if $p < 0.01$, *** if $p < 0.001$, and **** if $p < 0.0001$ for comparing each exposure and stimulation condition. Statistical significance was determined by unpaired t-tests with p-values shown as ns $p > 0.05$, # if $p < 0.05$, or ## $p < 0.01$.

TIGIT blockade also restored most of the ability of PM21-NK cells to degranulate upon PVR$^+$ cell restimulation post-tumor-co-culture. Surface CD107a expression, a marker for degranulation, increased in unexposed PM21-NK cells upon stimulation with K562 cells where the frequencies of degranulating, CD107a$^+$ NK cells increased from 6 ± 3% in unstimulated to 53 ± 9% ($p < 0.0001$) in cells stimulated with PVR$^-$K562, and to 44 ± 5% ($p < 0.0001$) after PVR$^+$-K562 cell stimulation (Figure 6E). Tumor co-culture in the presence of isotype control antibodies decreased the frequency of CD107a$^+$ NK cells upon restimulation with K562 cells (37 ± 5% for PVR$^-$ ($p = 0.004$) and 19 ± 8% PVR$^+$ ($p < 0.0001$)) with a larger decrease with PVR$^+$-K562 cells compared to PVR$^-$ cells ($p = 0.005$). TIGIT blockade during tumor co-culture only restored CD107a expression for PVR$^+$-K562-restimulated NK cells; resulting in an increase in the frequency of CD107a$^+$ NK cells compared to isotype control conditions (41% with TIGIT blockade vs. 19% with isotype control; $p < 0.0001$), resulting in comparable frequencies of CD107a$^+$ NK cells to those observed for PVR$^-$-K562-restimulated NK cells, which remained unchanged after TIGIT blockade (41% with PVR$^+$ cell restimulation vs. 39% with PVR$^-$).

In summary, evidence of NK cell exhaustion upon tumor exposure was observed, resulting in decreased frequencies of NK cells degranulating and producing IFNγ and TNFα after re-stimulation with K562 cells compared to K562 stimulation of unexposed NK cells, and these decreases were greater when restimulated with PVR$^+$-K562 cells. TIGIT blockade restored the ability of NK cells to produce IFNγ and TNFα and degranulate (based on CD107a surface expression) upon restimulation with PVR$^+$ cells in tumor-exposed PM21-NK cells back to levels comparable to re-stimulation with PVR$^-$-K562 cells, and for TNFα and degranulation to levels observed for unexposed NK cells stimulated with PVR$^+$-K562 cells.

In order to determine if the protective effect of TIGIT blockade on the effector functions of PM21-NK cells post-exposure occurs on a transcriptional level, NK cells were selected after co-culture with A549 spheroids for 7 days and RNA extracted for sequencing and transcriptomic analysis (schematically depicted in Figure 6A). Gene set enrichment analysis revealed that TIGIT blockade upregulated hallmark gene sets including TNFα signaling via NFκB, inflammatory response, IFNγ response, and IFNα response gene sets (Figure 6F, Supplementary Figure S9). These enrichments in the transcriptome indicate a more activated state [70] of PM21-NK cells upon TIGIT blockade during A549 co-culture. Altogether, these observations from functional and transcriptomic analyses demonstrated that TIGIT blockade restored PM21-NK cell anti-tumor functions against PVR$^+$ cancer cells after exposure to cancer cell spheroids.

3.5. Translational Importance of Activated NK Cells and PVR/TIGIT Axis

To assess if there is a correlation between NK cell levels and/or the PVR/TIGIT axis and outcomes, the lung adenocarcinoma (LUAD) cohort of The Cancer Genome Atlas (TCGA) was analyzed using the TIMER2.0 webserver. TIGIT was significantly upregulated in tumor tissue compared to adjacent normal tissue in the LUAD cohort (Figure 7A). While PVR was not upregulated, TIGIT ligands PVRL2 and PVRL4 had significantly increased expression levels (Figure 7A). Further, TIGIT expression positively correlated with infiltrated activated NK cells, but not resting NK cells (Figure 7B), indicating that the presence of activated NK cells in the tissue may lead to higher overall levels of TIGIT expression in tumors, including associated infiltrating immune cells, likely including activated NK cells. Most importantly, higher levels of activated NK cell infiltration correlated to better survival (Figure 7C) while higher levels of PVR on tumors correlated with poorer survival (Figure 7D). There was no correlation between the levels of resting NK cells and outcomes (Supplementary Materials Figure S10). Taken together, these results corroborate the importance of the in vitro findings and show that there is a correlation between levels of activated NK cells, TIGIT tumor tissue expression, and better outcomes. On the other hand, the presence of PVR on tumors would likely result in TIGIT engagement and progression to a more exhausted state correlated with poorer outcomes and also suggest that combining the adoptive transfer of highly activated NK cells with TIGIT blockade could enhance response rates and improve outcomes by preventing exhaustion and prolonging NK-cell activation state.

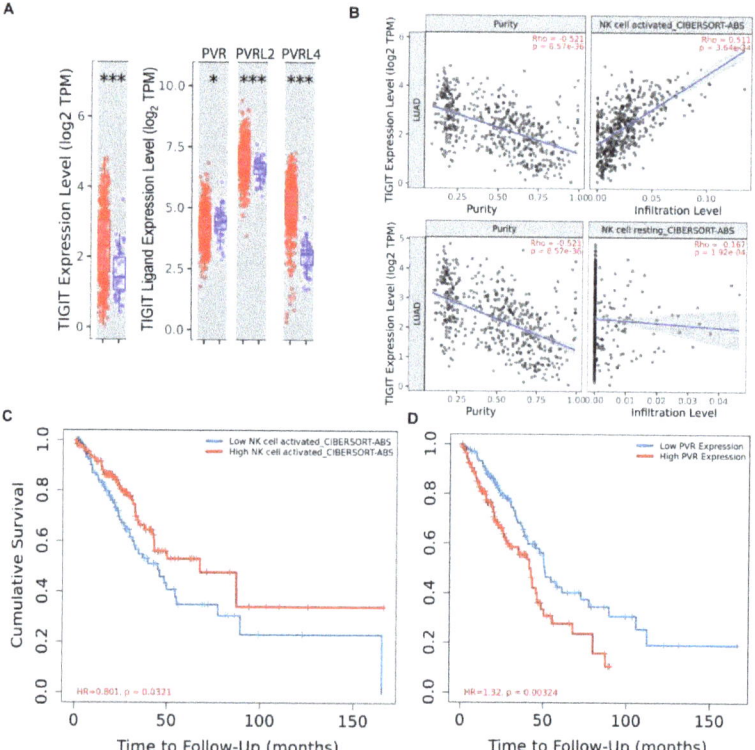

Figure 7. Activated NK cells infiltrated into LUAD tumors upregulate TIGIT and correlate with better survival. The TIMER2.0 webserver was used to analyze the lung adenocarcinoma (LUAD) cohort of The Cancer Genome Atlas (TCGA) (n = 515) to determine if there are correlations between NK cell levels, TIGIT/PVR expression, and outcomes. The analysis revealed that TIGIT and its ligands PVRL2 and PVRL4 are significantly upregulated in LUAD tumors compared to normal tissue (**A**). TIGIT expression positively correlated with activated NK cells, but not resting NK cells, based on absolute CIBSORT deconvolution of immune infiltrates and gene expression in the cohort (**B**). Additionally, higher levels of activated NK cell infiltration correlated with better survival (**C**) while higher levels of PVR on tumors correlated with poorer survival (**D**). Statistical significance in (**A**) was determined by the Wilcoxon test; p-values are shown as * if p < 0.05 or *** if p <0.001). Scatter plots with purity-adjusted spearman's rho and p-value are shown in (**B**). The hazard ratio (HR) and p-value for Kaplan-Meier curves are shown in (**C**,**D**).

4. Discussion

TIGIT has received a tremendous amount of attention in recent years as a promising target with the potential to match or exceed the success of anti-PD-(L)1 therapies. Based on the exciting preclinical and early clinical data, there are currently over 60 active trials of therapies targeting TIGIT in different cancer settings and in various combinations [71]. There are also more than 20 additional TIGIT-targeting modalities, including antibody–drug conjugates and bi- and tri-specifics, that are currently under development [72]. This high enthusiasm has been recently quenched by the release of data from larger phase III trials in NSCLC (SKYSCRPER-01) and ES-SCLC (SKYSCRAPER-02) that failed to meet primary endpoints in terms of reaching target improvement in progression-free survival or overall survival. Thus, there is a great need to gain a better understanding of TIGIT function in the cell populations that are behind tumor control to realize the potential shortcomings. NK cells are one of those populations that not only kill but also set the stage for other components of the immune system. NK cells also constitutively express TIGIT [13,18,21,22,73–75], and, under some circumstances, the levels of TIGIT expression were found to be higher than on any of the T cell subtypes, including CD8 T cells and Tregs [24]. Yet, NK cells are also largely ignored when investigating potential reasons behind the failure of TIGIT therapeutics. This study was designed to provide a more detailed understanding of TIGIT function on activated human NK cells derived from healthy donors prior to, and after, exposure to PVR-expressing lung cancer spheroids. The results were further compared with the analysis of patient data from the LUAD-TCGA database, and together, provide important findings that should be considered when using TIGIT therapeutics as well as adoptive NK cell therapies to potentially improve outcomes.

In the current study, TIGIT was found to be highly expressed on the surface of activated NK cells irrespective of the activation method used. Activation of NK cells with the methods used clinically for the generation of cells for adoptive NK cell therapy, such as cytokines, IL-12/15/18, or through expansion with PM21 particles, resulted in the upregulation of TIGIT expression. TIGIT expression marked NK cells that had increased expression of major activating receptors (CD16, NKG2D, NKp46, and NKp30) and some inhibitory receptors, such as CD96 and TIM-3. TIGIT$^+$ NK cells had enhanced cytotoxic function, resulting in a greater level of degranulation and effector cytokine secretion after exposure to tumor targets, suggesting that TIGIT is a marker of NK cell activation. Previous studies have similarly reported that IL-15 stimulation can increase TIGIT expression on NK cells, while other cytokines tested, such as IL-7 and IL-21, resulted in only minor increases (<15%) or no change (such as with IL-12) in the MFI of TIGIT-stained cells [3,25]. In contrast to our findings, the functional performance of TIGIT$^+$ NK cells was reported to be lower as compared to TIGIT$^-$, although most of the studies examined NK cells derived from tumor-bearing mice or patients either with chronic infection or cancer, which were likely already exhausted [22,26,28,76]. For example, TIGIT expression trended higher in early melanoma but was downregulated in metastatic melanoma [21]. TIGIT$^+$ NK cells from melanoma patients were found to have higher lytic potential, as determined by higher levels of perforins and granzyme, but lower lytic function, resulting in lower degranulation and specific lysis. In murine models, TIGIT$^+$ NK cells recovered from either spleen or tumors of tumor-bearing mice had a lower frequency of IFNγ-, TNFα-, or DNAM-expressing cells as compared to TIGIT$^-$ NK cells [28]. Wang et al. reported that TIGIT$^+$ NK cells from healthy individuals had decreased function resulting in lower degranulation and cytokine production, although the stimulation method used was either with IL-12 or lipopolysaccharide (LPS) [24]. Similarly, we did not observe any difference in IFNγ or TNFα production between TIGIT$^+$ and TIGIT$^-$ NK cells in response to cytokine stimulation, suggesting that these TIGIT$^+$ NK cells have greater anti-tumor but not general responsiveness. Thus, the observed differences are likely due to differences in the activation method used for testing the function or the cell source (healthy vs. tumor-derived NK cells). The present study demonstrated that freshly activated and/or expanded NK cells appear to have higher TIGIT expression, which also correlates to a more activated phenotype and enhanced anti-tumor function. Surprisingly, TIGIT blockade also did not affect PM21-NK cell cytotoxicity in short-term assays with 2D lung cancer monolayers. This suggests that activation, likely involving DNAM-1-PVR binding and/or NKG2D, overpowers TIGIT inhibitory signaling in the highly cytotoxic PM21-NK cells [55] in the short term. PM21 NK cells have high expression of major activating receptors such as DNAM-1, NKG2D, NKp46, and NKp30. This also suggests that the observed higher cytotoxicity of expanded cells may also be the result of lower sensitivity to inhibitory signaling.

To address if expanded cells are still susceptible to exhaustion after prolonged tumor exposure, a novel in vitro spheroid model was developed. This model was utilized in combination with blocking antibodies to assess the effect of TIGIT engagement on the function of expanded NK cells after chronic tumor exposure. In this chronic exposure model, TIGIT blockade had no effect within the first 48 h but thereafter gradually improved PM21-NK-cell cytotoxicity against multiple lung cancer spheroids. This suggests that during long-term exposure to tumors, TIGIT signaling can inhibit and/or downregulate NK-cell-mediated killing. Furthermore, chronic tumor exposure had a negative impact on general NK-cell anti-tumor function, resulting in reduced degranulation and decreased expression of effector cytokines IFNγ and TNFα in NK cells exposed to tumors and re-challenged with either PVR$^+$ and PVR$^-$ K562 cells. Combining TIGIT blockade during tumor exposure with either PVR$^+$ or PVR$^-$ restimulation allowed us to decern which function was negatively impacted by the engagement of the TIGIT/PVR pathway, and to what extent. PVR/TIGIT interaction was the main mechanism leading to the decline in TNFα production, whereas TIGIT blockade and/or absence of PVR resulted in the retention of full function at the level of unexposed cells. Additional factors contributed to decreased IFNγ production and degranulation in this system, preventing the full restoration of these functions with TIGIT blockade or in the absence of PVR engagement. Although in the present study, the blockade was applied concurrently with tumor exposure and as such likely prevented functional decline, the effect of TIGIT could also be reversing the loss of function, as others have shown when applying anti-TIGIT to cells recovered from tumor microenvironments either from patients or mice [22]. However, in those studies, it is difficult to assess how much of the function is recovered since starting levels are not easy to evaluate. In some of those studies, TIGIT blockade itself was not sufficient to enhance the function of exhausted cells but rather had to be combined with cytokine activation [21,22]. Interestingly, in the present study, no significant changes in the surface phenotype were observed after tumor exposure, including similar DNAM-1 expression, and a trend toward decreased expression was only observed for NKG2D, with some improvement with TIGIT blockade. Transcriptomic analysis of NK cells after exposure to the A549 spheroids demonstrated that chronic TIGIT engagement results in NK cell reprogramming associated with the functional decline, and blocking TIGIT resulted in the upregulation of gene sets involved in inflammatory responses and TNFα signaling, consistent with the functional results. These gene sets could be upregulated by applying TIGIT blockade and suggested a more activated state of NK cells when combined with anti-TIGIT.

These findings agree with previous reports from murine models that showed that in tumor-challenged mice, TIGIT deficiency or blockade resulted in better tumor control and that the recovered tumor-infiltrating NK cells had more than double the frequency of TNFα-producing cells and more CD107$^+$ and DNAM$^+$ cells within the tumor-infiltrating NK cell populations. There was either small or no change observed in the frequency of IFNγ-producing NK cells dependent on the model, which is somewhat different from the findings presented in this study, although in the current study, the decline observed in IFNγ production appears to be largely mediated by mechanisms other then TIGIT/PVR engagement, where only a minor component was restored with TIGIT blockade and a large decrease was observed with restimulation with PVR$^-$ cells. Another difference between the present study and others is in the lack of downregulation of DNAM-1 expression after tumor exposure. Several studies have reported that NK cells obtained from cancer patients or patients with chronic infections had lower expression of DNAM-1 and/or TIGIT [22,77,78].

Moreover, in the tumor-bearing murine models, TIGIT blockade or deficiency resulted in more DNAM-1$^+$ cells (~15% more) [28]. This is different from the present study and may be either due to shorter exposure time (7 days vs. >14 days) or due to the greater activation state of the expanded cells that renders the DNAM-1 expression more stable and resistant to downregulation upon TIGIT engagement and/or exhaustion. The cells also retained their function after exposure even in the absence of TIGIT blockade, supporting their utility for adoptive cell therapies.

As mentioned earlier, NK cells are the critical component of anti-tumor immunity. The efficacy of anti-TIGIT antibodies was dependent on NK cells and NK cells were shown to regulate CD8 T cell anti-tumor immunity, including preventing their exhaustion and helping with memory formation [28]. Thus, the presence of functional, TIGIT$^+$ NK cells is critical to the efficacy of anti-TIGIT therapies and adoptive NK cell therapy may further improve the efficacy of anti-TIGIT antibodies by boosting overall T cell immune response against cancer cells in cancer patients frequently lacking the NK cell compartment.

NK cells are critically important for the efficacy of anti-TIGIT therapies. Yet, the majority of current therapeutic anti-TIGIT antibodies in development, including tiragolumab that recently failed in PhIII trials, are Fc-competent and can engage FcγR on effector cells, e.g., macrophages, and potentially lead to clearance of TIGIT$^+$ cells. Depletion of TIGIT$^+$ populations including Tregs has been reported in tumor samples obtained from patients treated with Fc-optimized TIGIT antibodies and was considered important for the therapeutic effects of the antibodies [79,80]. Given that TIGIT is highly expressed on activated, tumor-infiltrating NK cells and at lower levels on resting non-activated NK cells (Figures 1 and 7), Fc-competent anti-TIGIT antibodies could lead to the depletion of this critical population through FcR-dependent mechanisms. The effect of an Fc-competent anti-TIGIT antibody on the function of NK cells has been examined in a short-term assay and shown to increase the percentage of CD107a$^+$ NK cells [81]; however, long-term assays or in-depth analyses of the effects on NK cell amount were not performed. Although blocking TIGIT could help prevent NK cell exhaustion and/or restore NK cell function, Fc-competent anti-TIGIT antibodies may negatively affect the efficacy of treatment by removal of this critical effector population. Further studies are warranted to probe this potential consequence of Fc-competent antibody use and its effect on treatment outcomes.

5. Conclusions

In summary, this study provides insight into mechanisms of TIGIT blockade in ex vivo-expanded human NK cells. TIGIT is highly expressed on activated NK cells and correlates with higher anti-tumor function, although during prolonged tumor exposure, its engagement can result in a decrease in NK cell function (Figure 8). Anti-TIGIT antibodies have the potential to improve the efficacy of PM21-NK cell tumor immunity, and adoptive PM21-NK cells and anti-TIGIT antibodies should be explored in future preclinical studies and clinical trials as a combination therapy against lung tumors.

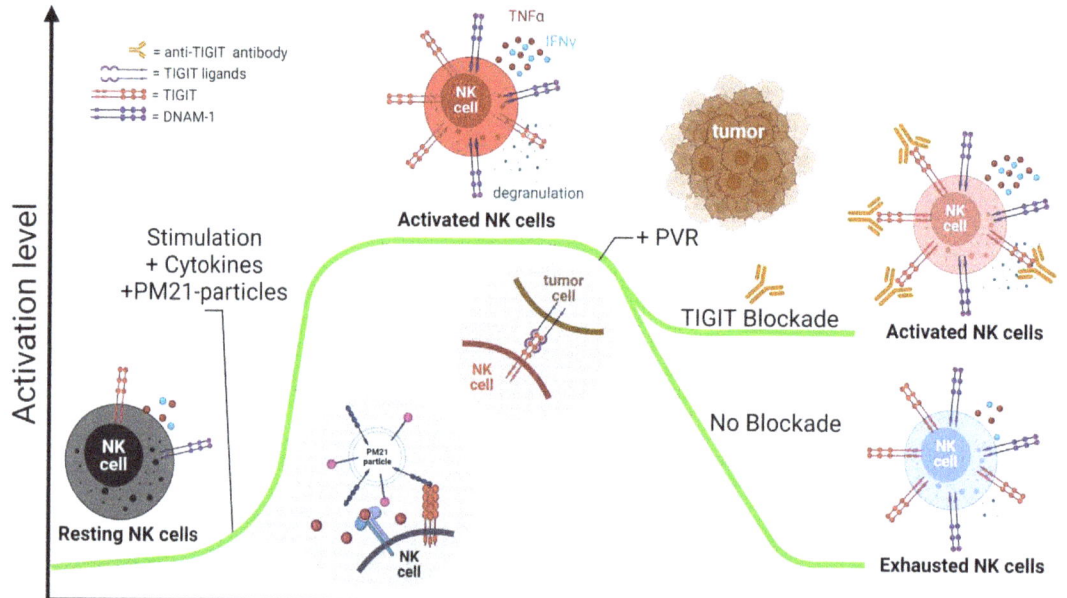

Figure 8. TIGIT expression in the context of NK cell activation state and TIGIT blockade. TIGIT expression is increased on activated NK cells compared to resting. Activated TIGIT$^+$ NK cells have a better anti-tumor response as compared to TIGIT$^-$ NK cells. However, chronic TIGIT engagement with its ligands in the tumor microenvironment leads to the functional decline of NK cells, which can be prevented with anti-TIGIT.

Supplementary Materials: The following supporting information can be downloaded at: https://www.mdpi.com/article/10.3390/cancers15102712/s1, Supplemental Methods, Figure S1: Example gating strategy for counting viable NK by flow cytometry; Figure S2: PM21-NK cell expansion; Figure S3: Cytokine-preactivated TIGIT$^+$ NK cells have increased TNFα and degranulation in response to K562 cells compared to TIGIT$^-$ cytokine-preactivated NK cells; Figure S4: TIGIT$^+$ PM21-NK cells have the same response as TIGIT$^-$ PM21-NK cells when exposed to cytokine stimulation; Figure S5: TIGIT ligand expression on cancer cells, Figure S6: Kinetic live-cell imaging cytotoxicity assay; Figure S7: PM21-NK cell phenotype does not change after tumor exposure in the presence of anti-TIGIT; Figure S8: Short-term TIGIT blockade does not further enhance PM21-NK cell function; Figure S9: Supplemental RNA-seq data; Figure S10: LUAD patient outcomes stratified by resting NK cell infiltration.

Author Contributions: Conceptualization, M.F.H. and A.J.C.; methodology, M.F.H. and A.J.C.; validation, M.F.H., T.J.C.-P., J.L.O. and A.J.C.; formal analysis, M.F.H., T.J.C.-P. and J.L.O.; investigation, M.F.H., T.J.C.-P., J.L.O., T.A.D., L.D.R.-C., J.E.E., S.K. and B.W.A.; resources, A.J.C.; data curation, M.F.H.; writing—original draft preparation, M.F.H., T.J.C.-P. and A.J.C.; writing—review and editing, M.F.H., T.J.C.-P., J.L.O., T.A.D, L.D.R.-C., J.E.E., S.K., B.W.A. and A.J.C.; visualization, M.F.H. and T.J.C.-P.; supervision, A.J.C.; project administration, A.J.C.; funding acquisition, A.J.C. All authors have read and agreed to the published version of the manuscript.

Funding: This research was funded by the FL DOH James and Ester King Program (Grant No. 9JK04) and the University of Central Florida Preeminent Postdoctoral Program.

Institutional Review Board Statement: This study was conducted in accordance with the University of Central Florida Institutional Biosafety Committee and all biological materials used were approved under BARA #19-27 (approved 7/17/2019-02/28/2023) and Safety Protocol ID: SPROTO202200000044 (approved 3/1/2023). No animal or human studies were included in the manuscript.

Data Availability Statement: Raw RNA sequencing data are deposited in the NCBI SRA database under submission number SUB12437119 and data will be made public and accession numbers provided prior to publication.

Acknowledgments: The graphics were created with BioRender.com. The results published here are in part based upon data generated by the TCGA Research Network: https://www.cancer.gov/tcga.

Conflicts of Interest: A.J.C.: licensed IP to, consultancy, and research support from Kiadis Pharma, a Sanofi company; J.L.O.: licensed IP to and consultancy with Kiadis Pharma, a Sanofi company. The funders had no role in the design of the study; in the collection, analyses, or interpretation of data; in the writing of the manuscript; or in the decision to publish the results.

References

1. Harjunpää, H.; Guillerey, C. TIGIT as an Emerging Immune Checkpoint. *Clin. Exp. Immunol.* **2020**, *200*, 108–119. [CrossRef] [PubMed]
2. Chauvin, J.M.; Zarour, H.M. TIGIT in Cancer Immunotherapy. *J. Immunother. Cancer* **2020**, *8*, e000957. [CrossRef] [PubMed]
3. Manieri, N.A.; Chiang, E.Y.; Grogan, J.L. TIGIT: A Key Inhibitor of the Cancer Immunity Cycle. *Trends Immunol.* **2017**, *38*, 20–28. [CrossRef] [PubMed]
4. Yusa, S.; Catina, T.L.; Campbell, K.S. KIR2DL5 Can Inhibit Human NK Cell Activation Via Recruitment of Src Homology Region 2-Containing Protein Tyrosine Phosphatase-2 (SHP-2). *J. Immunol.* **2004**, *172*, 7385–7392. [CrossRef]
5. Ren, X.; Peng, M.; Xing, P.; Wei, Y.; Galbo, P.M., Jr.; Corrigan, D.; Wang, H.; Su, Y.; Dong, X.; Sun, Q.; et al. Blockade of the Immunosuppressive KIR2DL5/PVR Pathway Elicits Potent Human NK Cell–Mediated Antitumor Immunity. *J. Clin. Investig.* **2022**, *132*, e163620. [CrossRef]
6. Sanchez-Correa, B.; Valhondo, I.; Hassouneh, F.; Lopez-Sejas, N.; Pera, A.; Bergua, J.M.; Arcos, M.J.; Bañas, H.; Casas-Avilés, I.; Durán, E.; et al. DNAM-1 and the TIGIT/PVRIG/TACTILE Axis: Novel Immune Checkpoints for Natural Killer Cell-Based Cancer Immunotherapy. *Cancers* **2019**, *11*, 877. [CrossRef]
7. Fuchs, A.; Cella, M.; Giurisato, E.; Shaw, A.S.; Colonna, M. Cutting Edge: CD96 (Tactile) Promotes NK Cell-Target Cell Adhesion by Interacting with the Poliovirus Receptor (CD155). *J. Immunol.* **2004**, *172*, 3994–3998. [CrossRef]
8. Georgiev, H.; Ravens, I.; Papadogianni, G.; Bernhardt, G. Coming of Age: CD96 Emerges as Modulator of Immune Responses. *Front. Immunol.* **2018**, *9*, 1072. [CrossRef]
9. Fujito, T.; Ikeda, W.; Kakunaga, S.; Minami, Y.; Kajita, M.; Sakamoto, Y.; Monden, M.; Takai, Y. Inhibition of cell movement and proliferation by cell–cell contact-induced interaction of Necl-5 with nectin-3. *J. Cell Biol.* **2005**, *171*, 165–173. [CrossRef]
10. Reches, A.; Ophir, Y.; Stein, N.; Kol, I.; Isaacson, B.; Charpak Amikam, Y.; Elnekave, A.; Tsukerman, P.; Kucan Brlic, P.; Lenac, T.; et al. Nectin4 Is a Novel TIGIT Ligand Which Combines Checkpoint Inhibition and Tumor Specificity. *J. Immunother. Cancer* **2020**, *8*, e000266. [CrossRef]
11. Sun, H.; Sun, C. The Rise of Nk Cell Checkpoints as Promising Therapeutic Targets in Cancer Immunotherapy. *Front. Immunol.* **2019**, *10*, 2354. [CrossRef] [PubMed]
12. Florou, V.; Garrido-Laguna, I. Clinical Development of Anti-TIGIT Antibodies for Immunotherapy of Cancer. *Curr. Oncol. Rep.* **2022**, *24*, 1107–1112. [CrossRef] [PubMed]
13. Chiang, E.Y.; Mellman, I. TIGIT-CD226-PVR Axis: Advancing Immune Checkpoint Blockade for Cancer Immunotherapy. *J. Immunother. Cancer* **2022**, *10*, e004711. [CrossRef] [PubMed]
14. Genentech: Press Releases | Tuesday. 10 May 2022. Available online: https://www.gene.com/media/press-releases/14951/2022-05-10/genentech-reports-interim-results-for-ph (accessed on 2 August 2022).
15. Genentech: Press Releases | Tuesday. 29 March 2022. Available online: https://www.gene.com/media/press-releases/14947/2022-03-29/genentech-provides-update-on-phase-iii-s (accessed on 24 January 2023).
16. Liu, S.; Zhang, H.; Li, M.; Hu, D.; Li, C.; Ge, B.; Jin, B.; Fan, Z. Recruitment of Grb2 and SHIP1 by the ITT-like Motif of TIGIT Suppresses Granule Polarization and Cytotoxicity of NK Cells. *Cell Death Differ.* **2013**, *20*, 456–464. [CrossRef]
17. Stanietsky, N.; Simic, H.; Arapovic, J.; Toporik, A.; Levy, O.; Novik, A.; Levine, Z.; Beiman, M.; Dassa, L.; Achdout, H.; et al. The Interaction of TIGIT with PVR and PVRL2 Inhibits Human NK Cell Cytotoxicity. *Proc. Natl. Acad. Sci. USA* **2009**, *106*, 17858–17863. [CrossRef]
18. Xu, F.; Sunderland, A.; Zhou, Y.; Schulick, R.D.; Edil, B.H.; Zhu, Y. Blockade of CD112R and TIGIT Signaling Sensitizes Human Natural Killer Cell Functions. *Cancer Immunol. Immunother.* **2017**, *66*, 1367–1375. [CrossRef] [PubMed]
19. González-Ochoa, S.; Tellez-Bañuelos, M.C.; Méndez-Clemente, A.S.; Bravo-Cuellar, A.; Hernández Flores, G.; Palafox-Mariscal, L.A.; Haramati, J.; Pedraza-Brindis, E.J.; Sánchez-Reyes, K.; Ortiz-Lazareno, P.C. Combination Blockade of the IL6R/STAT-3 Axis with TIGIT and Its Impact on the Functional Activity of NK Cells against Prostate Cancer Cells. *J. Immunol. Res.* **2022**, *2022*, 1810804. [CrossRef]
20. Brauneck, F.; Seubert, E.; Wellbrock, J.; Wiesch, J.S.Z.; Duan, Y.; Magnus, T.; Bokemeyer, C.; Koch-Nolte, F.; Menzel, S.; Fiedler, W. Combined Blockade of TIGIT and CD39 or A2AR Enhances NK-92 Cell-Mediated Cytotoxicity in AML. *Int. J. Mol. Sci.* **2021**, *22*, 12919. [CrossRef]

21. Chauvin, J.M.; Ka, M.; Pagliano, O.; Menna, C.; Ding, Q.; DeBlasio, R.; Sanders, C.; Hou, J.; Li, X.Y.; Ferrone, S.; et al. IL15 Stimulation with TIGIT Blockade Reverses CD155-Mediated NK-Cell Dysfunction in Melanoma. *Clin. Cancer Res.* **2020**, *26*, 5520–5533. [CrossRef]
22. Maas, R.J.; Hoogstad-van Evert, J.S.; van der Meer, J.M.; Mekers, V.; Rezaeifard, S.; Korman, A.J.; de Jonge, P.K.; Cany, J.; Woestenenk, R.; Schaap, N.P.; et al. TIGIT Blockade Enhances Functionality of Peritoneal NK Cells with Altered Expression of DNAM-1/TIGIT/CD96 Checkpoint Molecules in Ovarian Cancer. *Oncoimmunology* **2020**, *9*, 1843247. [CrossRef]
23. Holder, K.A.; Burt, K.; Grant, M.D. TIGIT Blockade Enhances NK Cell Activity against Autologous HIV-1-infected CD4+ T Cells. *Clin Transl Immunol.* **2021**, *10*, e1348. [CrossRef]
24. Wang, F.; Hou, H.; Wu, S.; Tang, Q.; Liu, W.; Huang, M.; Yin, B.; Huang, J.; Mao, L.; Lu, Y.; et al. TIGIT Expression Levels on Human NK Cells Correlate with Functional Heterogeneity among Healthy Individuals. *Eur. J. Immunol.* **2015**, *45*, 2886–2897. [CrossRef] [PubMed]
25. Judge, S.J.; Darrow, M.A.; Thorpe, S.W.; Gingrich, A.A.; O'Donnell, E.F.; Bellini, A.R.; Sturgill, I.R.; Vick, L.V.; Dunai, C.; Stoffel, K.M.; et al. Analysis of Tumor-Infiltrating NK and T Cells Highlights IL-15 Stimulation and TIGIT Blockade as a Combination Immunotherapy Strategy for Soft Tissue Sarcomas. *J. Immunother. Cancer* **2020**, *8*, e001355. [CrossRef] [PubMed]
26. Hoogstad-Van Evert, J.S.; Maas, R.J.; Van Der Meer, J.; Cany, J.; Van Der Steen, S.; Jansen, J.H.; Miller, J.S.; Bekkers, R.; Hobo, W.; Massuger, L.; et al. Peritoneal NK Cells Are Responsive to IL-15 and Percentages Are Correlated with Outcome in Advanced Ovarian Cancer Patients. *Oncotarget* **2018**, *9*, 34810. [CrossRef] [PubMed]
27. Zhang, C.; Wang, H.; Li, J.; Hou, X.; Li, L.; Wang, W.; Shi, Y.; Li, D.; Li, L.; Zhao, Z.; et al. Involvement of TIGIT in Natural Killer Cell Exhaustion and Immune Escape in Patients and Mouse Model With Liver Echinococcus Multilocularis Infection. *Hepatology* **2021**, *74*, 3376–3393. [CrossRef]
28. Rodriguez-Abreu, D.; Johnson, M.L.; Hussein, M.A.; Cobo, M.; Patel, A.J.; Secen, N.M.; Lee, K.H.; Massuti, B.; Hiret, S.; Yang, J.C.-H.; et al. Primary Analysis of a Randomized, Double-Blind, Phase II Study of the Anti-TIGIT Antibody Tiragolumab (Tira) plus Atezolizumab (Atezo) versus Placebo plus Atezo as First-Line (1L) Treatment in Patients with PD-L1-Selected NSCLC (CITYSCAPE). *J. Clin. Oncol.* **2020**, *38*, 9503. [CrossRef]
29. Zhang, Q.; Bi, J.; Zheng, X.; Chen, Y.; Wang, H.; Wu, W.; Wang, Z.; Wu, Q.; Peng, H.; Wei, H.; et al. Blockade of the Checkpoint Receptor TIGIT Prevents NK Cell Exhaustion and Elicits Potent Anti-Tumor Immunity. *Nat. Immunol.* **2018**, *19*, 723–732. [CrossRef]
30. Paul, S.; Lal, G. The Molecular Mechanism of Natural Killer Cells Function and Its Importance in Cancer Immunotherapy. *Front. Immunol.* **2017**, *8*, 1124. [CrossRef]
31. Morvan, M.G.; Lanier, L.L. NK Cells and Cancer: You Can Teach Innate Cells New Tricks. *Nat. Rev. Cancer* **2016**, *16*, 7–19. [CrossRef]
32. Myers, J.A.; Miller, J.S. Exploring the NK Cell Platform for Cancer Immunotherapy. *Nat. Rev. Clin. Oncol.* **2021**, *18*, 85–100. [CrossRef]
33. Vivier, E.; Tomasello, E.; Baratin, M.; Walzer, T.; Ugolini, S. Functions of Natural Killer Cells. *Nat. Immunol.* **2008**, *9*, 503–510. [CrossRef] [PubMed]
34. Shaver, K.A.; Croom-Perez, T.J.; Copik, A.J. Natural Killer Cells: The Linchpin for Successful Cancer Immunotherapy. *Front. Immunol.* **2021**, *12*, 679117. [CrossRef] [PubMed]
35. Shimasaki, N.; Jain, A.; Campana, D. NK Cells for Cancer Immunotherapy. *Nat. Rev. Drug Discov.* **2020**, *19*, 200–218. [CrossRef]
36. Roda, J.M.; Parihar, R.; Magro, C.; Nuovo, G.J.; Tridandapani, S.; Carson, W.E. Natural Killer Cells Produce T Cell-Recruiting Chemokines in Response to Antibody-Coated Tumor Cells. *Cancer Res.* **2006**, *66*, 517–526. [CrossRef] [PubMed]
37. Barry, K.C.; Hsu, J.; Broz, M.L.; Cueto, F.J.; Binnewies, M.; Combes, A.J.; Nelson, A.E.; Loo, K.; Kumar, R.; Rosenblum, M.D.; et al. A Natural Killer–Dendritic Cell Axis Defines Checkpoint Therapy–Responsive Tumor Microenvironments. *Nat. Med.* **2018**, *24*, 1178–1191. [CrossRef]
38. Böttcher, J.P.; Bonavita, E.; Chakravarty, P.; Blees, H.; Cabeza-Cabrerizo, M.; Sammicheli, S.; Rogers, N.C.; Sahai, E.; Zelenay, S.; Reis e Sousa, C. NK Cells Stimulate Recruitment of CDC1 into the Tumor Microenvironment Promoting Cancer Immune Control. *Cell* **2018**, *172*, 1022–1037. [CrossRef] [PubMed]
39. Kalinski, P.; Mailliard, R.B.; Giermasz, A.; Zeh, H.J.; Basse, P.; Bartlett, D.L.; Kirkwood, J.M.; Lotze, M.T.; Herberman, R.B. Natural Killer-Dendritic Cross-Talk in Cancer Immunotherapy. *Expert Opin. Biol. Ther.* **2005**, *5*, 1303–1315. [CrossRef]
40. Silla, L.; Valim, V.; Pezzi, A.; da Silva, M.; Wilke, I.; Nobrega, J.; Vargas, A.; Amorin, B.; Correa, B.; Zambonato, B.; et al. Adoptive Immunotherapy with Double-Bright (CD56 Bright /CD16 Bright) Expanded Natural Killer Cells in Patients with Relapsed or Refractory Acute Myeloid Leukaemia: A Proof-of-Concept Study. *Br. J. Haematol.* **2021**, *195*, 710–721. [CrossRef]
41. Oyer, J.L.; Croom-Perez, T.J.; Dieffenthaller, T.A.; Robles-Carillo, L.D.; Gitto, S.B.; Altomare, D.A.; Copik, A.J. Cryopreserved PM21-Particle-Expanded Natural Killer Cells Maintain Cytotoxicity and Effector Functions in Vitro and in Vivo. *Front. Immunol.* **2022**, *13*, 861681. [CrossRef]
42. Oh, E.; Min, B.; Li, Y.; Lian, C.; Hong, J.; Park, G.M.; Yang, B.; Cho, S.Y.; Hwang, Y.K.; Yun, C.O. Cryopreserved Human Natural Killer Cells Exhibit Potent Antitumor Efficacy against Orthotopic Pancreatic Cancer through Efficient Tumor-Homing and Cytolytic Ability. *Cancers* **2019**, *11*, 966. [CrossRef]

43. Min, B.; Choi, H.; Her, J.H.; Jung, M.Y.; Kim, H.J.; Jung, M.Y.; Lee, E.K.; Cho, S.Y.; Hwang, Y.K.; Shin, E.C. Optimization of Large-Scale Expansion and Cryopreservation of Human Natural Killer Cells for Anti-Tumor Therapy. *Immune Netw.* **2018**, *18*, e31. [CrossRef] [PubMed]
44. Holubova, M.; Miklikova, M.; Leba, M.; Georgiev, D.; Jindra, P.; Caprnda, M.; Ciccocioppo, R.; Kruzliak, P.; Lysak, D. Cryopreserved NK Cells in the Treatment of Haematological Malignancies: Preclinical Study. *J. Cancer Res. Clin. Oncol.* **2016**, *142*, 2561–2567. [CrossRef] [PubMed]
45. Ruggeri, L.; Capanni, M.; Urbani, E.; Perruccio, K.; Shlomchik, W.D.; Tosti, A.; Posati, S.; Rogaia, D.; Frassoni, F.; Aversa, F.; et al. Effectiveness of Donor Natural Killer Cell Alloreactivity in Mismatched Hematopoietic Transplants. *Science* **2002**, *295*, 2097–2100. [CrossRef] [PubMed]
46. Miller, J.S.; Soignier, Y.; Panoskaltsis-Mortari, A.; McNearney, S.A.; Yun, G.H.; Fautsch, S.K.; McKenna, D.; Le, C.; Defor, T.E.; Burns, L.J.; et al. Successful Adoptive Transfer and in Vivo Expansion of Human Haploidentical NK Cells in Patients with Cancer. *Blood* **2005**, *105*, 3051–3057. [CrossRef] [PubMed]
47. Cooley, S.; He, F.; Bachanova, V.; Vercellotti, G.M.; DeFor, T.E.; Curtsinger, J.M.; Robertson, P.; Grzywacz, B.; Conlon, K.C.; Waldmann, T.A.; et al. First-in-Human Trial of RhIL-15 and Haploidentical Natural Killer Cell Therapy for Advanced Acute Myeloid Leukemia. *Blood Adv.* **2019**, *3*, 1970–1980. [CrossRef] [PubMed]
48. Oyer, J.L.; Pandey, V.; Igarashi, R.Y.; Somanchi, S.S.; Zakari, A.; Solh, M.; Lee, D.A.; Altomare, D.A.; Copik, A.J. Natural Killer Cells Stimulated with PM21 Particles Expand and Biodistribute in Vivo: Clinical Implications for Cancer Treatment. *Cytotherapy* **2016**, *18*, 653–663. [CrossRef]
49. Oyer, J.L.; Igarashi, R.Y.; Kulikowski, A.R.; Colosimo, D.A.; Solh, M.M.; Zakari, A.; Khaled, Y.A.; Altomare, D.A.; Copik, A.J. Generation of Highly Cytotoxic Natural Killer Cells for Treatment of Acute Myelogenous Leukemia Using a Feeder-Free, Particle-Based Approach. *Biol. Blood Marrow Transplant.* **2015**, *21*, 632–639. [CrossRef]
50. Lee, D.A. Cellular Therapy: Adoptive Immunotherapy with Expanded Natural Killer Cells. *Immunol. Rev.* **2019**, *290*, 85–99. [CrossRef]
51. Xie, G.; Dong, H.; Liang, Y.; Ham, J.D.; Rizwan, R.; Chen, J. CAR-NK Cells: A Promising Cellular Immunotherapy for Cancer. *EBioMedicine* **2020**, *59*, 102975. [CrossRef]
52. Suen, W.C.W.; Lee, W.Y.W.; Leung, K.T.; Pan, X.H.; Li, G. Natural Killer Cell-Based Cancer Immunotherapy: A Review on 10 Years Completed Clinical Trials. *Cancer Investig.* **2018**, *36*, 431–457. [CrossRef]
53. Minnie, S.A.; Kuns, R.D.; Gartlan, K.H.; Zhang, P.; Wilkinson, A.N.; Samson, L.; Guillerey, C.; Engwerda, C.; MacDonald, K.P.A.; Smyth, M.J.; et al. Myeloma Escape after Stem Cell Transplantation Is a Consequence of T-Cell Exhaustion and Is Prevented by Tigit Blockade. *Blood* **2018**, *132*, 1675–1688. [CrossRef] [PubMed]
54. Wu, L.; Mao, L.; Liu, J.F.; Chen, L.; Yu, G.T.; Yang, L.L.; Wu, H.; Bu, L.L.; Kulkarni, A.B.; Zhang, W.F.; et al. Blockade of TIGIT/CD155 Signaling Reverses t-Cell Exhaustion and Enhances Antitumor Capability in Head and Neck Squamous Cell Carcinoma. *Cancer Immunol. Res.* **2019**, *7*, 1700–1713. [CrossRef] [PubMed]
55. Guillerey, C.; Harjunpää, H.; Carrié, N.; Kassem, S.; Teo, T.; Miles, K.; Krumeich, S.; Weulersse, M.; Cuisinier, M.; Stannard, K.; et al. TIGIT Immune Checkpoint Blockade Restores CD8$^+$ T-Cell Immunity against Multiple Myeloma. *Blood* **2018**, *132*, 1689–1694. [CrossRef] [PubMed]
56. Oyer, J.L.; Gitto, S.B.; Altomare, D.A.; Copik, A.J. PD-L1 Blockade Enhances Anti-Tumor Efficacy of NK Cells. *Oncoimmunology* **2018**, *7*, e1509819. [CrossRef]
57. Livak, K.J.; Schmittgen, T.D. Analysis of Relative Gene Expression Data Using Real-Time Quantitative PCR and the $2^{-\Delta\Delta CT}$ Method. *Methods* **2001**, *25*, 402–408. [CrossRef]
58. Croom-Perez, T.J.; Robles-Carillo, L.D.; Oyer, J.L.; Dieffenthaller, T.A.; Hasan, M.F.; Copik, A.J. Kinetic, Imaging Based Assay to Measure NK Cell Cytotoxicity against Adherent Cells. *Methods Cell Biol.* **2022**, *In Press, Corrected Proof.* [CrossRef]
59. Varudkar, N.; Oyer, J.L.; Copik, A.; Parks, G.D. Original Research: Oncolytic Parainfluenza Virus Combines with NK Cells to Mediate Killing of Infected and Non-Infected Lung Cancer Cells within 3D Spheroids: Role of Type I and Type III Interferon Signaling. *J. Immunother. Cancer* **2021**, *9*, e002373. [CrossRef]
60. Andrews, S. FastQC: A Quality Control Tool for High Throughput Sequence Data. Available online: https://www.bioinformatics.babraham.ac.uk/projects/fastqc/ (accessed on 6 May 2023).
61. Bolger, A.M.; Lohse, M.; Usadel, B. Trimmomatic: A Flexible Trimmer for Illumina Sequence Data. *Bioinformatics* **2014**, *30*, 2114–2120. [CrossRef]
62. Pertea, M.; Kim, D.; Pertea, G.M.; Leek, J.T.; Salzberg, S.L. Transcript-Level Expression Analysis of RNA-Seq Experiments with HISAT, StringTie and Ballgown. *Nat. Protoc.* **2016**, *11*, 1650–1667. [CrossRef]
63. Zhang, Y.; Parmigiani, G.; Johnson, W.E. ComBat-Seq: Batch Effect Adjustment for RNA-Seq Count Data. *NAR Genom. Bioinform.* **2020**, *2*, lqaa078. [CrossRef]
64. Robinson, M.D.; McCarthy, D.J.; Smyth, G.K. EdgeR: A Bioconductor Package for Differential Expression Analysis of Digital Gene Expression Data. *Bioinformatics* **2009**, *26*, 139–140. [CrossRef]
65. Subramanian, A.; Tamayo, P.; Mootha, V.K.; Mukherjee, S.; Ebert, B.L.; Gillette, M.A.; Paulovich, A.; Pomeroy, S.L.; Golub, T.R.; Lander, E.S.; et al. Gene Set Enrichment Analysis: A Knowledge-Based Approach for Interpreting Genome-Wide Expression Profiles. *Proc. Natl. Acad. Sci. USA* **2005**, *102*, 15545–15550. [CrossRef] [PubMed]

66. Li, B.; Severson, E.; Pignon, J.C.; Zhao, H.; Li, T.; Novak, J.; Jiang, P.; Shen, H.; Aster, J.C.; Rodig, S.; et al. Comprehensive Analyses of Tumor Immunity: Implications for Cancer Immunotherapy. *Genome Biol.* **2016**, *17*, 174. [CrossRef] [PubMed]
67. Li, T.; Fan, J.; Wang, B.; Traugh, N.; Chen, Q.; Liu, J.S.; Li, B.; Liu, X.S. TIMER: A Web Server for Comprehensive Analysis of Tumor-Infiltrating Immune Cells. *Cancer Res.* **2017**, *77*, e108–e110. [CrossRef] [PubMed]
68. Li, T.; Fu, J.; Zeng, Z.; Cohen, D.; Li, J.; Chen, Q.; Li, B.; Liu, X.S. TIMER2.0 for Analysis of Tumor-Infiltrating Immune Cells. *Nucleic Acids Res.* **2020**, *48*, W509–W514. [CrossRef] [PubMed]
69. Bi, J.; Tian, Z. NK Cell Exhaustion. *Front. Immunol.* **2017**, *8*, 760. [CrossRef]
70. Blackburn, S.D.; Shin, H.; Haining, W.N.; Zou, T.; Workman, C.J.; Polley, A.; Betts, M.R.; Freeman, G.J.; Vignali, D.A.A.; Wherry, E.J. Coregulation of CD8+ T Cell Exhaustion by Multiple Inhibitory Receptors during Chronic Viral Infection. *Nat. Immunol.* **2009**, *10*, 29–37. [CrossRef]
71. Yang, C.; Siebert, J.R.; Burns, R.; Gerbec, Z.J.; Bonacci, B.; Rymaszewski, A.; Rau, M.; Riese, M.J.; Rao, S.; Carlson, K.S.; et al. Heterogeneity of Human Bone Marrow and Blood Natural Killer Cells Defined by Single-Cell Transcriptome. *Nat. Commun.* **2019**, *10*, 3931. [CrossRef]
72. Search of: TIGIT | Recruiting, Active, Not Recruiting Studies–List Results–ClinicalTrials.Gov. Available online: https://clinicaltrials.gov/ct2/results?term=TIGIT&Search=Apply&recrs=a&recrs=d&age_v=&gndr=&type=&rslt= (accessed on 26 January 2023).
73. Liu, G.; Zhang, Q.; Yang, J.; Li, X.; Xian, L.; Li, W.; Lin, T.; Cheng, J.; Lin, Q.; Xu, X.; et al. Increased TIGIT Expressing NK Cells with Dysfunctional Phenotype in AML Patients Correlated with Poor Prognosis. *Cancer Immunol. Immunother.* **2022**, *71*, 277–287. [CrossRef]
74. Yin, X.; Liu, T.; Wang, Z.; Ma, M.; Lei, J.; Zhang, Z.; Fu, S.; Fu, Y.; Hu, Q.; Ding, H.; et al. Expression of the Inhibitory Receptor Tigit Is Up-Regulated Specifically on Nk Cells with Cd226 Activating Receptor from HIV-Infected Individuals. *Front. Immunol.* **2018**, *9*, 2341. [CrossRef]
75. Luo, Q.; Li, X.; Fu, B.; Zhang, L.; Deng, Z.; Qing, C.; Su, R.; Xu, J.; Guo, Y.; Huang, Z.; et al. Decreased Expression of TIGIT in NK Cells Correlates Negatively with Disease Activity in Systemic Lupus Erythematosus. *Int. J. Clin. Exp. Pathol.* **2018**, *11*, 2408.
76. Peng, Y.P.; Xi, C.H.; Zhu, Y.; Yin, L.D.; Wei, J.S.; Zhang, J.J.; Liu, X.C.; Guo, S.; Fu, Y.; Miao, Y. Altered Expression of CD226 and CD96 on Natural Killer Cells in Patients with Pancreatic Cancer. *Oncotarget* **2016**, *7*, 66586. [CrossRef] [PubMed]
77. Sanchez-Correa, B.; Gayoso, I.; Bergua, J.M.; Casado, J.G.; Morgado, S.; Solana, R.; Tarazona, R. Decreased Expression of DNAM-1 on NK Cells from Acute Myeloid Leukemia Patients. *Immunol. Cell Biol.* **2012**, *90*, 109–115. [CrossRef] [PubMed]
78. Hattori, N.; Kawaguchi, Y.; Sasaki, Y.; Shimada, S.; Murai, S.; Abe, M.; Baba, Y.; Watanuki, M.; Fujiwara, S.; Arai, N.; et al. Monitoring TIGIT/DNAM-1 and PVR/PVRL2 Immune Checkpoint Expression Levels in Allogeneic Stem Cell Transplantation for Acute Myeloid Leukemia. *Biol. Blood Marrow Transplant.* **2019**, *25*, 861–867. [CrossRef] [PubMed]
79. Preillon, J.; Cuende, J.; Rabolli, V.; Garnero, L.; Mercier, M.; Wald, N.; Pappalardo, A.; Denies, S.; Jamart, D.; Michaux, A.C.; et al. Restoration of T-Cell Effector Function, Depletion of Tregs, and Direct Killing of Tumor Cells: The Multiple Mechanisms of Action of a-TIGIT Antagonist Antibodies. *Mol. Cancer* **2021**, *20*, 121–131. [CrossRef]
80. ITeos Presents New Data for Anti-TIGIT Antibody, EOS-448/GSK4428859A, at the AACR Annual Meeting 2022. Available online: https://finance.yahoo.com/news/iteos-presents-data-anti-tigit-170000345.html?guce_referrer=aHR0cHM6Ly93d3cuZ29vZ2xlLmNvbS8&guce_referrer_sig=AQAAAJYWXKCTML13lbl3lrecbFrJl37qWFj33vNp1ZmkVPyDSI5gl2Xt84wo-TeYuQ29Mg4xy7jT5dodQxhDxPewTQ_PeUVXK9BFT037hZn-6VYyt4zK-aKdjs0W0mQK358pTnOmxVFRjk0zjGKlNPFMOl_MhPXxTpym56uehz-mpcJD&guccounter=2 (accessed on 26 January 2023).
81. Chen, X.; Xue, L.; Ding, X.; Zhang, J.; Jiang, L.; Liu, S.; Hou, H.; Jiang, B.; Cheng, L.; Zhu, Q.; et al. An Fc-Competent Anti-Human TIGIT Blocking Antibody Ociperlimab (BGB-A1217) Elicits Strong Immune Responses and Potent Anti-Tumor Efficacy in Pre-Clinical Models. *Front. Immunol.* **2022**, *13*, 828319. [CrossRef] [PubMed]

Disclaimer/Publisher's Note: The statements, opinions and data contained in all publications are solely those of the individual author(s) and contributor(s) and not of MDPI and/or the editor(s). MDPI and/or the editor(s) disclaim responsibility for any injury to people or property resulting from any ideas, methods, instructions or products referred to in the content.

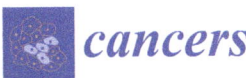

Article

Treatment with Anti-HER2 Chimeric Antigen Receptor Tumor-Infiltrating Lymphocytes (CAR-TILs) Is Safe and Associated with Antitumor Efficacy in Mice and Companion Dogs

Elin M. V. Forsberg [1,†], Rebecca Riise [1,†], Sara Saellström [2,†], Joakim Karlsson [1,3], Samuel Alsén [1], Valentina Bucher [1], Akseli E. Hemminki [4,5], Roger Olofsson Bagge [1], Lars Ny [1], Lisa M. Nilsson [1,3], Henrik Rönnberg [2] and Jonas A. Nilsson [1,3,*]

1. Sahlgrenska Translational Melanoma Group, Sahlgrenska Center for Cancer Research, Departments of Surgery and Oncology, Institute of Clinical Sciences, University of Gothenburg, Sahlgrenska University Hospital, 40530 Gothenburg, Sweden
2. Department of Clinical Sciences, Swedish University of Agricultural Sciences, 75007 Uppsala, Sweden
3. Harry Perkins Institute of Medical Research, University of Western Australia, Perth, WA 6009, Australia
4. Cancer Gene Therapy Group, Translational Immunology Research Program, Faculty of Medicine, University of Helsinki, 00290 Helsinki, Finland
5. Department of Oncology, Comprehensive Cancer Centre, Helsinki University Hospital, 00290 Helsinki, Finland
* Correspondence: jonas.a.nilsson@surgery.gu.se or jonas.nilsson@perkins.org.au; Tel.: +61-08-6151-0979
† These authors contributed equally to this work.

Simple Summary: CAR-T cells are immune cells equipped with a claw that enable them to bind cancer cells. Usually, CAR-T cells are made using immune cells from blood. Here, we tested the hypothesis that also immune cells that reside in the tumor, so called tumor-infiltrating lymphocytes, can also be modified to carry the claw. This may mean that these cells, called CAR-TILs, will be able to attack cancer cells in two ways, using the claw or binding using its normal protein on the cell surface, the so-called T cell receptor. We show that CAR-TILs can be generated, and that they can kill melanoma cells in cell culture and in mice. Finally, to prepare for clinical trials, we also assess if CAR-TILs can be safe in a human cancer patient-like model, a companion dog suffering from cancer. Our data suggest that CAR-TILs may be a way to treat patients with melanoma but human clinical trials are needed.

Abstract: Patients with metastatic melanoma have a historically poor prognosis, but recent advances in treatment options, including targeted therapy and immunotherapy, have drastically improved the outcomes for some of these patients. However, not all patients respond to available treatments, and around 50% of patients with metastatic cutaneous melanoma and almost all patients with metastases of uveal melanoma die of their disease. Thus, there is a need for novel treatment strategies for patients with melanoma that do not benefit from the available therapies. Chimeric antigen receptor-expressing T (CAR-T) cells are largely unexplored in melanoma. Traditionally, CAR-T cells have been produced by transducing blood-derived T cells with a virus expressing CAR. However, tumor-infiltrating lymphocytes (TILs) can also be engineered to express CAR, and such CAR-TILs could be dual-targeting. To this end, tumor samples and autologous TILs from metastasized human uveal and cutaneous melanoma were expanded in vitro and transduced with a lentiviral vector encoding an anti-HER2 CAR construct. When infused into patient-derived xenograft (PDX) mouse models carrying autologous tumors, CAR-TILs were able to eradicate melanoma, even in the absence of antigen presentation by HLA. To advance this concept to the clinic and assess its safety in an immune-competent and human-patient-like setting, we treated four companion dogs with autologous anti-HER2 CAR-TILs. We found that these cells were tolerable and showed signs of anti-tumor activity. Taken together, CAR-TIL therapy is a promising avenue for broadening the tumor-targeting capacity of TILs in patients with checkpoint immunotherapy-resistant melanoma.

Citation: Forsberg, E.M.V.; Riise, R.; Saellström, S.; Karlsson, J.; Alsén, S.; Bucher, V.; Hemminki, A.E.; Olofsson Bagge, R.; Ny, L.; Nilsson, L.M.; et al. Treatment with Anti-HER2 Chimeric Antigen Receptor Tumor-Infiltrating Lymphocytes (CAR-TILs) Is Safe and Associated with Antitumor Efficacy in Mice and Companion Dogs. *Cancers* 2023, *15*, 648. https://doi.org/10.3390/cancers15030648

Academic Editor: Vita Golubovskaya

Received: 10 January 2023
Revised: 17 January 2023
Accepted: 18 January 2023
Published: 20 January 2023

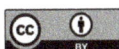

Copyright: © 2023 by the authors. Licensee MDPI, Basel, Switzerland. This article is an open access article distributed under the terms and conditions of the Creative Commons Attribution (CC BY) license (https:// creativecommons.org/licenses/by/ 4.0/).

Keywords: metastatic melanoma; uveal melanoma; patient-derived xenograft mouse model; adoptive T cell therapy; chimeric antigen receptor T cells; immunotherapy; canine; companion dog; comparative oncology; HER2

1. Introduction

Patients with metastatic melanoma have a historically poor prognosis; however [1], recent advances in treatment options have drastically improved patient prognosis. Targeted therapies using inhibitors of BRAF alone [2,3] or in combination with MEK inhibitors [4,5] have shown good response rates in patients with metastatic cutaneous melanoma. However, most patients treated with these inhibitors develop drug resistance. Immunotherapies, including checkpoint inhibitors targeting PD1 and CTLA4 or LAG3, can result in more durable response rates among patients with melanoma [6–9]. Adoptive T cell transfer (ACT) with tumor-infiltrating lymphocytes (TILs) has also been used to treat metastatic melanoma in clinical trials, with response rates of approximately 50% [10–12]. Importantly, not all patients with metastatic malignant melanoma respond to current treatment strategies; therefore, alternative and/or combination therapies are currently being explored in preclinical experiments and trials.

Uveal melanoma (UM) is a rare form of melanoma [13] arising in the uveal tract of the eye, i.e., the iris, ciliary body, and choroid. UM is treated with brachytherapy or enucleation with very good local control (97%) [14]. However, approximately 50% of patients will later present with metastatic disease [15], mainly to the liver, but also to other sites [16]. Patients with spread UM rarely respond to systemic chemotherapy or targeted therapies, [17] and combined immune checkpoint inhibitors have not shown the same promising effect in UM [18,19] as in cutaneous melanoma [20]. Benchmark data suggest an average progression-free and overall survival of approximately 3.3 and 10.2 months, respectively [21]. Loco-regional treatment with isolated hepatic perfusion or percutaneous hepatic perfusion demonstrates high response rates and prolonged progression-free survival in randomized trials, but mature survival data are still pending [22,23]. The combined treatment with PD-1 inhibitor pembrolizumab and the HDAC inhibitor entinostat exhibited durable responses in a fraction of patients, including one with an iris melanoma with a high mutation burden and patients with tumors exhibiting a wildtype *BAP1* tumor suppressor gene [24]. ACT with TILs was tested in patients with UM in a clinical trial, with a response rate of 35% [25]. Finally, for patients with the HLA-A2 genotype, the bispecific T cell engager tebentafusp can activate anti-tumor immune responses [26] and prolong the survival of patients with UM [27], despite surprisingly low response rates [28]. Hence, although recent progress has been made, metastatic UM remains a medical challenge.

Immunotherapies aim to overcome tumor immune evasion strategies to re-activate the patient's own immune system to attack and kill the tumor. However, some tumors downregulate the antigen presentation pathway [29,30], rendering these tumor cells insensitive to TCR-mediated recognition and cytotoxicity, thereby disarming both immune checkpoint inhibition and ACT. One way to overcome this problem is to equip T cells with a chimeric antigen receptor (CAR) designed to recognize a specific protein expressed on the surface of tumor cells irrespective of antigen presentation. CAR-T therapy has not yet been approved for use in any solid cancer; however, CD19 CAR-T therapy is used in young patients with acute lymphocytic leukemia (ALL) [31]. The reason why CAR-T therapy has not yet been successful in solid cancers is not fully understood, but includes heterogeneous expression of antigens, expression of checkpoint proteins, poor homing and tissue penetrance of CAR-T cells, an immune suppressive tumor microenvironment (TME), and CAR-T cell endurance [32].

Mouse models are useful for studying the antitumor efficacy of human CAR-T cells, but there are limitations. Patient-derived xenograft (PDX) models are immunodeficient [33], and in both PDX models and cell line-derived xenograft models, the tumor stroma and off-target tissues of CAR-T cells are of mouse origin. Therefore, these models cannot be readily used for TME or toxicity studies without additional genetic engineering. Neither xenograft nor syngeneic transplant models are spontaneous tumor models; therefore, tumor architecture can also be suboptimal. Companion dogs are an emerging and complementary model to study toxicity and anti-cancer treatment efficacy [34]. Dogs live and socialize with their human owners, share their habits and microbiota, and develop lifestyle diseases, such as cardiovascular problems, joint problems, diabetes, and cancer, with age [35]. Malignancies range from leukemia and lymphoma to solid tumors such as mammary or squamous cell carcinoma of the head and neck [36]. Melanoma is a particularly aggressive form of cancer in some breeds of dogs [37]. It is not associated with solar damage and most often develops in mucosal areas such as the mouth or under the nail bed. Similar to human mucosal melanoma, the spectrum and driver mutations of canine melanoma are different from those of human cutaneous and uveal melanoma [38,39].

We previously reported good antitumor efficacy of CAR-T cells directed against HER2 in PDX models of cutaneous and uveal melanoma [40]. We demonstrated that the elicited effect of CAR-T cells was target-specific, as CRISPR/Cas9-mediated disruption of HER2 abolished the sensitivity of melanoma cells to anti-HER2 CAR-T cells. Importantly, CAR-T cells were also able to eradicate tumors that were refractory to ACT. Current CAR-T therapies use CAR-transduced T-cells from blood as drug substances. This T cell pool largely consists of naïve and memory T cells carrying a TCR with irrelevant affinity. Naïve T cells generally do not express molecules that facilitate homing to inflamed peripheral tissues. TILs, on the other hand, can home to tumors; therefore [41,42], they could potentially serve as good starting materials for the generation of CAR-T cells. The aim of this study was to assess whether CAR expression in TILs can boost tumor cell death. We also assessed whether the CAR-TILs were safe and tolerable in mice and companion dogs.

2. Materials and Methods

2.1. Human Patient Samples

Tumor samples were obtained from patients treated at the Department of Surgery, Sahlgrenska University Hospital, Gothenburg, Sweden, following informed consent (Regional Human Ethics Board of Västra Götaland, Sweden approval #288-12 and #44-18). Tumor cells were extracted from tumor samples and used for patient-derived xenograft establishment, as previously described [43]. Young TILs (y-TILs) were extracted from the same tumor samples, cultured, and expanded, as previously described [42].

2.2. Cell Experiments

Patient-derived melanoma cell lines were maintained in RPMI with 10% fetal bovine serum and were either described previously [UM22, MM2, MM3, MM4 [42,44]] or generated by culturing melanoma samples in RPMI with 10% FCS (MM5, MM6). 92-1 Uveal melanoma cells were a kind gift from the European Collection of Authenticated Cell Cultures (ECACC, UK, or available from Sigma-Aldrich), and the HER2 knockout line was established previously [40]. The canine tumor cell lines D17.os and CF41.mg were purchased from ATCC (Manassas, VA, USA).

For CRISPR/Cas9 inactivation of *B2M*, the Cas9:crRNA:tracrRNA ribonucleoprotein (RNP) complex was assembled according to the manufacturer's recommendations (IDT DNA) and transfected into the cells using Lipofectamine RNAiMAX reagent (Invitrogen, Thermo Fisher, Carlsbad, CA, USA). Negative cells were sorted based on the absence of B2M-PE antibody staining (clone 2M2, BioLegend, San Diego, CA, USA) using magnetic separation with PE-beads (Miltenyi, Bergisch, Germany), confirmed negative by staining with the same antibody, and analyzed using an Accuri C6 flow cytometer (BD, Franklin Lakes, NJ, USA) equipped with the BD Accuri C6 softwaren (v1.0).

2.3. Generation of TILs and CAR-TILs

Young TILs (yTILs) were made by cutting 2–3 mm^3 pieces from tumors and placing these in a 24-well plate containing RPMI medium supplemented with 10% human AB serum (Sigma-Aldrich, St. Louis, MO, USA), 6000 IU/mL human recombinant IL2 (Peprotech, East Windsor, NJ, USA), 1 mM sodium pyruvate (Gibco, Thermo Fisher, Carlsbad, CA, USA), and 50 µM 2-Mercaptoethanol (Gibco). After 10–14 days, the yTILs were either expanded or cryopreserved for future use. For the rapid expansion (REP) of TILs, yTILs (1×10^5) were mixed with irradiated (40 Gy) feeder cells (20×10^6), CD3 antibody (clone OKT3, 30 ng/mL, Miltenyi), and a medium containing 50% RPMI and 50% AIM-V (Invitrogen) supplemented with 10% human AB serum (Sigma-Aldrich) and 6000 IU/mL IL-2 (Peprotech).

A HER2 CAR-expressing lentiviral vector that was previously shown to be specific for HER2 was purchased from ProMab (Richmond, CA, USA) [40]. The second-generation CAR expressed from this vector contains a CD8 leader, a Herceptin-like scFV binding domain, a CD8 transmembrane region and the intracellular signaling domains from CD3ζ and CD28. CAR-TILs were produced by transducing TILs on days 1 and 2 of the REP with the HER2 CAR lentiviral vector in the presence of Vectofusin-1 (Miltenyi). After five days of culture at 37 °C in 5% CO$_2$, half of the medium was replenished. From day six onwards, the flasks were inspected daily and split when necessary to maintain cell densities of approximately $1-2 \times 10^6$/mL. After 14 days in culture, the cells were harvested, resuspended in PBS with 300 IU/mL of IL-2, and intravenously transplanted into mice (20×10^6 cells per mouse in 100 µL).

Alternatively, REP-TILs were transfected with anti-HER2 CAR mRNA via electroporation using a 4D nucleofector (Lonza, Basel, Switzerland). This mRNA was generated by PCR amplification of the coding sequence of anti-HER2-CAR [40] using primers that carried a T7 RNA polymerase recognition sequence at the 5′-end. The resulting PCR product was used in an in vitro transcription reaction with the T7 mScript Standard mRNA Production System (Cellscript, Madison, WI, USA). The TILs were resuspended in P3 primary cell solution with supplement (Lonza), and mRNA was added before pulsing using the DN100 program.

2.4. CAR Detection

For qPCR detection, genomic DNA was prepared from TILs and CAR-TILs 10–14 days after the start of REP by lysing in Direct PCR Lysis Reagent (Nordic BioSite, Stockholm, Sweden) and proteinase K. Quantitative PCR was performed in triplicate using a qPCR SyGreen mix (Techtum Lab AB, Stockholm, Sweden), and the PCR reaction was performed with a CFX cycler (Bio-Rad, Hercules, CA, USA). Data analysis comparing ΔCT values normalized to a reference gene (β-actin) was performed to determine the CAR copies/cell.

For analysis of the HER2 protein binding capacity of CAR-TILs, 100,000 cells were incubated with 1 µg biotinylated HER2 protein (Abcam, Cambridge, UK) for 30 min at 4 °C, followed by incubation with an allophycocyanin-conjugated streptavidin antibody (Jackson Immuno Research, West Grove, PA, US) for 25 min at 4 °C, and flow cytometry analysis was performed.

2.5. Cytotoxicity Experiments

Melanoma cells were infected with a lentivirus made using pHAGE-PGK-GFP-IRES-LUC-W (Addgene # 46793) containing coding sequences for green-fluorescent protein and firefly luciferase. To assess the cytotoxicity of T cells, patient-derived melanoma cell lines expressing luciferase were plated at 20,000 cells/well in black 96-well plates (Corning, Corning NY, USA) and cultured in the presence or absence of different ratios of T cells per well. After 48 h, the medium was aspirated for IFN-γ secretion analysis using an ELISA kit (Diaclone, Besancon Cedex, France), and the viability of the cancer cells was assessed by measuring luminescence with a GloMax Discover plate reader (Promega, Madison, WI, USA) or an IVIS Lumina III XR (Perkin-Elmer, Waltham, MA, USA) after adding luciferin (150 µg/mL) to the cells. For degranulation analysis, TILs and CAR-TILs were co-cultured with cancer cells for 4–6 h in RPMI supplemented with human AB serum (Sigma-Aldrich) and CD107a antibody (clone H4A3, BD), followed by washing in PBS and the detection of bound CD107a antibody by flow cytometry (BD Accuri C6 Plus). For the IFN-γ secretion assay, the degranulation assay was followed by additional staining procedures according to the manufacturer's instructions (Miltenyi Biotech), and bound IFN-γ was detected using flow cytometry. For the detection of cleaved caspase 3 (CC3), cancer cells were co-cultured with TILs and CAR-TILs for 24 h, followed by fixation and permeabilization using Cytofix/Cytoperm solution for 25 min (554714, BD), washed twice with supplemented Wash/Perm buffer (554714, BD), and stained with a CC3 antibody (clone C92-605, BD) at 1:10 dilution in Wash/Perm buffer. Finally, the cells were washed and analyzed using flow cytometry.

2.6. Mouse Experiments

All mouse experiments were performed in accordance with EU Directive 2010/63 (Regional Animal Ethics Committee of Gothenburg #2014-36, #2016-100, and #2018-1183). Non-obese diabetic-severe combined immune-deficient interleukin-2 chain receptor γ chain knockout mice (NOG mice, Taconic, Ry, Denmark) and human IL-2 transgenic NOG (hIL2-NOG) mice (Taconic) were used for the engraftment of tumor samples. Tumor size was monitored by caliper measurements, alternatively bioluminescent signals, using the IVIS imaging system (Perkin-Elmer). When tumor growth was confirmed by two consecutive measurements, hIL2-NOG mice were treated with autologous human tumor-infiltrating lymphocytes (TILs; 20 million cells per mouse) by intravenous injection into the tail vein. NOG mice served as untreated controls.

2.7. Canine CAR-TIL Expansion

For canine yTIL expansion, 2–3 mm^3 tumor pieces were cut and placed in a 24-well plate containing RPMI medium supplemented with 10% human AB serum (Sigma-Aldrich), 6000 IU/mL human recombinant IL2 (Peprotech), 1 mM sodium pyruvate (Gibco), and 50 µM 2-Mercaptoethanol (Gibco). After seven days, the yTILs were harvested, washed in PBS, and resuspended in PBS supplemented with 10% fetal bovine serum. Cells were stained with a CD5-PE antibody (clone YKIX322.3, eBioscience) diluted 1:50 for 20 min at 4 °C, washed in PBS, and stained with PE microbeads (Miltenyi) according to the manufacturer's protocol. Finally, cells were washed and CD5 positive cells were sorted using MACS separation with LD columns (Miltenyi) using a QuadroMACS Separator (Miltenyi) according to the manufacturer's instructions. CD5 positivity was confirmed by analyzing PE expression using flow cytometry (BD Accuri C6 Plus). CD5 positive yTILs were either cryopreserved for later expansion or directly expanded using a rapid-expansion protocol (REP). For REP of canine TILs, CD5 positive yTILs (1×10^5) were mixed with 20×10^6 irradiated (40 Gy) feeder cells from healthy dog blood donors (three different donors) and human CD3 antibody (clone OKT3, 30 ng/mL, Miltenyi) and expanded for 14 days in RPMI supplemented with 10% human AB serum (Sigma-Aldrich), 6000 IU/mL human IL2 (Peprotech), 1 mM sodium pyruvate (Gibco), and 50 µM 2-Mercaptoethanol (Gibco). For CAR-TIL production, cells were electroporated with anti-HER2 CAR mRNA after expansion and used to treat the patient the next day. Alternatively, anti-HER2 CAR lentivirus was added after 1, 2, and 12 d of culture.

2.8. First-in-Dog (FIDO) Trial

Four client-owned dogs with HER-2 positive aggressive tumors were recruited at the University Animal Hospital (Uppsala, Sweden) between November 2019 and April 2021. All the dogs had recurrent spontaneous cancers with metastases. The CAR-TIL FIDO study and sample collection were approved by the Swedish Animal Ethical Committee and Swedish Animal Welfare Agency (#2019-2435). Written consent was obtained from dog owners.

The study design was as follows: at the initial visit, blood samples were collected and the hematology and biochemistry were analyzed. The dogs were screened with a whole-body CT scan (dogs 1 and 4) or thoracic X-rays and ultrasound of the local lymph nodes and abdomen (dogs 2 and 3). As soon as possible, surgical extirpation of the primary tumor was performed in three dogs (dogs 1–3) and of the metastasized local lymph nodes in one dog (dog 4). The tumors were sent to a pathology laboratory for diagnostic purposes. Parts of the tumors were sent in sterile PBS containing Primocin (InVivoGen, San Diego, CA, USA) to the laboratory in Gothenburg for expansion of autologous TILs. The TILs were modified, grown, and harvested as described below.

Before the first dose of CAR-TILs, each dog was treated for 10–14 days with oral Toceranib phosphate (Hospital pharmacy, brand name Palladia™) 2.3–2.5 mg/kg qd to suppress regulatory T-cells. Treatment was stopped five days before CAR-TIL transfusion. The dogs were sedated with subcutaneous injections of medetomidine:butorphanol (0.01 mg/kg:0.1 mg/kg). Transfusion of CAR-TILs was performed via a peripheral venous catheter for 30 min using a protocol that included monitoring vital signs (body temperature, breathing, mucous membrane heart rate, blood pressure, and pulses). After the transfusion, the sedated dogs were reverted with an intramuscular injection of atipamezol (0.05 mg/kg). Dogs stayed at the clinic for at least one hour after transfusion for supervision. Three dogs were treated with amoxicillin 9.5–11.5 mg/kg bidaily (BID) for 10 days and 1 (dog 2) was treated with clindamycin 12 mg/kg BID for 10 days, after each CAR-TIL treatment. Human IL-2 (a kind gift from the NCI) was administered by subcutaneous injections.

Blood samples were collected at visits for treatment and revisits. A complete blood count, standard clinical chemistry profile, and immunoglobulin gel electrophoresis were performed. Response to therapy was categorized in accordance with veterinary-adjusted RECIST criteria [45] as CR (complete regression of measurable soft tissue disease), PR (partial response of at least 30% reduction in the sum of diameters of target lesions, taking as reference the baseline sum), PD (progression of the disease by either the appearance of one or more new lesions or at least a 20% increase in the sum of diameters of target lesions, taking as reference the smallest sum on study), and SD (less than 30% reduction or 20% increase in the sum of diameters of target lesions, taking as reference the smallest sum of diameters while on the study). The best overall response was defined as the best response recorded from the start of treatment to disease progression or recurrence. Macroscopic tumor lesions were measured using a caliper and documented using photographs. In addition, dogs were followed up with diagnostic imaging (computed tomography, radiography, and/or ultrasound), using the most suitable modality for each case. Adverse events were graded according to VCOG-CTCAE version 2 [46].

2.9. Protein Analysis

For immunohistochemistry, dog tumor tissues were fixed in 4% formalin, dehydrated, and embedded in paraffin. Sections (4 µm were mounted onto positively charged glass slides and dried at 60 °C for 1 h. The slides were rehydrated, and antigen retrieval was performed by heat-induced epitope retrieval (HIER) in Dako PT Link with a high pH buffer (Dako, Glostrup, Denmark). The staining was performed with an autostainer (Autostainer Link 48, Dako) using the following protocol: Endogenous Enzyme Block for 5 min (FLEX Peroxidase Block, Dako), primary antibody (HER2 A0485 and Melan-A IR633; both from Dako) staining for 60 min at room temperature, secondary reagent staining (FLEX + Rabbit LINKER, K8009, Dako) for 15 min, FLEX HRP for 20 min, diaminobenzidine (DAB) chromogen development for 10 min, and counterstaining with hematoxylin for 12 min. The slides were dehydrated and mounted using a Pertex.

2.10. Statistical Analyses of Experimental Data

Statistical analysis was performed using GraphPad software, ordinary one-way ANOVA, multiple comparisons with Tukey's correction (Figure 1 and Figure 3b,c), and alternatively unpaired t tests (Figures 2 and 3a). P values are represented as * $p < 0.05$, ** $p < 0.01$, *** $p < 0.001$, and **** $p < 0.0001$. All mouse experiments contained 3–4 mice per group.

2.11. Single Cell Gene Expression Analysis

Single-cell RNA-seq from two recent studies [24,44] was used to compare the gene expression profiles of CD8$^+$ and CD4$^+$ T cells found in tumors (TILs) and blood from patients with uveal melanoma. Alignment and estimation of gene expression levels were performed using Cell Ranger (v. 3.0.2, 10× Genomics). The specific commands used were *cellranger count* (with the 10× Genomics version of the GRCh38 reference transcriptome; v. 3.0.0) and *cellranger vdj* (with the 10× Genomics GRCh38 VDJ reference dataset, v. 2.0.0). After identifying cell types, the remaining analyses were performed using the *Seurat* R package (v. 4.0.3) [47], and data were imported and normalized using the *NormalizeData* function with default settings. Cells predicted to be duplicates were excluded from statistical tests using R package *DoubletFinder* (v. 2.0.3, parameters: PCs = 1:15, pN = 0.25). Cells with more than one TCR alpha or beta chain were also excluded; however, not all cells were duplicates. An approach described by Karlsson et al. [44] was used to classify the cell types in both datasets. Differential expression was assessed using the Seurat FindMarkers function (test.use = "LR," logfc.threshold = $-$Inf) between the same cell type in the two datasets. Note that the batch effects cannot be excluded from the analysis. FindMarkers were run at three different times with or without accounting for the cell cycle (derived from the Seurat function CellCycleScoring) and sex, and only genes commonly identified as differentially expressed in all three analyses were retained (Supplementary Table S3).

2.12. RNA-Sequencing

RNA was prepared from companion dog tumors using the RNA/DNA kit from Qiagen. RNA was sequenced at the Clinical Genetics Center at Sahlgrenska University Hospital using a Novaseq sequencer. Reads were aligned to the CanFam3.1 genome (http://ngi-igenomes.s3.amazonaws.com/igenomes/Canis_familiaris/Ensembl/CanFam3.1/Sequence/WholeGenomeFasta/genome.fa, accessed on 5 February, 2021) with STAR (v. 2.7.10a) [48], with a matching reference genome annotation supplied from AWS iGenomes (http://ngi-igenomes.s3.amazonaws.com/igenomes/Canis_familiaris/Ensembl/CanFam3.1/Annotation/Genes/genes.gtf, accessed on 5 February 2021), using the parameters "twopassMode Basic" and "setting—sjdbOverhang" equal to read length 1. Gene expression levels were quantified from name-sorted and non-duplicate marked alignment files using htseq-count (v. 1.99.2) [49], with the parameters "-s reverse -m intersection-strict".

2.13. Transcriptomic Classification

TCGA data, downloaded and processed as described previously [50], were used for the classification of canine tumors relative to human cancer types. Pairwise Spearman correlation coefficients were calculated between our sample and each TCGA sample for all coding genes. Classification was performed using a k-nearest neighbor approach based on these correlation coefficients, using $k = 6$, as previously found to be optimal based on leave-one-out cross-validation in TCGA cohort [50].

3. Results

3.1. TILs Differentially Express Chemokine Receptors and Selectins

CAR-T cells were approved for clinical use against some B-cell malignancies; however, no CAR-T cell therapy has been approved for solid tumors. To investigate the difference in the expression of cell surface molecules involved in T cell trafficking and homing, we performed single-cell sequencing of blood-derived T cells and young TILs that had grown out uveal melanoma metastases in the presence of the T cell growth factor interleukin-2 (IL-2) [44]. Focusing on differentially expressed genes in the category of 'chemokine receptors' or 'adhesion molecules' we find that genes like ITGA4 (CD49D), ITGB2 (CD18), ITGAL (CD11a), ITGAE (CD103), PECAM1 (CD31), and CXCR3 are all more highly expressed on

TILs compared to on blood-derived T cells (Supplementary Figure S1a). Since TILs are cultured, we validated the finding at the protein level using flow cytometry. Although it confirmed the differential expressions, it also demonstrated that at least some of this differential expression could be caused by the IL-2 used in the culture medium of TILs (Supplementary Figure S1b,c).

3.2. CAR-TILs Can Kill Melanoma Cells In Vitro

CAR-T cell manufacturing is performed by modifying blood-derived T cells from leukapheresis with a chimeric antigen receptor (CAR) that binds to a surface antigen on the tumor cell. To investigate whether anti-HER2 CAR-expressing TILs, hereafter called CAR-TILs, are capable of recognizing melanoma cells, we used TILs from human patients with melanoma and transfected these cells with an mRNA encoding a HER2 CAR consisting of a single-chain variable fragment (scFv) to detect HER2 fused with the signaling domains of CD3 epsilon and the CD28 co-stimulatory molecule [40]. We consistently observed HER2 CAR expression in these cells which peaked at 5–16 h but lasted for at least 24 h, as assessed by recombinant HER2 binding to CAR-TILs (Figure 1a and Supplementary Figure S2). CAR was functional and specific because the CAR-TILs (but not mock-transfected TILs) from patient MM1 degranulated, released, and caused accumulation of interferon gamma (IFN-γ) in the medium when co-cultured with the HER2 positive uveal melanoma cell line 92-1 (Figure 1b–d). This was dependent on HER2 expression since CRISPR-generated 92-1 HER2 knockout cells [40] were not able to activate CAR-TILs. This demonstrates that anti-HER2 CAR-TILs can react with HER2 on the surface of melanoma cells.

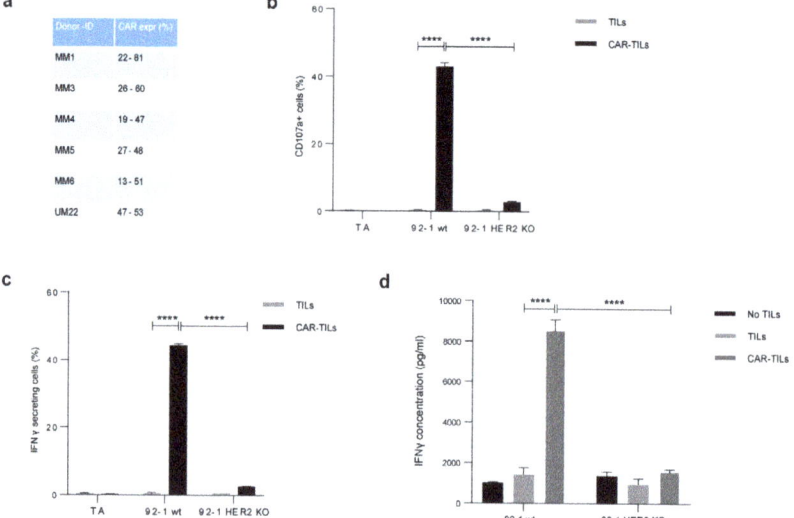

Figure 1. TILs can be activated by equipping them with a CAR construct. mRNA encoding anti-HER2 CAR was electroporated into TILs from five cutaneous melanomas (MM1, MM3, MM4, MM5, and MM6) and one uveal melanoma (UM22) to produce CAR-TILs. CAR expression was detected by HER2-biotin binding at 5–16 h post-transfection (**a**). MM1 TILs and CAR-TILs were co-cultured with the parental or HER2 KO 92-1 uveal melanoma cell line for 4–6 h, followed by flow cytometry to measure degranulation (CD107a expression) (**b**) or IFN-γ-secreting cells (**c**). TILs and CAR-TILs not co-cultured with 92-1 cells (TILs alone; TA) were used as controls in (**b,c**). Alternatively, cells were co-cultured for 48 h, and the supernatant was collected for analysis of secreted IFN-γ by ELISA (**d**). 92-1 cells not co-cultured with TILs (no TILs) were used as a control. Data are presented as mean ± standard deviation (SD) of duplicates. The experiments were performed twice, and representative results are shown. *p* values are represented as **** $p < 0.0001$.

Next, we co-cultured MM1 or CAR-TILs with 92-1 cells and stained them with an antibody directed against cleaved caspase-3. 92-1 cells cultured with CAR-TILs, but not TILs, were positive for intracellular cleaved caspase-3, suggesting that the cells underwent apoptosis (Figure 2a). We also generated patient-derived cell lines, TILs, and CAR-TILs from MM5 cells. CAR expression in autologous MM5 TILs enhanced their ability to kill melanoma cells (Figure 2b). Four out of five patient-derived cell lines were more sensitive to increasing amounts of CAR-TILs than to TILs in the co-culture experiments (Figure 2c–g). This correlated with the greater degranulation of CAR-TILs than mock-transfected TILs (Supplementary Figure S3).

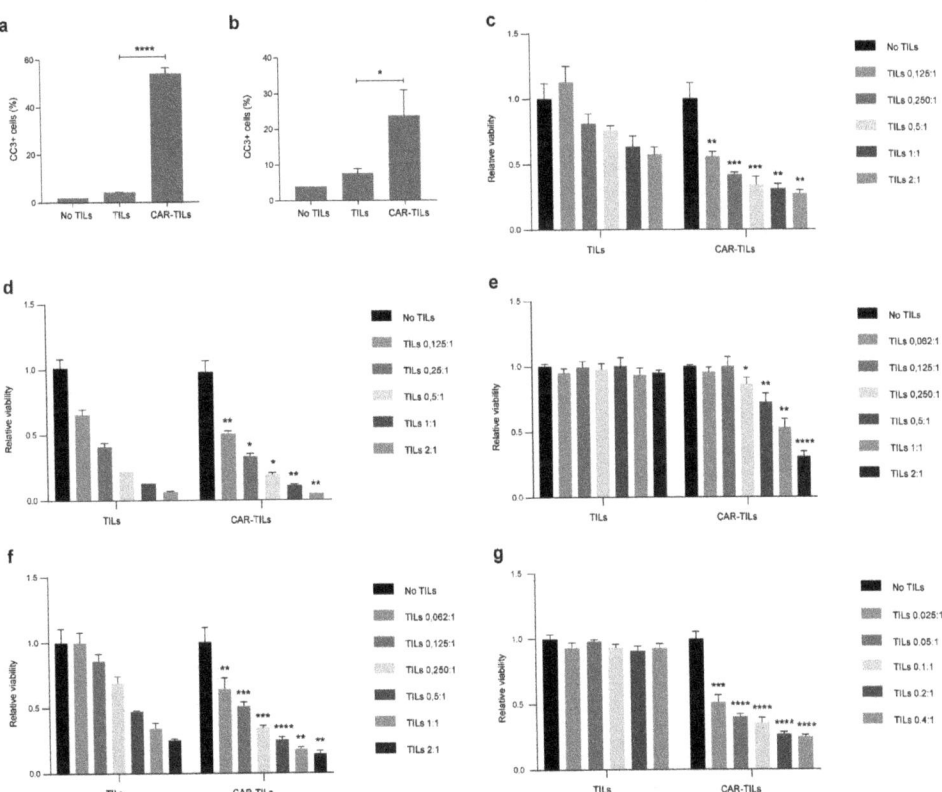

Figure 2. CAR-TILs kill tumor cells more efficiently than TILs. (**a**,**b**) TILs and CAR-TILs from MM1 were co-cultured with the parental or HER2 KO 92-1 uveal melanoma cell line for 24 h, followed by cleaved caspase 3 (CC3) detection in the tumor cells using flow cytometry (**a**). Additionally, TILs and CAR-TILs from MM5 were co-cultured with autologous cancer cells for 24 h, followed by cleaved CC3 detection using flow cytometry (**b**). Cancer cells not treated with TILs were used as a control (no TILs). (**c**–**g**) Viability of autologous cancer cells was measured by luciferase signal detected after 48 h co-culture with increasing doses of TILs and CAR-TILs from UM22 (**c**), MM3 (**d**), MM4 (**e**), MM5 (**f**), and MM6 (**g**) in the indicated ratios (TILs:cancer cells). Data are presented as mean with SD of triplicates. Asterisks represent p-values of difference between similar doses of TILs and CAR-TILs. The experiments were performed twice, and representative data from one experiment is shown. P values are represented as * $p < 0.05$, ** $p < 0.01$, *** $p < 0.001$, and **** $p < 0.0001$.

3.3. CAR-TILs Can Kill Melanoma Cells In Vivo

The mRNA transfection of CAR into TILs allowed for a fast way to assess the efficacy of CAR in TILs, but the expression was not durable. TILs kill via the binding of the

T-cell receptor (TCR) to the MHC class I complex, which is loaded with peptides. The MHC complex consists of one alpha chain (encoded by HLA A/B/C) and one beta-2-microglobulin (B2M) chain (encoded by B2M). To challenge the TILs, we deleted B2M by CRISPR/Cas9 (B2M KO; Supplementary Figure S4) in a cell line from patient MM3, rendering the tumor cells resistant to the cytotoxic activity of autologous TILs but not to anti-HER2 CAR mRNA-transfected CAR-TILs (Figure 3a).

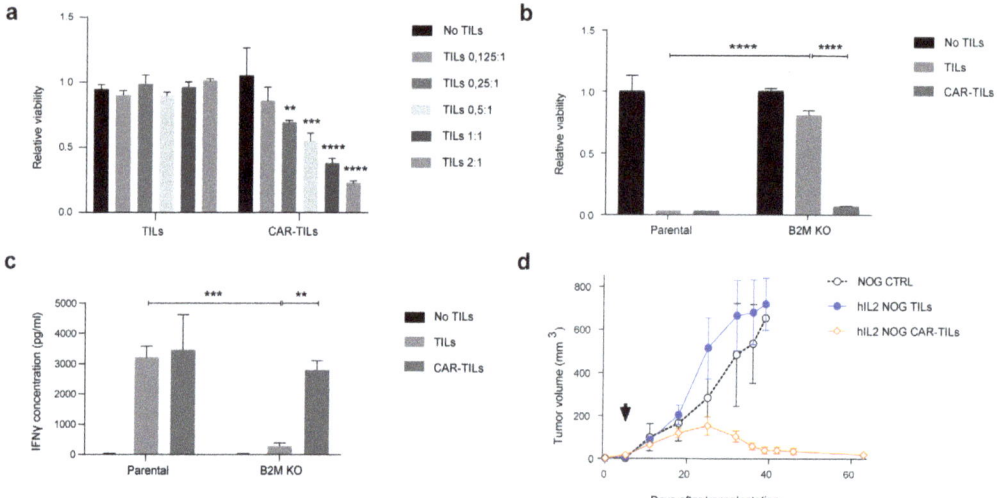

Figure 3. Anti-HER2 CAR-TILs eradicate autologous tumor cells refractory to TCR-mediated cytotoxicity. Parental MM3 melanoma and MM3 cells with CRISPR-Cas9 disruption of β-2-Microglobulin (B2M KO, Supplementary Figure S5) were cultured with autologous TILs or CAR-TILS. (**a**,**b**) Viability was measured by luciferase activity in melanoma cells after 48 h of co-culture with TILs or mRNA generated (**a**) or virus generated (**b**) CAR-TILs. (**c**) IFNγ was measured in the culture supernatant from the same experiment as in (**b**). (**d**) Mice bearing B2M CRISPR knockout MM3 melanoma cells were treated with PBS ($n = 3$), 20×10^6 TILs ($n = 3$), or 20×10^6 CAR-TILs ($n = 3$). Arrow indicates treatment start. Data are presented as mean ± standard error of the mean. p values are represented as ** $p < 0.01$, *** $p < 0.001$, and **** $p < 0.0001$.

To study the effect of CAR-TILs in vivo we used a lentivirus expressing the same anti-HER2 CAR mRNA [40]. CAR expression was much lower in lentivirus-transduced cells than in those transfected with CAR mRNA and only 1–10% of TILs were susceptible to lentivirus transduction (Supplementary Figure S5). Nevertheless, this modification of MM3 TILs enabled the cytotoxicity of both parental MM3 cells and B2M KO tumor cells in vitro (Figure 3b), which correlated with IFN-γ secretion into the medium.

We previously showed that TILs and blood-derived HER2 CAR-T cells can eradicate PDX tumor models in the human IL-2 transgenic NOG/NSG mouse strain (hIL2-NOG). We transplanted B2M KO MM3 cells into hIL2-NOG cells and treated them with TILs or anti-HER2 CAR-TILs. As expected from the in vitro experiments (Figure 3a–c), TILs were not able to eradicate B2M deficient melanoma in the PDXv2 model, but CAR-TILs could (Figure 3d). In PDX models from UM1, MM2, and MM7, the added value of lentiviral CAR expression in TILs was only visible in MM2, since unmodified TILs could eradicate tumors in UM1 and MM7 PDX models (Supplementary Figure S6).

3.4. First-in-Dog (FIDO) Trial Suggests CAR-TIL Therapy Is Safe and May Have Anti-Tumoral Activity in Tumor-Bearing Companion Dogs

To assess the safety of anti-HER2 CAR-TILs in an immune-competent and spontaneous tumor model before the first-time-in-man trial (FTIM), we conducted a first-in-dog (FIDO) trial that recruited four companion dogs with high-grade cancer (two with squamous carcinoma and two with melanoma). In parallel with the recruitment and treatment of dogs, we also performed several analyses of the tumors and TILs. First, we assessed the expression of HER2 in the tumors of all dogs compared to blood leukocytes, canine D17.os osteosarcoma and CF41.mg mammary cell lines. The Dog 2 tumor had the highest HER2 mRNA expression, followed by the mammary cell line and the second melanoma dog (Dog 4). The tumors of dogs 1 and 3 had a similar expression as the osteosarcoma line, whereas blood leukocytes were practically negative for HER2 expression (Figure 4a). Immunohistochemistry demonstrated HER2 expression in all dog tumors (Figure 4b).

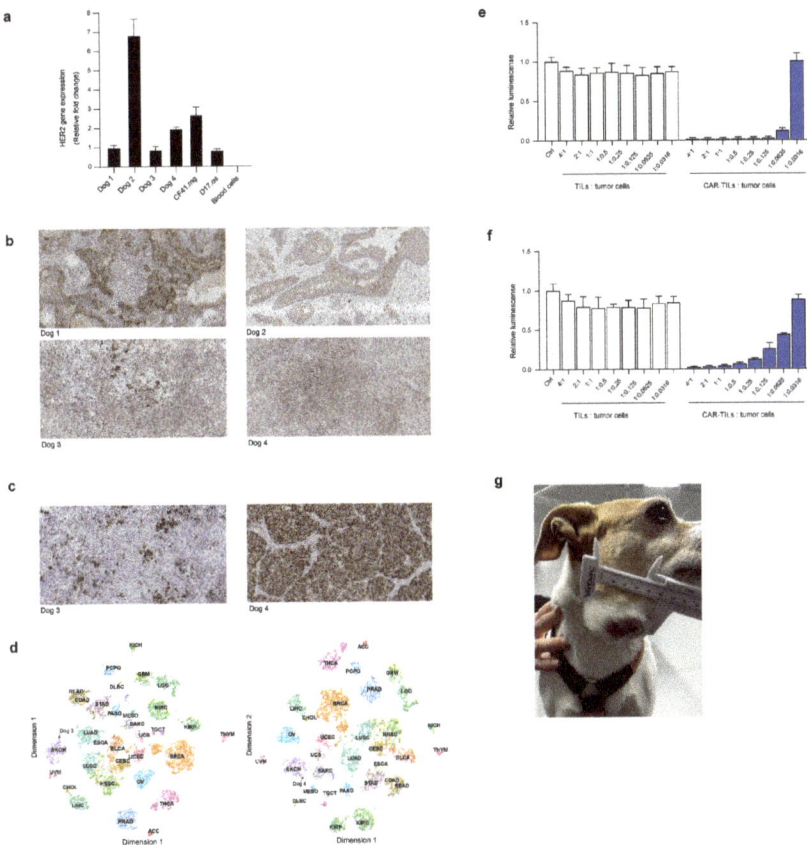

Figure 4. Dog tumor cells express HER2 and can be killed by anti-HER2 CAR-TILs. HER2 expression detected by qPCR (**a**) and immunohistochemistry (**b**) in tumors from four companion dogs (dogs 1-4). Canine cell lines D17.os and CF41.mg and canine PBMC were used as controls in a. (**c**) Expression of human melanoma marker Melan-a in tumors from dogs 3 and 4 with melanoma. (**d**) Classification of canine tumor biopsies from dogs 3 and 4 based on gene expression relative to TCGA cohort of >10,000 human tumor samples from 32 cancer types. The similarities between canine melanoma and samples in TCGA were visualized using tSNE dimensionality reduction. SKCM: melanoma cases. (**e**,**f**) TILs and mRNA electroporated CAR-TILs from dog 3 were co-cultured with the canine cell lines CF41.mg (**e**) and D17.os (**f**) for 24 h. The experiment was performed twice and representative data (n = 3, data ± SD) from one experiment are shown. (**g**) Photograph of Dog 3 with metastatic oral malignant melanoma enrolled in the FIDO trial evaluating the safety of CAR-TIL treatment in companion dogs.

We recruited two dogs with melanoma, Dog 3, which had a patchy expression, and Dog 4, which had a uniform expression of the melanoma marker Melan-a (Figure 4c). To compare the transcriptomes of canine and human cancers, we used an in-house bioinformatics pipeline developed to diagnose cancer of unknown primary origin [50]. By comparing the gene expression of around 10,000 human tumors in The Cancer Genome Atlas (TCGA) with those of the biopsies from dogs 3 and 4 using k-nearest neighbor analysis, we could analyze the similarities between the canine melanomas to other cancers. Of the 10 tumors whose transcriptome correlated to that of dog 3's tumor (Spearman correlation 0.8), 8 were melanomas. The other two tumors were those of breast cancer and bladder cancer. In total, 5 of the 10 most similar tumors to Dog 4's tumor were melanomas, the remaining being 2 sarcomas, 1 breast cancer, 1 bladder cancer, and 1 esophageal tumor. The similarity to human melanoma (SKCM) with all tumors in TCGA are also visible in tSNE plots (Figure 4d).

To evaluate whether our anti-HER2 CAR binder would bind to canine HER2, we transfected canine TILs with the mRNA encoding anti-HER2 CAR. We co-cultured the TILs or anti-HER2 CAR-TILs with the canine D17.os and CF41.mg cell lines labeled with firefly luciferase. Since luciferase requires ATP to glow, we were able to assess the viability of tumor cells exclusively by luciferase measurements when co-cultured with increasing amounts of TILs or CAR-TILs. None of the cell lines were sensitive to allogenic TILs, but both were killed by CAR-TILs in a dose-dependent manner (Figure 4e,f). The canine mammary carcinoma cell line was more sensitive than the osteosarcoma cell line, suggesting that the level of HER2 expression (Figure 4a) affects sensitivity to CAR-TILs.

The FIDO trial design was a dose-escalation study giving 0.1–10 million CAR-TILs/kg dog, without or with injections of human IL-2. All dogs received one dose of the lowest dose of CAR-TILs, and after safety monitoring, one or two additional doses with or without IL-2 were administered. The first two dogs had squamous cell carcinoma of the tongue and tonsils. The dogs initially tolerated the treatment well; however, the first dog developed pyometra, a common disease in female dogs of this breed. None of the other two female dogs in the study developed this disease, suggesting that it was not apparently related to treatment. The first dog experienced a slight reduction in tumor size, but this was not a durable response (Supplementary Table S1). Since the percentage of anti-HER2 CAR positive cells was very low in the CAR-TILs of the first dog, and the main purpose of the trial was to evaluate the safety of the anti-HER2 CAR binder, we used anti-HER2 CAR mRNA transfection for the next dog. We achieved approximately 30% of CAR-positive cells. The tumor size was not accurately measurable from the back of the tongue, but there was no apparent softening or decrease in size with treatment, and the dog was euthanized upon tumor progression because of deteriorating quality of life (Supplementary Table S2).

Dogs 3 and 4 suffer from melanoma, a debilitating disease in dogs because it often affects eating: it rapidly develops systemic metastases and, if untreated, is lethal. We were able to generate more TILs from dogs with melanoma and were therefore able to inject both mRNA-transfected and virus-transduced CAR-TILs, as well as treatment with IL-2. Initially, the tumor grew rapidly on Dog 3 (Figure 4g), but a transient decrease in tumor size (PR) was observed after the third CAR-TIL injection and first IL-2 injections. The dog experienced gastrointestinal side effects, such as loss of appetite, vomiting, and diarrhea (Table 1), which were resolved and did not appear after subsequent reduction in the dose of reminders of IL-2 injections. After the initial decrease in tumor size, the tumor progressed, and the dog was euthanized because of tumor progression.

Table 1. Clinical responses to CAR-TIL treatment of Dog 3. Abbreviations used: CRP, C-reactive protein, and WBC, white blood cell count.

Days after Treatment	Treatment	Number of Cells/kg	CAR Expression	Tumor Size (mm)	CRP (mg/L)	WBC (109/L)	Eosinophils (109/L)	Side Effects
0	Dose 1: CAR-TILs	0.1 million	70% (mRNA)		<7	5	0.3	
14	Dose 2: CAR-TILs	10 million	75% (mRNA)	15 × 13	<7	8.4	0.4	Diarrhea that resolved after one day
35				27 × 14	<7	7.9	0.5	
63				35 × 29	<7	7.4	0.4	
78	Dose 3: CAR-TILs	10 million	1–7% (virus)	42 × 24	<7	7.2	0.6	
78	IL-2 injections 30,000 IU/kg q12h							Diarrhea and vomiting, decreased appetite all grade 1
84	IL-2 injections 30,000 IU/kg q12h			36 × 22	58	10.5	1.3	Eosinophilia grade 1
89	IL-2 injections 30,000 IU/kg q12h			34 × 24	51	23.2	9.7	Eosinophilia grade 1
112				52 × 44	<7	11.2		
133	Euthanized due to tumor progression							

The fourth dog underwent surgery for subungual melanoma with metastasis to the prescapular lymph node, and no detectable tumor was detected after surgery. Nevertheless, since local recurrence or distant metastases invariably develop within 3–6 months in these cases, we treated the dog with both the lowest and therapeutic dose of CAR-TILs in an adjuvant setting. No acute side effects were observed with CAR-TIL treatment; however, after IL-2 treatment, gastrointestinal side effects and eosinophilia resolved with treatment discontinuation and re-emerged when reinitiating treatment (Table 2). IL-2 treatment ceased, and one year after surgery, the dog was still tumor-free.

Table 2. Clinical responses to CAR-TIL treatment of Dog 4.

Days after Treatment	Treatment	Number of Cells/kg	CAR Expression	CRP (mg/L)	WBC (109/L)	Eosinophils (109/L)	Side Effects
0	Dose 1: CAR-TILs	0.1 million	79% (mRNA)	<7	6.6	0.5	
20	Dose 2: CAR-TILs	10 million	9% (virus)	<7	4.4	0.3	
21–24	IL-2 injections 30,000 IU/kg q12h						Altered appetite, vomiting and diarreha all grade 1
27–32	IL-2 injections 30,000 IU/kg q24h			43	12.9	2.5	Eosinophilia, altered appetite, vomiting, diarreha and lethargy all grade 1
34				12	22.1	10.9	Eosinophilia grade 1
241							Revisit, in CR
290							Revisit, still in CR

Monitoring of safety in all four dogs throughout the treatment period did not reveal any apparent effects on blood pressure or cardiac, pulmonary, or endocrine functions. Liver and electrolyte levels were normal, but CRP was elevated in response to tumor progression, IL-2 administration, or infection (Supplementary Tables S1 and S2, and Tables 1 and 2).

4. Discussion

Immunotherapies with checkpoint blockade have revolutionized the treatment of metastatic melanoma, with durable and high response rates in patients who previously had a poor prognosis. However, some tumors pose a challenge for immunotherapies because of their low antigen load or different immune evasion strategies. A great challenge in the field is how to render these tumors immunogenic.

We posed the question of whether it would be possible to enhance the effect of TIL therapy by genetic engineering with CAR. Indeed, we showed that this therapeutic approach resulted in the activation of T cells that could not kill allogenic or immune-evaded autologous tumors. We observed complete tumor regression in PDX mice from tumors that lacked B2M and were treated with CAR-TILs (but not TILs). These responses were superior to those observed in a study published while writing this manuscript [51]. This can be explained by the use of different immunocompromised mouse strains. Our data confirm the importance of IL-2 supplementation for TIL and CAR-T activity in vivo as shown in hIL2-NOG mice [40,42]. On the other hand, Mills et al. [51] reported better transduction efficiencies using CAR-expressing retroviruses, although they selected cells to ensure high expression levels. This information is valuable for advancing the concept of CAR-TILs in the clinic.

CAR-TIL treatment could be used in patients with cancers that are normally not recognized by the immune system, for instance, due to downregulation of MHC or the antigen presentation machinery, lack of suitable neoantigens, or expression of any inhibitory receptors (including but not limited to PD1 and CTLA-4). One PDX model, which is a poor responder to TIL therapy (MM2), was rendered more responsive to T-cell cytotoxicity after equipping the TILs with a CAR construct. However, tumors that respond to ACT treatment with autologous TILs (e.g., UM1 and MM7 in this study) may not be eradicated more efficiently by CAR-TIL treatment. Hence, a potential target population for a trial could consist of patients with immune checkpoint inhibitor-resistant metastatic cutaneous, mucosal, or uveal melanoma.

A challenge for immunotherapy research is to utilize good preclinical models to study human tumors and to generate preclinical efficacy and safety data that can warrant the start of clinical trials. Most preclinical advances have depended on in vitro studies of human tumors and immune cells, mouse tumor models, and mouse immune cells. In vitro systems do not always recapitulate the in vivo setting in a satisfactory manner, highlighting the importance of using in vivo models to develop novel treatment strategies for cancer patients. Mouse models used to study mouse tumors and immune cells accurately recapitulate the complex truth [52], but with limitations attributed to differences between mouse and human biology. The hIL2-NOG mouse model used here [42] has the advantage of recapitulating the heterogeneous nature of TIL therapy in cancer patients, which is not possible in NOG mice. Unfortunately, for the rare form of melanoma arising in the eye, uveal melanoma, there is a lack of models, and those that we have developed [40,44] most often grow slower in NSG/NOG mice than in cutaneous melanoma.

Companion dogs are emerging models for human diseases because their etiologies are very similar [34,36]. In this study, we utilized the fact that solid tumors in companion dogs express the dog variant of HER2, which was also similar to the human protein, so that we could generate CAR-expressing T cells using our human-specific construct. The primary aim of the FIDO trial was to generate safety data for a planned FTIM study, as a previous trial with HER2 CAR-T cells reported a lethal incident [53]. All adverse events were mild and exclusively associated with IL-2 treatment. Toxicity was concentrated in the GI tract, with loose stool, decreased appetite, and vomiting. The eosinophilia observed has been described previously and is likely due to the release of IL-5 and GM-CSF release by IL-2-stimulated CD4-positive lymphocytes [54]. Reduced dosing of IL-2 resulted in control of toxicity, which was completely resolved after the termination of IL-2 administration.

In the safety FIDO trial, we also observed some signs of anti-tumoral activity, as evidenced by a near partial response in a dog with melanoma and potentially a delay in recurrence in a second dog. We are cautiously optimistic about these early signs of efficacy, although mindful of the pitfalls and caveats of the experiments. First, since our mouse data comparing the efficacy of TILs and CAR-T cells in NOG vs. hIL2-NOG mice undeniably indicated that IL-2 is essential for the efficacy of these therapies, we treated the dogs with subcutaneous injections of IL-2. It is therefore not inconceivable that some of the therapeutic effects observed were mediated by this factor, or that the gastrointestinal adverse events resulted in metabolic effects on the tumor. Second, we could not detect CAR-TILs in the blood of dogs using PCR. This could be due to the CAR-TILs not surviving or expanding, but it could also be due to them leaving the bloodstream because they express homing receptors for inflamed areas, such as tumors [41,42]. A future study protocol will need to include metastasectomy or biopsy after CAR-TIL therapy to evaluate whether CAR-TILs reach the target, as they commonly do in humans.

5. Conclusions

We present a novel approach to treating metastatic cancer in mice and dogs by combining CAR-T cell therapy and adoptive T cell transfer, called CAR-TIL treatment. CAR-TILs elicited complete eradication of tumors in immune-humanized PDX mouse models of melanoma, even in the absence of antigen presentation, indicating the potential usefulness of this strategy for treating melanomas that do not respond to existing therapies. This regimen should be tested in patients with metastatic melanoma to assess the potential of this therapy. Since owners and veterinarians of companion dogs with melanoma have difficulty accessing effective immunotherapies when they progress on approved therapies, the data here provide an interesting avenue for future trial activities. Companion dogs also contribute to 3R by reducing (and long-term replacing) the use of healthy beagles for safety studies and refining, since companion dogs have spontaneous tumor formation and are therefore more representative of patients in FTIM studies than using beagles.

Supplementary Materials: The following supporting information can be downloaded at: https://www.mdpi.com/article/10.3390/cancers15030648/s1, Figure S1: Differential expression of chemokine and adhesion between TILs and blood-derived T cells.; Figure S2: anti-HER2 CAR-expression after mRNA electroporation; Figure S3: Cytotoxicity of CAR-TILs and TILs on autologous tumor cells; Figure S4: Flow analysis of B2M in KO cells; Figure S5: Expression of anti-HER2 CAR in virus transduced melanoma TILs; Figure S6: CAR-TIL activity against melanoma xenografts in IL2 transgenic NOG mice; Tables S1 and S2: Clinical responses to CAR-TIL treatment of Dog 1 and 2.

Author Contributions: Conceptualization, J.A.N.; methodology, E.M.V.F., R.R., S.S., S.A. and V.B.; software, J.K.; formal analysis, J.K.; investigation, J.K.; resources, R.O.B.; data curation, E.M.V.F., R.R. and J.K.; writing—original draft preparation, E.M.V.F. and J.A.N.; writing—review and editing, J.K.; visualization, E.M.V.F., J.A.N. and J.K.; supervision, L.M.N., L.N., H.R. and A.E.H.; project administration, J.A.N.; funding acquisition, J.A.N. All authors have read and agreed to the published version of the manuscript.

Funding: This work was supported by the Swedish Cancer Society, Swedish Research Council, EU Horizon 2020 (ERA PerMed), Region Västra Götaland (ALF-grant), Knut and Alice Wallenberg Foundation, Sjöberg Foundation, Familjen Erling Persson Foundation, IngaBritt and Arne Lundberg Foundation (to J.A.N.), Assar Gabrielsson Foundation, and Sahlgrenska Universitetssjukhusets stiftelse (Sahlgrenska University Hospital, Gothenburg) (to E.M.V.F.). S.S. and H.R. were supported by the Johansson Family Swedish Boxer Club Cancer Donation, and A.E.H. was supported by the Jane and Aatos Erkko Foundation. J.A.N., L.M.N., and J.K. were supported by the Kirkbride Melanoma Discovery Lab at the Harry Perkins Institute of Medical Research.

Institutional Review Board Statement: Approvals for human studies were obtained from Regional Human Ethics Board of Västra Götaland, Sweden (approval #288-12 and #44-18), for mouse studies from the Regional Animal Ethics Committee of Gothenburg (approvals #2014-36, #2016-100 and #2018-1183) and for dog studies from the Swedish Animal Ethical Committee in Uppsala (approval #2019-2435).

Informed Consent Statement: Informed consent was obtained from all humans and the owners of all the dogs involved in the study.

Data Availability Statement: All sequencing data was deposited to the European Genome Archives and made available under controlled data access.

Acknowledgments: We wish to thank Carina Karlsson for technical support and Larissa Rizzo, Sofia Stenqvist, and Mona Svedman for assistance with animal experiments. We want to thank NIH/NCI preclinical repository for the kind donation of human IL-2.

Conflicts of Interest: The authors declare no conflict of interest with regards to this study.

References

1. Balch, C.M.; Gershenwald, J.E.; Soong, S.-J.; Thompson, J.F.; Atkins, M.B.; Byrd, D.R.; Buzaid, A.C.; Cochran, A.J.; Coit, D.G.; Ding, S.; et al. Final Version of 2009 AJCC Melanoma Staging and Classification. *J. Clin. Oncol.* **2009**, *27*, 6199–6206. [CrossRef]
2. Hauschild, A.; Grob, J.J.; Demidov, L.V.; Jouary, T.; Gutzmer, R.; Millward, M.; Rutkowski, P.; Blank, C.U.; Miller Jr., W. H.; Kaempgen, E.; et al. Dabrafenib in BRAF-mutated metastatic melanoma: A multicentre, open-label, phase 3 randomised controlled trial. *Lancet* **2012**, *380*, 358–365. [CrossRef]
3. Sosman, J.A.; Kim, K.B.; Schuchter, L.; Gonzalez, R.; Pavlick, A.C.; Weber, J.S.; McArthur, G.A.; Hutson, T.E.; Moschos, S.J.; Flaherty, K.T.; et al. Survival in BRAF V600-mutant advanced melanoma treated with vemurafenib. *N. Engl. J. Med.* **2012**, *366*, 707–714. [CrossRef] [PubMed]
4. Flaherty, K.T.; Infante, J.R.; Daud, A.; Gonzalez, R.; Kefford, R.F.; Sosman, J.; Hamid, O.; Schuchter, L.; Cebon, J.; Ibrahim, N.; et al. Combined BRAF and MEK inhibition in melanoma with BRAF V600 mutations. *N. Engl. J. Med.* **2012**, *367*, 1694–1703. [CrossRef] [PubMed]
5. Long, G.V.; Stroyakovskiy, D.; Gogas, H.; Levchenko, E.; de Braud, F.; Larkin, J.; Garbe, C.; Jouary, T.; Hauschild, A.; Grob, J.J.; et al. Combined BRAF and MEK inhibition versus BRAF inhibition alone in melanoma. *N. Engl. J. Med.* **2014**, *371*, 1877–1888. [CrossRef] [PubMed]
6. Hodi, F.S.; O'Day, S.J.; McDermott, D.F.; Weber, R.W.; Sosman, J.A.; Haanen, J.B.; Gonzalez, R.; Robert, C.; Schadendorf, D.; Hassel, J.C.; et al. Improved Survival with Ipilimumab in Patients with Metastatic Melanoma. *N. Engl. J. Med.* **2010**, *363*, 711–723. [CrossRef]
7. Robert, C.; Thomas, L.; Bondarenko, I.; O'Day, S.; Weber, J.; Garbe, C.; Lebbe, C.; Baurain, J.-F.; Testori, A.; Grob, J.-J.; et al. Ipilimumab plus Dacarbazine for Previously Untreated Metastatic Melanoma. *N. Engl. J. Med.* **2011**, *364*, 2517–2526. [CrossRef]
8. Robert, C.; Long, G.v.; Brady, B.; Dutriaux, C.; Maio, M.; Mortier, L.; Hassel, J.C.; Rutkowski, P.; McNeil, C.; Kalinka-Warzocha, E.; et al. Nivolumab in previously untreated melanoma without BRAF mutation. *N. Engl. J. Med.* **2015**, *372*, 320–330. [CrossRef]
9. Tawbi, H.A.; Schadendorf, D.; Lipson, E.J.; Ascierto, P.A.; Matamala, L.; Gutiérrez, E.C.; Rutkowski, P.; Gogas, H.J.; Lao, C.D.; De Menezes, J.J.; et al. Relatlimab and Nivolumab versus Nivolumab in Untreated Advanced Melanoma. *N. Engl. J. Med.* **2022**, *386*, 24–34. [CrossRef]
10. Andersen, R.; Donia, M.; Ellebaek, E.; Borch, T.H.; Kongsted, P.; Iversen, T.Z.; Hölmich, L.R.; Hendel, H.W.; Met, O.; Andersen, M.H.; et al. Long-Lasting Complete Responses in Patients with Metastatic Melanoma after Adoptive Cell Therapy with Tumor-Infiltrating Lymphocytes and an Attenuated IL2 Regimen. *Clin. Cancer Res.* **2016**, *22*, 3734–3745. [CrossRef]
11. Rosenberg, S.A.; Yang, J.C.; Sherry, R.M.; Kammula, U.S.; Hughes, M.S.; Phan, G.Q.; Citrin, D.E.; Restifo, N.P.; Robbins, P.F.; Wunderlich, J.R.; et al. Durable complete responses in heavily pretreated patients with metastatic melanoma using T-cell transfer immunotherapy. *Clin. Cancer Res.* **2011**, *17*, 4550–4557. [CrossRef] [PubMed]
12. Rosenberg, S.A.; Packard, B.S.; Aebersold, P.M.; Solomon, D.; Topalian, S.L.; Toy, S.T.; Simon, P.; Lotze, M.T.; Yang, J.C.; Seipp, C.A.; et al. Use of Tumor-Infiltrating Lymphocytes and Interleukin-2 in the Immunotherapy of Patients with Metastatic Melanoma. *N. Engl. J. Med.* **1988**, *319*, 1676–1680. [CrossRef]
13. Chang, A.E.; Karnell, L.H.; Menck, H.R. The national cancer data base report on cutaneous and noncutaneous melanoma: A summary of 84,836 cases from the past decade. *Cancer* **1998**, *83*, 1664–1678. [CrossRef]
14. Seibel, I.; Cordini, D.; Rehak, M.; Hager, A.; Riechardt, A.I.; Böker, A.; Heufelder, J.; Weber, A.; Gollrad, J.; Besserer, A.; et al. Local Recurrence After Primary Proton Beam Therapy in Uveal Melanoma: Risk Factors, Retreatment Approaches, and Outcome. *Am. J. Ophthalmol.* **2015**, *160*, 628–636. [CrossRef] [PubMed]
15. Kujala, E.; Mäkitie, T.; Kivelä, T. Very Long-Term Prognosis of Patients with Malignant Uveal Melanoma. *Investig. Ophthalmol. Vis. Sci.* **2003**, *44*, 4651–4659. [CrossRef]
16. Diener-West, M.; Reynolds, S.M.; Agugliaro, D.J.; Caldwell, R.; Cumming, K.; Earle, J.D.; Hawkins, B.S.; Hayman, J.A.; Jaiyesimi, I.; Jampol, L.M.; et al. Development of metastatic disease after enrollment in the COMS trials for treatment of choroidal melanoma: Collaborative Ocular Melanoma Study Group Report No. 26. *Arch. Ophthalmol.* **2005**, *123*, 1639–1643. [PubMed]
17. Leyvraz, S.; Konietschke, F.; Peuker, C.; Schütte, M.; Kessler, T.; Ochsenreither, S.; Ditzhaus, M.; Sprünken, E.D.; Dörpholz, G.; Lamping, M.; et al. Biomarker-driven therapies for metastatic uveal melanoma: A prospective precision oncology feasibility study. *Eur. J. Cancer* **2022**, *169*, 146–155. [CrossRef] [PubMed]
18. Piulats, J.M.; Espinosa, E.; de la Cruz, M.L.; Varela, M.; Alonso, C.L.; Martin-Algarra, S.; Lopez Castro, R.; Curiel, T.; Rodriguez-Abreu, D.; Redrado, M.; et al. Nivolumab Plus Ipilimumab for Treatment-Naive Metastatic Uveal Melanoma: An Open-Label, Multicenter, Phase II Trial by the Spanish Multidisciplinary Melanoma Group (GEM-1402). *J. Clin. Oncol.* **2021**, *39*, 586–598. [CrossRef]

19. Pelster, M.S.; Gruschkus, S.K.; Bassett, R.; Gombos, D.S.; Shephard, M.; Posada, L.; Glover, M.S.; Simien, R.; Diab, A.; Hwu, P.; et al. Nivolumab and Ipilimumab in Metastatic Uveal Melanoma: Results from a Single-Arm Phase II Study. *J. Clin. Oncol.* **2021**, *39*, 599–607. [CrossRef]
20. Wolchok, J.D.; Chiarion-Sileni, V.; Gonzalez, R.; Rutkowski, P.; Grob, J.-J.; Cowey, C.L.; Lao, C.D.; Wagstaff, J.; Schadendorf, D.; Ferrucci, P.F.; et al. Overall Survival with Combined Nivolumab and Ipilimumab in Advanced Melanoma. *N. Engl. J. Med.* **2017**, *377*, 1345–1356. [CrossRef]
21. Khoja, L.; Atenafu, E.; Suciu, S.; Leyvraz, S.; Sato, T.; Marshall, E.; Keilholz, U.; Zimmer, L.; Patel, S.; Piperno-Neumann, S.; et al. Meta-analysis in metastatic uveal melanoma to determine progression free and overall survival benchmarks: An international rare cancers initiative (IRCI) ocular melanoma study. *Ann. Oncol.* **2019**, *30*, 1370–1380. [CrossRef]
22. Olofsson, B.R.; Nelson, A.; Shafazand, A.; All-Ericsson, C.; Cahlin, C.; Elander, N.; Helgadottir, H.; Kiilgaard, J.F.; Kinhult, S.; Ljuslinder, I.; et al. Isolated hepatic perfusion as a treatment for uveal melanoma liver metastases, first results from a phase III randomized controlled multicenter trial (the SCANDIUM trial). *J. Clin. Oncol.* **2022**, LBA9509. [CrossRef]
23. Zager, J.S.; Orloff, M.M.; Ferrucci, P.F.; Glazer, E.S.; Ejaz, A.; Richtig, E.; Ochsenreither, S.; Lowe, M.C.; Reddy, S.A.; Beasley, G.; et al. FOCUS phase 3 trial results: Percutaneous hepatic perfusion (PHP) with melphalan for patients with ocular melanoma liver metastases (PHP-OCM-301/301A). *J. Clin. Oncol.* **2022**, 9510. [CrossRef]
24. Ny, L.; Jespersen, H.; Karlsson, J.; Alsén, S.; Filges, S.; All-Eriksson, C.; Andersson, B.; Carneiro, A.; Helgadottir, H.; Levin, M.; et al. The PEMDAC phase 2 study of pembrolizumab and entinostat in patients with metastatic uveal melanoma. *Nat. Commun.* **2021**, *12*, 1–10. [CrossRef]
25. Chandran, S.S.; Somerville, R.P.T.; Yang, J.C.; Sherry, R.M.; Klebanoff, C.A.; Goff, S.L.; Wunderlich, J.R.; Danforth, D.N.; Zlott, D.; Paria, B.C.; et al. Treatment of metastatic uveal melanoma with adoptive transfer of tumour-infiltrating lymphocytes: A single-centre, two-stage, single-arm, phase 2 study. *Lancet Oncol.* **2017**, *18*, 792–802. [CrossRef]
26. Middleton, M.R.; McAlpine, C.; Woodcock, V.K.; Corrie, P.; Infante, J.R.; Steven, N.M.; Evans, T.R.J.; Anthoney, A.; Shoushtari, A.N.; Hamid, O.; et al. Tebentafusp, a TCR/anti-CD3 bispecific fusion protein targeting gp100, potently activated anti-tumor immune responses in patients with metastatic melanoma. *Clin. Cancer Res.* **2020**, *26*, 5869–5878. [CrossRef]
27. Nathan, P.; Hassel, J.C.; Rutkowski, P.; Baurain, J.-F.; Butler, M.O.; Schlaak, M.; Sullivan, R.J.; Ochsenreither, S.; Dummer, R.; Kirkwood, J.M.; et al. Overall Survival Benefit with Tebentafusp in Metastatic Uveal Melanoma. *N. Engl. J. Med.* **2021**, *385*, 1196–1206. [CrossRef]
28. Olivier, T.; Prasad, V. Tebentafusp in first-line melanoma trials: An outperforming outlier. *Transl. Oncol.* **2022**, *20*, 101408. [CrossRef]
29. Slingluff, C.L.; Colella, T.A.; Thompson, L.; Graham, D.D.; Skipper, J.C.; Caldwell, J.; Brinckerhoff, L.; Kittlesen, D.J.; Deacon, D.H.; Oei, C.; et al. Melanomas with concordant loss of multiple melanocytic differentiation proteins: Immune escape that may be overcome by targeting unique or undefined antigens. *Cancer Immunol. Immunother.* **2000**, *48*, 661–672. [CrossRef]
30. Drake, C.G.; Jaffee, E.; Pardoll, D.M. Mechanisms of Immune Evasion by Tumors. *Adv Immunol.* **2006**, *90*, 51–81.
31. Maude, S.L.; Laetsch, T.W.; Buechner, J.; Rives, S.; Boyer, M.; Bittencourt, H.; Bader, P.; Verneris, M.R.; Stefanski, H.E.; Myers, G.D.; et al. Tisagenlecleucel in Children and Young Adults with B-Cell Lymphoblastic Leukemia. *N. Engl. J. Med.* **2018**, *378*, 439–448. [CrossRef] [PubMed]
32. Majzner, R.G.; Mackall, C.L. Clinical lessons learned from the first leg of the CAR T cell journey. *Nat. Med.* **2019**, *25*, 1341–1355. [CrossRef]
33. Aparicio, S.; Hidalgo, M.; Kung, A. Examining the utility of patient-derived xenograft mouse models. *Nat. Rev. Cancer* **2015**, *15*, 311–316. [CrossRef] [PubMed]
34. Paoloni, M.; Khanna, C. Translation of new cancer treatments from pet dogs to humans. *Nat. Rev. Cancer* **2008**, *8*, 147–156. [CrossRef]
35. Bonnett, B.N.; Egenvall, A.; Hedhammar, A.; Olson, P. Mortality in over 350,000 insured Swedish dogs from 1995-2000: I. Breed-, gender-, age- and cause-specific rates. *Acta Veter Scand.* **2005**, *46*, 105–120. [CrossRef]
36. Gordon, I.; Paoloni, M.; Mazcko, C.; Khanna, C. The Comparative Oncology Trials Consortium: Using Spontaneously Occurring Cancers in Dogs to Inform the Cancer Drug Development Pathway. *PLOS Med.* **2009**, *6*, e1000161. [CrossRef]
37. Pazzi, P.; Steenkamp, G.; Rixon, A.J. Treatment of Canine Oral Melanomas: A Critical Review of the Literature. *Vet. Sci.* **2022**, *9*, 196. [CrossRef] [PubMed]
38. Wong, K.; van der Weyden, L.; Schott, C.R.; Foote, A.; Constantino-Casas, F.; Smith, S.; Dobson, J.M.; Murchison, E.P.; Wu, H.; Yeh, I.; et al. Cross-species genomic landscape comparison of human mucosal melanoma with canine oral and equine melanoma. *Nat. Commun.* **2019**, *10*, 353. [CrossRef]
39. Prouteau, A. Canine Melanomas as Models for Human Melanomas: Clinical, Histological, and Genetic Comparison. *Genes* **2019**, *10*, 501. [CrossRef]
40. Forsberg, E.; Lindberg, M.F.; Jespersen, H.; Alsén, S.; Bagge, R.O.; Donia, M.; Svane, I.M.; Nilsson, O.; Ny, L.; Nilsson, L.M.; et al. HER2 CAR-T Cells Eradicate Uveal Melanoma and T-cell Therapy-Resistant Human Melanoma in IL2 Transgenic NOD/SCID IL2 Receptor Knockout Mice. *Cancer Res.* **2019**, *79*, 899–904. [CrossRef]
41. Dudley, M.E.; Wunderlich, J.R.; Robbins, P.F.; Yang, J.C.; Hwu, P.; Schwartzentruber, D.J.; Topalian, S.L.; Sherry, R.; Restifo, N.P.; Hubicki, A.M.; et al. Cancer regression and autoimmunity in patients after clonal repopulation with antitumor lymphocytes. *Science* **2002**, *298*, 850–854. [CrossRef]

42. Jespersen, H.; Lindberg, M.F.; Donia, M.; Söderberg, E.M.V.; Andersen, R.; Keller, U.; Ny, L.; Svane, I.M.; Nilsson, L.M.; Nilsson, J.A. Clinical responses to adoptive T-cell transfer can be modeled in an autologous immune-humanized mouse model. *Nat. Commun.* **2017**, *8*, 707. [CrossRef]
43. Einarsdottir, B.O.; Bagge, R.O.; Bhadury, J.; Jespersen, H.; Mattsson, J.; Nilsson, L.M.; Truvé, K.; López, M.D.; Naredi, P.; Nilsson, O.; et al. Melanoma patient-derived xenografts accurately model the disease and develop fast enough to guide treatment decisions. *Oncotarget* **2014**, *5*, 9609–9618. [CrossRef]
44. Karlsson, J.; Nilsson, L.M.; Mitra, S.; Alsén, S.; Shelke, G.V.; Sah, V.R.; Forsberg, E.M.V.; Stierner, U.; All-Eriksson, C.; Einarsdottir, B.; et al. Molecular profiling of driver events in metastatic uveal melanoma. *Nat. Commun.* **2020**, *11*, 1894. [CrossRef]
45. Nguyen, S.M.; Thamm, D.; Vail, D.M.; London, C.A. Response evaluation criteria for solid tumours in dogs (v1.0): A Veterinary Cooperative Oncology Group (VCOG) consensus document. *Vet. Comp. Oncol.* **2013**, *13*, 176–183. [CrossRef]
46. LeBlanc, A.K.; Atherton, M.; Bentley, R.T.; Boudreau, C.E.; Burton, J.H.; Curran, K.M.; Dow, S.; Giuffrida, M.A.; Kellihan, H.B.; Mason, N.J.; et al. Veterinary Cooperative Oncology Group—Common Terminology Criteria for Adverse Events (VCOG-CTCAE v2) following investigational therapy in dogs and cats. *Vet. Comp. Oncol.* **2021**, *19*, 311–352.
47. Butler, A.; Hoffman, P.; Smibert, P.; Papalexi, E.; Satija, R. Integrating single-cell transcriptomic data across different conditions, technologies, and species. *Nat. Biotechnol.* **2018**, *36*, 411–420. [CrossRef]
48. Dobin, A.; Davis, C.A.; Schlesinger, F.; Drenkow, J.; Zaleski, C.; Jha, S.; Batut, P.; Chaisson, M.; Gingeras, T.R. STAR: Ultrafast universal RNA-seq aligner. *Bioinformatics* **2013**, *29*, 15–21. [CrossRef]
49. Anders, S.; Pyl, P.T.; Huber, W. HTSeq—A Python framework to work with high-throughput sequencing data. *Bioinformatics* **2015**, *31*, 166–169. [CrossRef]
50. Bagge, R.O.; Demir, A.; Karlsson, J.; Alaei-Mahabadi, B.; Einarsdottir, B.O.; Jespersen, H.; Lindberg, M.F.; Muth, A.; Nilsson, L.M.; Persson, M.; et al. Mutational Signature and Transcriptomic Classification Analyses as the Decisive Diagnostic Tools for a Cancer of Unknown Primary. *JCO Precis. Oncol.* **2018**, *2*, 1–25. [CrossRef]
51. Mills, J.K.; Henderson, M.A.; Giuffrida, L.; Petrone, P.; Westwood, J.A.; Darcy, P.K.; Neeson, P.J.; Kershaw, M.H.; Gyorki, D.E. Generating CAR T cells from tumor-infiltrating lymphocytes. *Ther. Adv. Vaccines Immunother.* **2021**, *9*, 25151355211017119. [CrossRef] [PubMed]
52. Sharpless, N.E.; DePinho, R. The mighty mouse: Genetically engineered mouse models in cancer drug development. *Nat. Rev. Drug Discov.* **2006**, *5*, 741–754. [CrossRef] [PubMed]
53. Morgan, R.A.; Yang, J.C.; Kitano, M.; E Dudley, M.; Laurencot, C.M. A Rosenberg. Case Report of a Serious Adverse Event Following the Administration of T Cells Transduced with a Chimeric Antigen Receptor Recognizing ERBB2. *Mol. Ther.* **2010**, *18*, 843–851. [CrossRef] [PubMed]
54. Macdonald, D.; Gordon, A.A.; Kajitani, H.; Enokihara, H.; Barrett, A.J. Interleukin-2 treatment-associated eosinophilia is mediated by interleukin-5 production. *Br. J. Haematol.* **1990**, *76*, 168–173. [CrossRef] [PubMed]

Disclaimer/Publisher's Note: The statements, opinions and data contained in all publications are solely those of the individual author(s) and contributor(s) and not of MDPI and/or the editor(s). MDPI and/or the editor(s) disclaim responsibility for any injury to people or property resulting from any ideas, methods, instructions or products referred to in the content.

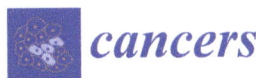

Article

Humoral Responses to Repetitive Doses of COVID-19 mRNA Vaccines in Patients with CAR-T-Cell Therapy

Simona Gössi [1], Ulrike Bacher [2], Claudia Haslebacher [1], Michael Nagler [3], Franziska Suter [4], Cornelia Staehelin [5], Urban Novak [1] and Thomas Pabst [1,*]

1. Department of Medical Oncology, Inselspital, Bern University Hospital, 3010 Bern, Switzerland; simona.goessi@students.unibe.ch (S.G.); claudia.haslebacher@insel.ch (C.H.); urban.novak@insel.ch (U.N.)
2. Department of Hematology, Inselspital, Bern University Hospital, 3010 Bern, Switzerland; veraulrike.bacher@insel.ch
3. University Institute of Clinical Chemistry (UKC), Inselspital, Bern University Hospital, 3010 Bern, Switzerland; michael.nagler@insel.ch
4. Institute for Infectious Diseases (IFIK), Inselspital, University of Bern, 3010 Bern, Switzerland; franziska.suter@ifik.unibe.ch
5. Department of Infectiology, Inselspital, University of Bern, 3010 Bern, Switzerland; cornelia.staehelin@insel.ch
* Correspondence: thomas.pabst@insel.ch; Tel.: +41-31-632-8430; Fax: +41-31-632-3410

Simple Summary: Data on the efficacy of SARS-CoV-2 mRNA vaccinations in patients with CAR-T-cell therapy is very limited. We analyzed patients (predominantly DLBCL) undergoing CAR-T-cell therapy and receiving BNT162b2 (Pfizer-BioNTech) or mRNA-1273 (Moderna) vaccination. This single center retrospective analysis aimed to evaluate the number of B-cells and CAR-T-cell copies as prognostic factors of humoral antibody test results as well as the effects of a third and fourth dose on humoral antibody response. Our results demonstrate that patients with more B-cells and fewer CAR-T-cells at vaccination were more likely to produce a positive antibody test result. Overall, we found very poor humoral antibody responses, while additional doses increased rates of seroconversion and antibody titers.

Abstract: *Background*: Due to B-cell aplasia following CAR-T-cell therapy, patients are at risk of severe SARS-CoV-2 course. *Methods*: COVID-19 vaccines were assessed by IgG antibody tests against SARS-CoV-2 spike protein (anti-S1/S2). Vaccination procedures: group (1): CAR-T-cells followed by two to four vaccine doses; group (2): Two vaccine doses prior to CAR-T-cells, followed by doses 3 or 4. *Results*: In group 1 (n = 32), 7/30 patients (23.2%) had positive antibody tests after a second dose, 9/23 (39.1%) after a third dose, and 3/3 patients after a fourth dose. A third dose led to seroconversion in 5 of 21 patients (23.8%) with available data, while a fourth dose did so in 2/3 patients. Higher B-cells (AUC: 96.2%, CI: 89–100, p = 0.0006) and lower CAR-T-cell copies (AUC: 77.3%, CI: 57–97, p = 0.0438) were predictive of positive humoral vaccine response. In group 2 (n = 14), 6/14 patients (42.9%) had a positive antibody test after a second dose, 3/8 patients (37.5%) after a third dose, and 3/4 patients after a fourth dose. A third dose led to seroconversion in 1/8 patients (12.5%), while a fourth dose did so in 3/4 patients. *Conclusion*: Additional vaccine doses increased seroconversion rates whilst high B-cell counts and low CAR-T-cell copy numbers were associated with positive antibody response.

Keywords: CAR-T-cell therapy; mRNA COVID-19 vaccines; humoral antibody responses; diffuse large B-cell lymphoma (DLBCL)

Citation: Gössi, S.; Bacher, U.; Haslebacher, C.; Nagler, M.; Suter, F.; Staehelin, C.; Novak, U.; Pabst, T. Humoral Responses to Repetitive Doses of COVID-19 mRNA Vaccines in Patients with CAR-T-Cell Therapy. *Cancers* 2022, 14, 3527. https://doi.org/10.3390/cancers14143527

Academic Editor: Vita Golubovskaya

Received: 2 June 2022
Accepted: 20 July 2022
Published: 20 July 2022

Publisher's Note: MDPI stays neutral with regard to jurisdictional claims in published maps and institutional affiliations.

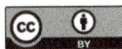

Copyright: © 2022 by the authors. Licensee MDPI, Basel, Switzerland. This article is an open access article distributed under the terms and conditions of the Creative Commons Attribution (CC BY) license (https://creativecommons.org/licenses/by/4.0/).

1. Introduction

CAR-T-cell therapy is a highly promising therapeutic option in the treatment of advanced lymphoproliferative neoplasms such as diffuse large B-cell lymphoma (DLBCL), acute lymphatic leukemia (ALL), and mantle cell lymphoma [1–4]. CD19-directed

CAR-T-cells have an impact on malignant B-cell tissues as well as the healthy B-cell compartment and thus lead to B-cell depletion and hypogammaglobulinemia [5,6]. Frequent complications are Cytokine release syndrome (CRS) in more than 60% and CAR-T-Related Encephalopathy Syndrome (CRES) in more than 30% of the patients, according to the literature [7]. Increased serum IL-6 levels and clinical CRS symptoms can contribute to the indication of therapeutic interventions [8]. Tocilizumab should be administered to patients with CRS, while corticosteroids are used in patients with CRES and CRS not responsive to tocilizumab [6].

Patients with CAR-T-cell therapy suffer from severe immunosuppression and thus are particularly vulnerable to infectious diseases, such as COVID-19. This is due to the prolonged cytopenias with B-cell aplasia and hypogammaglobulinemia caused by CAR-T-cell therapy. Also, treatment of CAR-T-cell complications with tocilizumab and steroids has been shown to further increase these patients' vulnerability [9]. Spanjaart et al. have found that patients diagnosed with a COVID-19 infection after B-cell targeted CAR-T-cell therapy have a COVID-19 attributable mortality rate of 41%. Therefore, in the context of the COVID-19 pandemic, it is crucial to protect the patients undergoing CAR-T-cell therapy with an effective vaccination against COVID-19. The mRNA-COVID-19 vaccines of Pfizer/BioNTech Comirnaty (BNT162b2) and Moderna (mRNA-1273) were approved by the European Medicines Agency and are widely used [10]. The European Society for Blood and Marrow Transplantation (EBMT) recommends maintaining a period of 6 months between CAR-T-cell therapy and vaccination, due to delayed B-cell reconstitution. After this interval, three doses are recommended as a primary series, at 4 week intervals [11]. However, data on the efficacy of the vaccinations for CAR-T-cell patients are sparse.

Dhakal et al. have reported a seropositivity rate of only 21% (3/14 patients) after two doses of the mRNA vaccine in patients with CAR-T-cell therapy [12]. Similarly low percentages have been reported by Ram et al. with a positive serology of 36% (5/14 patients) in patients after CAR-T-cell therapy and two doses of the BNT162b2 mRNA COVID-19 vaccine [13]. However, the efficacy of a third dose in patients with CAR-T-cell therapy has yet to be examined. A small study identified patients who had no humoral response after two vaccine doses and eventually achieved a positive serology after a third vaccine dose in 40% (4/10 patients) of patients post allogeneic HCT and in 17% (1/6 patients) post CAR-T-cell therapy [14]. Currently, there is no data on the efficacy of a fourth dose of a COVID-19 vaccine in patients with CAR-T-cell therapy. Additionally, patients vaccinated before CAR-T-cell therapy face another problem, as the therapy procedures often wipe out all immune memory of other vaccines. It is therefore recommended by the EBMT to re-vaccinate these individuals as if they had never received a COVID-19 vaccine [11]. This recommendation is based on evidence from other vaccines, where revaccination after CAR-T-cell therapy is also recommended [15].

There are still many open questions regarding optimal timing of vaccination after CAR-T-cell therapy as well as the efficacy of different amounts of vaccine doses. In addition, re-vaccination strategies of patients with vaccination prior to CAR-T-cell therapy have yet to be clarified. This analysis attempted to provide further details to this limited data, analyzing humoral antibody responses to COVID-19 vaccines in CAR-T-cell therapy patients. In this real-world retrospective approach, we studied two consecutive cohorts: (A) patients who received two to four doses of the vaccine after CAR-T-cell therapy since vaccination was simply not yet available at CAR-T treatment, and (B) patients with two doses before CAR-T-cell therapy and subsequent re-vaccination after CAR-T treatment. Finally, the impacts of B-cell and CAR-T-cell levels in patients' peripheral blood were assessed at the time of the first vaccination as well as the relevance of the interval between CAR-T-cell infusion and subsequent vaccination.

2. Materials and Methods

2.1. Methods

We conducted a retrospective single-center study at the University Hospital Inselspital, Bern, Switzerland. Patients (predominantly DLBCL, mantle cell lymphoma, B-ALL) undergoing CAR-T-cell therapy between January 2019 and December 2021 were analyzed. They received two to four doses of COVID-19 mRNA vaccines between January 2021 and February 2022. We assessed the COVID-19 vaccines using IgG antibodies against SARS-CoV-2 spike protein (anti-S1/S2) (Clia Diasorin; cut-off > 12 AU/mL for minimal positive results and cut-off > 100 AU/mL for clear positive results). IgG antibody test results were compared after the second, third, and fourth dose of the mRNA COVID-19 vaccine. In patients with CAR-T-cell therapy before vaccination, the number of B-cells and CAR-T-cells in peripheral blood at the time of first vaccination and the interval between CAR-T-cell infusion and first vaccination were analyzed. Additionally, we analyzed the effect of age at the time of vaccination on the antibody response to control for any bias due to the substantial age range in our cohort. The purpose of this analysis was to assess the possible influence of these parameters related to CAR-T-cell therapy before vaccination on the results of the IgG antibody test. The infection rate of the patients is based on medical history and anamnesis. Data on eventual COVID-19 PCR test results were not available for this analysis.

2.2. Patients

Patients received vaccinations depending on availability of the vaccines throughout the evolution of the pandemic, as well as the treating decisions of the attending physicians. Retrospectively, we analyzed the vaccination procedure. To this end, we divided the patients retrospectively into two groups depending on their vaccination status prior to CAR-T-cell therapy. This allowed a more differentiated analysis of the data in these two different vaccination settings. In group 1, which will be called "CAR-T before VAC", vaccines were not yet available before the CAR-T-cell therapy. The procedure in these patients was as follows: Administration of CAR-T-cell therapy followed by either two, three, or four doses of the COVID-19 vaccine. In group 2, which will be called "CAR-T after VAC", the procedure was as follows: Administration of two doses of COVID-19 vaccines, followed by CAR-T-cell therapy, and then re-vaccination with doses 3 or 4 of the COVID-19 vaccine. Figure 1 is an illustration of these vaccination procedures. Informed consent was obtained from all subjects involved in the study.

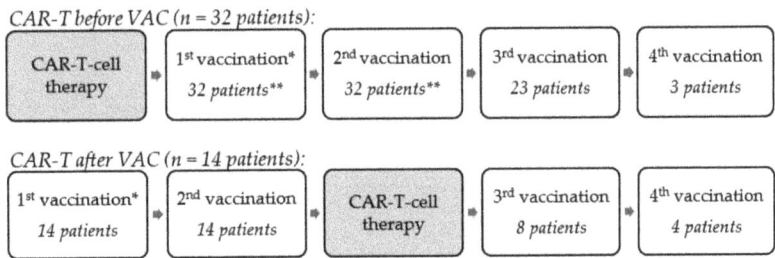

Figure 1. Illustration of vaccination procedures. * No antibody determination after the 1st vaccination. ** In the group "CAR-T before VAC", 32 patients had a 1st and 2nd vaccination, but data on antibody determination after 2nd vaccination were only available for 30 patients.

2.3. Laboratory Analysis

2.3.1. Antibody Determination

The quantitative analysis of anti-S1 and anti-S2 IgG against SARS-CoV-2 in human serum was based on an indirect chemiluminescence immuno assay (CLIA).

In the first step, human serum is incubated with recombinant S1- and S2-coated magnetic beads. Anti-SARS-CoV-2 IgG antibodies present in human serum bind to S1 and S2 antigens. Unbound antibodies are removed by washing cycles. In the second step, isoluminol-conjugated mouse anti-human antibodies are added to bind immobilized anti-SARS-CoV-2 IgG captured in the solid phase. Unbound isoluminol-conjugated antibodies are removed by washing cycles. In the last step, starter reagents are added to evoke a chemiluminescence light reaction. Luminescence is measured in relative light units (RLU) and converted to antibody concentrations in arbitrary units per milliliter (AU/mL) by the automated immunoassay analyzer Liaison® XL by DiaSorin, Saluggia, Italy. CLIA is very similar to an ELISA. The difference is that in an ELISA, the readout is based on a colorimetric reaction and subsequent quantification by absorption, whereas in a CLIA, the readout is based on measuring luminescence signal. Sensitivity of the assay was as follows: ≤5 days: 25% (14.6–39.4%); 5–15 days: 90.4% (79.4–95.8%); and >15 days: 97.4% (86.8–99.5%). The specificity of the assay was 98.9 % (94.0–99.8 %). Of note, in this assay, it is not possible to distinguish between anti-S1 and anti-S2 IgG. RBD is part of the S1 subunit of the SARS-CoV-2 spike protein; therefore, binding to RBD is also considered. Meanwhile, there are tests commercially available specifically targeting RBD alone or the whole trimer of the spike protein.

2.3.2. B-Cells

B-cells were measured by multiparameter flow cytometry using the TBNK Multitest kit (including CD4/CD8, CD19, CD16+/CD56+) on the Lyrics platform (kit and platform, both from BD Biosciences, Allschwil, Switzerland). For absolute cell count measurement, this system includes tubes with a defined number of fluorescent Latex beads ("TruCOUNT"). Alternatively, for some samples, we used the BD OneFlowTM Lymphoid Screening Tube (LST), which includes mature lymphocyte populations of B, T, and NK lineages (including the B-cell antigens CD19, CD20, skappa/slambda) (previously Cytognos, now also BD Biosciences, Allschwil, Switzerland). SARS-CoV-2 specific memory B-cells had not been determined in these patients, as B-cells were only analyzed before vaccination.

2.4. Statistical Analyses

For the statistical analyses, we used GraphPad Prism and we performed One-Way ANOVA in a mixed effect model with a follow-up Tukey test for the comparison of the IgG antibody test results. For the analysis of prognostic parameters, we used simple logistic regression.

3. Results

3.1. Clinical Characteristics of the Patients

The clinical characteristics of the 46 patients are presented in Table 1. Median age of patients at time of diagnosis was 58.5 years, and the male/female ratio was 1.6. The initial diagnosis was de novo DLBCL (52%; 24/46), transformed DLBCL (24%; 11/46), mantle cell lymphoma (15%; 7/46), and B-ALL (9%; 4/46). Previous autologous stem cell transplantation before CAR-T-cell therapy had been conducted in 21 patients (46%) and allogeneic stem cell transplantation before CAR-T-cell therapy in 1 patient (2%). The median age at the time of CAR-T-cell therapy was 64 years. A total of 25 patients had the CAR-T-cell therapy tisagenlecleucel (61%; 28/46), 10 patients had axicabtagene ciloleucel (22%; 10/46), and 8 patients had brexucabtagen autoleucel (17%; 8/46). A total of 30 patients suffered from a Cytokine release syndrome (grade I–III) (65%; 30/46), while 12 patients suffered from a CAR-T-Related Encephalopathy Syndrome (grade I-IV) (26%; 12/46). A total of 21 patients were treated with Tocilizumab (46%; 21/46), and 16 with steroids (35%; 16/46). A total of 10 patients had a relapse after CAR-T-cell therapy (22%; 10/46), and 3 patients died during the follow-up of this study (7%; 3/46).

Table 1. Clinical characteristics of the patients.

Parameter	Total (46 Patients)
Demographic characteristics	
Males: females (ratio)	28:18 (1.6)
Median age at the time of diagnosis (range)	58.5 (17–78)
Initial diagnosis	
Primary (de novo) DLBCL	24 (52%)
Secondary/transformed DLBCL	11 (24%)
Mantle cell lymphoma	7 (15%)
B-ALL	4 (9%)
Previous hematopoietic SCT before CAR-T-cell therapy	
Autologous SCT	21 (46%)
Allogeneic SCT	1 (2%)
Median age at the time of CAR-T-cell therapy (range)	64 (18–80)
CAR-T-cell-therapy type	
tisagenlecleucel	28 (61%)
axicabtagene ciloleucel	10 (22%)
brexucabtagen autoleucel	8 (17%)
Clinical course after CAR-T-cell therapy	
CRS	30 (65%)
CRES	12 (26%)
Tocilizumab therapy	21 (46%)
Steroid therapy	16 (35%)
Relapse after CAR-T-cell therapy	10 (22%)
Death	3 (7%)

DLBCL—diffuse large B-cell lymphoma; B-ALL—B-cell acute lymphoblastic leukemia; SCT—hematopoietic stem-cell transplantation; CAR-T—chimeric antigen receptor T-cell; CRS—Cytokine release syndrome; CRES—CAR-T-related Encephalopathy Syndrome.

3.2. Vaccination Procedures

Retrospectively, we assessed the effectivity of the vaccinations of the CAR-T-cell patients. Overall, we identified two vaccination procedures. The retrospective distribution of patients into two groups is illustrated in Figure 1. We observed 32 patients with their CAR-T-cell therapy before a COVID-19 vaccination ("CAR-T before VAC"). In total, 32 patients were identified with two vaccinations after the CAR-T-cell therapy (but only 30 patients with an antibody test result after second vaccination, as in two patients, data was not available due to the retrospective data collection). In total, 23 of these patients also received a third vaccination and 3 patients a fourth vaccination. Finally, we identified 14 patients with their CAR-T-cell therapy after a COVID-19 vaccination ("CAR-T after VAC"). In total, 14 patients were identified with two vaccinations before the CAR-T-cell therapy; we found that 8 of these patients received a third dose after the CAR-T-cell therapy, and 4 patients received a fourth dose.

3.3. Parameters Concerning Vaccination

Table 2 shows all the parameters concerning vaccination. The first vaccine in 33 patients (72%; 33/46) was Moderna (mRNA-1273), while 13 patients (28%; 13/46) were administered the vaccine of Pfizer/BioNTech (BNT162b2). All patients, except for one, had the same vaccine for all following doses. Only one patient had the first two doses with Moderna and received the third booster dose with Pfizer/BioNTech. The remission status at the time of first vaccination was complete remission (46%; 21/46), partial remission (11%; 5/46), progressive disease (28%; 13/46), and not evaluated (15%; 7/46).

Table 2. Parameters concerning vaccination.

Parameter	Total [46 Patients]	CAR-T before VAC [32 Patients]	CAR-T after VAC [14 Patients]
Vaccine			
Moderna (mRNA-1273)	33 (72%)	22 (69%)	11 (78.6%)
Pfizer/BioNTech (BNT162b2)	13 (28%)	10 (31%)	3 (21.4%)
Remission Status at time of 1st vaccination			
CR	21 (46%)	21 (65.6%)	0 (0%)
PR	5 (11%)	4 (12.5%)	1 (7.1%)
SD	0 (0%)	0 (0%)	0 (0%)
PD	13 (28%)	3 (9.4%)	10 (71.4%)
NE	7 (15%)	4 (12.5%)	3 (21.4%)
Median interval between CAR-T and respective VAC in days (range)			
1st VAC (range)		286 (23–975) [32 patients]	−76 (−278; −34)) [14 patients]
2nd VAC (range)		317 (51–1003) [32 patients]	−37 (−239; −8) [14 patients]
3rd VAC (range)		531 (262–882) [23 patients]	102 (54–248) [8 patients]
4th VAC (range)		757 (610–1026) [3 patients]	274 (179–314) [4 patients]
Median interval of antibody determination after respective VAC in days (range)			
2nd VAC (range)		57 (24–203) [30 patients]	40 (5–289) [14 patients]
3rd VAC (range)		59 (14–162) [23 patients]	40 (6–90) [8 patients]
4th VAC (range)		48 (47–59) [3 patients]	59 (23–64) [4 patients]

CR—complete remission; PR—partial remission; SD—stable disease; PD—progressive disease; NE—not evaluated; CAR-T—chimeric antigen receptor T-cell therapy; VAC—vaccination.

In total, 32 patients with the "CAR-T before VAC" procedure were identified. The median time between CAR-T-cell therapy and the first vaccination was 286 days, while the median time between CAR-T-cell therapy and second vaccination was 317 days. The median time between second vaccination and antibody determination was 57 days.

In total, 14 patients with the "CAR-T after VAC" vaccination procedure were identified. The first vaccination had a median of 76 days and the second vaccination had a median of 37 days before CAR-T-cell therapy. The median time between second vaccination and antibody determination was 40 days. The third vaccination took place a median of 102 days after CAR-T-cell therapy.

3.4. Humoral Antibody Responses

3.4.1. CAR-T before VAC (n = 32 Patients)

The humoral antibody titers after second, third, and fourth vaccination in patients with CAR-T-cell therapy before vaccination are illustrated in Table 3. In patients with the procedure "CAR-T before VAC", we identified 32 patients who received at least two doses of the COVID-19 vaccination after their CAR-T-cell therapy. Two patients received no antibody determination after two vaccine doses. Negative antibodies were found in 23 patients (76.7%; 23/30), while 7 patients (23.3%; 7/30) had positive humoral antibody responses, among whom 5 patients (16.6%; 5/30) had clear positive antibody titers > 100 AU/mL.

Table 3. Outcome of humoral antibody determinations after CAR-T-cell therapy and COVID-19 mRNA vaccine in patients with "CAR-T before VAC".

	CAR-T before VAC (32 Patients): Anti-Spike Protein IgG Antibodies (AU/mL)		
	after 2nd VAC (30 Patients)	after 3rd VAC (23 Patients)	after 4th VAC (3 Patients)
	Results after 2 doses (no 3rd or 4th vaccination)		
Pat. 1–8	<12	x	x
Pat. 9	143	x	x
	Results after 3 doses (no data on 2nd dose and no 4th vaccination)		
Pat 10–11	x	<12	x
	Results after 2 and 3 doses (no 4th vaccination)		
Pat. 12–20	<12	<12	x
Pat. 21	<12	12.2	x
Pat. 22	<12	28.5	x
Pat. 23	<12	43.5	x
Pat. 24	<12	110	x
Pat. 25	<12	138	x
Pat. 26	17.2	20.2	x
Pat. 27	106	400	x
Pat. 28	129	<12	x
Pat. 29	152	>400	x
	Results after 2, 3, and 4 doses		
Pat. 30	<12	<12	24.3
Pat. 31	26.3	<12	22.1
Pat. 32	190	>400	302

All results are in AU/mL; <12 AU/mL: negative anti-spike protein IgG antibody test result; >12 AU/mL: positive anti-spike protein IgG antibody test result; >100 AU/mL: clear positive result; VAC—vaccination; x—no data available.

Furthermore, in 23 patients, data were available after a third dose of the COVID-19 vaccination after their CAR-T-cell therapy. Negative antibodies were found in 14 patients (60.8%; 14/23), while 9 patients (39.1%; 9/23) had positive humoral antibody responses (only 5 patients (21.7%; 5/23) with clear positive antibody titers > 100 AU/mL). In 21 of these patients, data were available after both the second and third dose of the vaccination. In total, 10 patients (47.6%; 10/21) stayed negative after the second and third dose, while in 5 patients (23.8%; 5/21), a negative result after the second vaccine could be turned into a positive result after the third dose (2 patients (9.5%; 2/21) with a clear positive result after third vaccination). Six patients (28.6%; 6/21) already had a positive test result after two doses, which increased due to third vaccination in four patients (19%; 4/21).

Finally, in three patients, data were available after a fourth vaccination after their CAR-T-cell therapy. All three patients evaluated with four vaccine doses had positive humoral antibody responses (only 1pt. (1/3) with clear positive antibody titers > 100 AU/mL). Two patients seroconverted after the fourth vaccination, while 1pt. stayed clear positive after the third and fourth vaccination.

3.4.2. CAR-T after VAC (14 Patients)

The humoral antibody titers after second, third, and fourth vaccination in patients with CAR-T-cell therapy after vaccination are illustrated in Table 4. In patients with the procedure

"CAR-T after VAC", there were 14 patients who received at least two doses of the COVID-19 vaccination before their CAR-T-cell therapy. Among these, eight patients had negative humoral antibody responses (57.1%; 8/14), while six patients (42.9%; 6/14) had positive humoral antibodies (only 1pt. (7.1%; 1/14) with clear positive antibody titers > 100 AU/mL).

Table 4. Outcome of humoral antibody determinations after CAR-T-cell therapy and the COVID-19 mRNA vaccine in patients with "CAR-T after VAC".

	CAR-T after VAC (14 Patients): Anti-Spike Protein IgG Antibodies (AU/mL)		
	after 2nd VAC (14 Patients)	after 3rd VAC (8 Patients)	after 4th VAC (4 Patients)
Results after 2 doses (no 3rd and 4th vacciantion)			
Pat. 1–3	<12	x	x
Pat. 4	80.2	x	x
Pat. 5	87	x	x
Pat. 6	>400	x	x
Results after 2 and 3 doses (no 4th vaccination)			
Pat. 7–8	<12	<12	x
Pat. 9	<12	47.6	x
Pat. 10	90.01	321	x
Results after 2, 3, and 4 doses			
Pat. 11	<12	<12	<12
Pat. 12	<12	<12	346
Pat. 13	25.5	42.9	30.4
Pat. 14	99.2	<12	400

All results are in AU/mL; <12 AU/mL: negative anti-spike protein IgG antibody test result; >12 AU/mL: positive anti-spike protein IgG antibody test result; >100 AU/mL: clear positive result; VAC—vaccination; x—no data available.

Of these patients, eight received a third dose of the COVID-19 vaccination after their CAR-T-cell therapy. Negative antibodies were found in five patients (62.5%; 5/8), while three patients (37.5%; 3/8) had positive humoral antibody responses (only 1pt. (12.5%; 1/8) with clear positive antibody titers > 100 AU/mL). In all of these eight patients, data were available after the second and third doses of the vaccination. Four patients (50%; 4/8) remained negative after the second and third dose, while 1 pt. (12.5%; 1/8) seroconverted after the third dose. Three patients (37.5%; 3/8) already had a positive test result after two doses, and this increased due to a third vaccination in two patients (25%; 2/8).

Finally, four patients received a fourth dose of the vaccination after their CAR-T-cell therapy. Negative antibodies were found in one patient (1/4), while three patients (3/4) had positive humoral antibody responses (only two patients (2/4) with clear positive antibody titers > 100 AU/mL). In three patients (3/4), we noted seroconversion after the fourth vaccination (two patients (2/4) with clear positive results after the fourth vaccination), while one patient (1/4) stayed negative after the third and fourth vaccinations.

3.5. Anti-Spike Protein IgG Antibody Titers

Due to our small sample size, we found distinct differences in the point estimates (mean differences of titer levels between specific vaccinations), but none of these showed statistical significance.

3.5.1. CAR-T before VAC (32 Patients)

In patients with "CAR-T before VAC", the third dose of the COVID-19 vaccination in comparison with the second dose led to an increase from 34.65 AU/mL to 74.8 AU/mL (mean diff. 40.15 AU/mL; SE of diff. 19.33; $p = 0.1202$). The fourth dose in comparison to the third dose led to an increase from 74.8 AU/mL to 116.1 AU/mL (mean diff. 41.3 AU/mL; SE of diff. 44.72 AU/mL; $p = 0.6804$). Comparing the second to the fourth dose of the vaccination, there was an increase from 34.65 AU/mL to 116.1 AU/mL (mean diff. 81.48; SE of diff. 34.6 AU/mL; $p = 0.2475$).

In Figure 2a, we illustrate IgG antibody titers after second ($n = 30$ patients), third ($n = 23$ patients), and fourth ($n = 3$ patients) vaccination in patients with CAR-T-cell therapy before vaccination. Each point in the columns shows data of one individual patient. We also illustrate the mean values with range after second (mean 34.65 AU/mL; range 12–190), third (mean 74.8 AU/mL; range 12–400), and fourth vaccination (mean 116.1 AU/mL; range 22.1–302). Please note that all patients with an antibody determination of <12 AU/mL are depicted at 12 AU/mL in this graph.

3.5.2. CAR-T after VAC ($n = 14$ Patients)

In patients with "CAR-T after VAC", the third dose of the COVID-19 vaccination in comparison with the second dose led to a slight decrease from 62.71 AU/mL to 58.94 AU/mL (mean diff. -3.77 AU/mL; SE of diff. 30 AU/mL; $p = 0.9913$). The fourth dose in comparison to the third dose led to an increase from 58.94 AU/mL to 197.1 AU/mL (mean diff. 138.2 AU/mL; SE of diff. 94.39 AU/mL; $p = 0.4196$). Comparing the second to the fourth dose of the vaccination, there was an increase from 62.71 to 197.1 AU/mL (mean diff. 134.4 AU/mL; SE of diff 74.05 AU/mL; $p = 0.3055$).

In Figure 2b, we illustrate IgG antibody titers after second ($n = 14$ patients), third ($n = 8$ patients), and fourth ($n = 4$ patients) vaccination in patients with CAR-T-cell therapy after vaccination. Each point in the columns shows data of one individual patient. The figure also illustrates the mean antibody levels with the corresponding ranges after second (mean 62.71 AU/mL; range 12–400), third (mean 58.94 AU/mL; range 12–321), and fourth vaccination (mean 197.1 AU/mL; range 12–400). Please note that all patients with an antibody level <12 AU/mL are depicted at 12 AU/mL in this graph.

3.6. Prognostic Factors on the Antibody Outcome (CAR-T before VAC; n = 32 Patients)

In this study, we examined the number of B-cells and CAR-T-cells at time of vaccination, the time interval between CAR-T-cell therapy and first vaccination, and the age at time of vaccination as prognostic factors on the antibody outcome.

In 28 of the 32 identified patients who received a vaccination after CAR-T-cell therapy, data regarding the amount of B-cells in the blood of the patients were available. This blood sample of B-cells was taken a median of 34 days before the first vaccination. All 21 patients with 0/uL B-cells in this blood sample at the time of the first vaccination had a negative antibody test result after the second vaccination. The more B-cells (optimal cutoff at >10/uL B-cells; PPV 85.7%; NPV 100%) in the patients' peripheral blood at the time of the first vaccination, the more likely patients were to develop a positive antibody test result after the second vaccination (area under the curve (AUC): 96.2%, CI: 89–100, $p = 0.0006$).

In 28 of the 32 identified patients who received a vaccination after CAR-T-cell therapy, data regarding the amount of CAR-T copies in the blood of the patients were available. This blood sample of CAR-T copies was taken a median of 30 days before the first vaccination. The fewer the CAR-T copies (optimal cutoff at <38/µg DNA CAR-T copies; PPV 94.7%; NPV 55.5%) in the patients' peripheral blood at the time of the first vaccination, the more likely patients were to develop a positive antibody test result after the second vaccination (area under the curve (AUC): 77.3%, CI: 57–97, $p = 0.0438$).

The influence of B-cells and CAR-T-cells at first vaccination on antibody outcome is shown in Figure 3. The distribution of B-cells and CAR-T-cell copies in patients with positive and negative antibodies is illustrated.

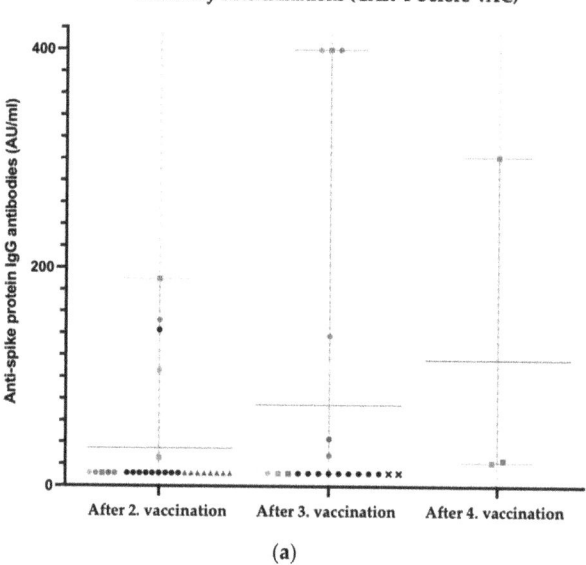

(a)

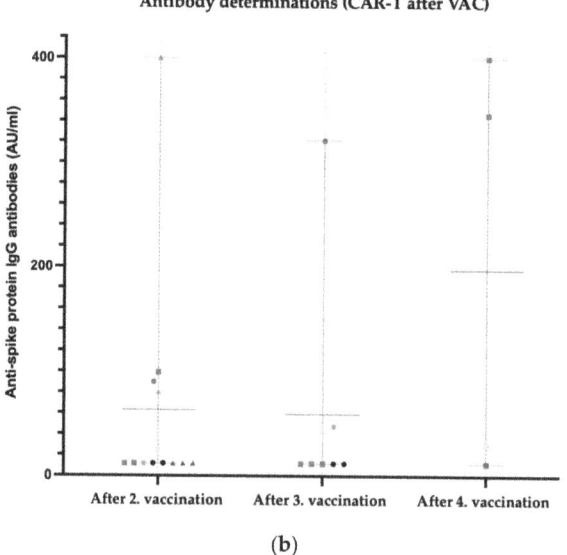

(b)

Figure 2. (a) Anti-spike protein IgG antibody titers after 2nd, 3rd, and 4th vaccination in patients with "CAR-T before VAC"; Square: In this patient, data after 2nd, 3rd, and 4th vaccination are available; Circle: in this patient, data after 2nd and 3rd vaccination are available; Triangle: in this patient, data after 2nd vaccination are available; X: in this patient, data only after third vaccination are available; eight patients had an antibody titer of <12AU/mL after 2nd vaccination (grey triangle) and nine patients had an antibody titer of <12AU/mL after 2nd and 3rd vaccination (black circle). (b) Anti-spike protein IgG antibody titers after 2nd, 3rd, and 4th vaccination in patients with "CAR-T after VAC". Square: in this patient, data after 2nd, 3rd, and 4th vaccination are available; Circle: in this patient, data after 2nd and 3rd vaccination are available; Triangle: in this patient data, after 2nd vaccination are available; three patients had an antibody titer of <12AU/mL after 2nd vaccination (grey triangle) and two patients had an antibody titer of <12AU/mL after 2nd and 3rd vaccination (black circle).

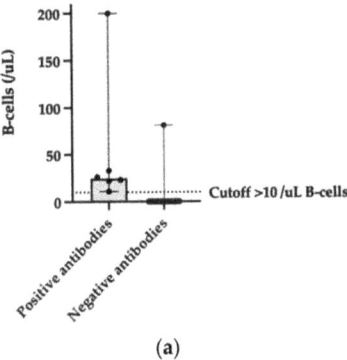

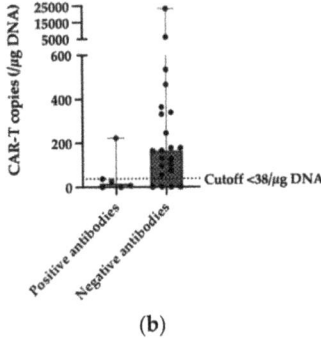

Figure 3. Scatter plot (median with range) depicting (**a**) number of B-cells at time of 1st vaccination and (**b**) number of CAR-T-cell copies at time of 1st vaccination in patients with positive anti-spike protein IgG antibody test result (>12AU/mL) compared to patients with a negative antibody test result. (**a**) n = 28 patients (21 patients with negative antibodies overlap at 0/uL B-cells); (**b**) n = 28 patients.

The time interval between CAR-T-cell therapy and first vaccination was tested as a prognostic parameter for the antibody outcome after the second vaccination. In 30 of the 32 patients with vaccination after CAR-T-cell therapy (2 patients had no antibody evaluation after second vaccination), we found no significant correlation between time interval and antibody outcome (AUC: 65.8%, CI: 41–89, p = 0.2112). The time interval between CAR-T-cell therapy and vaccination was ≤6 months in 8 patients, while it was >6 months in 22 patients. Overall, 1/8 patients with a time interval of ≤6 months had a positive antibody response, whereas 6/22 patients with a time interval of >6 months had a positive antibody response. These differences are not statistically significant.

Due to the substantial age range in patients, we also tested the age at time of first vaccination as a prognostic parameter for the antibody outcome after the second vaccination. In 30 of the 32 patients with vaccination after CAR-T-cell therapy (2 patients had no antibody evaluation after 2nd vaccination), we found no significant correlation between age at time of first vaccination and antibody outcome (AUC: 50.6%, CI: 27–73, p = 0.9609). Overall, 5 patients were under the age of 50 years, while 25 patients were more than 50 years old. Only 1/5 patients < 50 years in age had a positive antibody response, whereas 6/25 patients > 50 years of age had a positive antibody test result. These differences are not significant.

3.7. Infection Rate

Overall, 12 out of 46 patients reported a COVID-19 infection in their medical history. Eight patients had no detectable antibody response before the infection. Four patients had a positive antibody response before the infection (but only 1/4 with a strong positive result > 100 AU/mL). In seven patients, the infection took place after the second vaccination, in four patients after the third vaccination, and in one patient after the fourth vaccination.

Taking a closer look at the groups, 9/32 patients with CAR-T before VAC were infected. Four patients with reported infection were infected after second vaccination. These were 4/23 patients with negative antibodies and 0/7 patients with positive antibodies. Four patients were infected after third vaccination. These were 3/14 patients with negative antibodies and 1/9 patients with positive antibodies. One patient was infected after fourth vaccination. These were 1/3 patients with positive antibodies.

Overall, 3/14 patients with CAR-T after VAC were infected. All three patients with reported infection were infected after second vaccination. These were 1/8 patients with negative antibodies and 2/6 patients with positive antibodies (only 1 infected patient with a strong positive result > 100AU/mL) after second vaccination.

4. Discussion

In this retrospective real-world analysis, performed at a single tertiary academic center, we examined patients with CAR-T-cell therapy and two to four doses of COVID-19 vaccination and two different vaccination procedures.

In patients who underwent CAR-T-cell therapy before COVID-19 vaccination, we found a very low seropositivity rate of only seven patients (23.3%; 7/30) after two doses of the vaccine. Other studies have shown similar low results, with a seropositivity rate of 21% (3/14 patients) in the study from Dhakal et al. and 36% (5/14) in the study from Ram et. al. [12,13]. Administration of a third dose lead to seroconversion in five patients (23.8%; 5/21) and an increase of antibody titers in four patients (19%; 4/21). Ram et al. showed similar results with post CAR-T-cell patients who had no humoral response after two doses, in which 17% (1/6) of patients achieved a positive result after a third dose [14]. Our study showed that seroconversion could be achieved in two patients (66%; 2/3) due to the fourth vaccination, while 1pt. (33%; 1/3) stayed clearly positive after third and fourth vaccination. Currently, there is very limited data on a fourth dose in immunosuppressed patients, but a study from Alejo et al. with 18 solid organ transplant recipients showed that 50% of participants with negative and all with low-positive titers showed significant boosting to high-positive titers after the fourth dose [16]. Therefore, our study suggests a clear benefit from a third as well as a fourth vaccination in patients with prior CAR-T-cell therapy, as it could lead to an increase in the number of patients with a positive antibody result and an increase in anti-spike protein IgG antibody titers.

In this analysis, the number of B-cells and CAR-T copies in patients' peripheral blood at time of first vaccination and the time interval between CAR-T-cell therapy and first vaccination were investigated as a prognostic factor for the outcome of antibody tests in patients with prior CAR-T-cell therapy. We found that all 21 patients with 0/μL B-cells at the time of the first vaccination had a negative antibody test result. The more B-cells (optimal cutoff at >10/μL B-cells; PPV 85.7%; NPV 100%) in the patients' peripheral blood at the time of the first vaccination, the more likely patients were to develop a positive antibody test result (AUC: 96.2%, CI: 89–100, $p = 0.0006$). Also, the fewer the CAR-T copies (optimal cutoff at <38/μg DNA CAR-T copies; PPV 94.7%; NPV 55.5%) in the patients' peripheral blood at the time of the first vaccination, the more likely patients were to develop a positive antibody test result (AUC: 77.3%, CI: 57–97, $p = 0.0438$). However, no significant correlation between time interval from CAR-T-cell therapy to the first vaccination and antibody outcome was observed. We also found no significant correlation between the age at time of vaccination and the antibody outcome. These results suggest that patients' B-cells and CAR-T-cells are important prognostic parameters in order to find the optimal time for vaccination. An earlier study from Ram et al. produced similar results. They examined

66 hematopoietic cell transplantation patients and 14 patients with CAR-T-cell therapy and found that higher CD19+ cells were associated with positive humoral responses [13].

Patients with two doses of the vaccination before CAR-T-cell therapy (CAR-T after VAC) showed a slightly higher seropositivity rate after the second vaccine dose, as six patients (42.9%; 6/14) had positive humoral antibodies. However, it was only in one patient (12.5%; 1/8) that a negative result after the second vaccine could be turned into a positive result after the third dose, which took place as re-vaccination after CAR-T-cell therapy. Three patients (3/4) seroconverted after the fourth vaccination, while 1pt. (1/4) stayed negative after the third and fourth vaccinations. Therefore, our study suggests that patients with vaccination prior to CAR-T-cell therapy should receive two doses as re-vaccination after CAR-T-cell therapy. The reason for this is the higher benefit shown above in the administration of a fourth dose in comparison with only a third dose.

Given that patients were retrospectively divided into two groups (CAR-T before VAC/CAR-T after VAC), a comparison between these two groups is difficult as there were different amounts of patients in the two groups. Our study reflects a real-world scenario in which some of the patients had their CAR-T-cell therapy without the protection of a COVID-19 vaccination as vaccines were not available at the time. In these patients with CAR-T before VAC, only 23.3% (7/30) had a positive antibody test result after two vaccinations. In comparison, patients with CAR-T after VAC 42.9% (6/14) had a positive antibody test result after two vaccinations. Thus, we could assume that six patients with CAR-T after VAC had protection by a positive antibody test result as they went through the procedure of the CAR-T-cell therapy. We consider this as a benefit in vaccination before CAR-T-cell therapy.

Overall, 12 out of 46 patients reported a COVID-19 infection: 4 patients with positive antibody response and 8 patients with no detectable antibody response. Due to the limited patient count, no definite conclusions can be drawn as to the protection offered by different antibody levels.

Limitations to this study were the retrospective data collection and the limited number of patients, particularly at the fourth vaccination time point. Additionally, our study only examined the humoral antibody responses and not the cellular reactivity to COVID-19 vaccines. Currently, it also remains unclear which quantities of antibody titers are protective against severe courses of COVID-19 infection. It is also not conclusively clarified how long protection by high antibody titers lasts; more studies are needed to address this question. However, this study provides an important real-world analysis of COVID-19 vaccines in CAR-T-cell patients with two different vaccination procedures. This information shows the benefits of additional booster doses for these patients and can give guidance for the optimal time of vaccination. Our study is an important addition to the very limited data available in this group of patients. Further studies with more CAR-T-cell recipients, especially for third and fourth vaccination, are needed to conclusively confirm our results.

5. Conclusions

Our results indicate poor humoral antibody responses in patients with CAR-T-cell therapy and two doses of mRNA COVID-19 vaccines, which could be improved by administration of an additional third or fourth dose of the vaccine. Low B-cell counts and high CAR-T-cell numbers are associated with lacking antibody response and could therefore be an important parameter in choosing the optimal moment of vaccination. However, larger studies will be needed to ultimately clarify this question.

Author Contributions: Conceptualization, T.P.; data curation, C.H.; formal analysis, S.G.; investigation, S.G., michael Nagler, F.S., C.S. and T.P.; methodology, S.G., U.B., M.N., F.S., C.S. and T.P.; project administration, T.P.; resources, C.H., U.N. and T.P.; supervision, U.B., M.N. and T.P.; validation, T.P.; writing—original draft, S.G., U.B. and T.P.; writing—review and editing, U.B., C.H., M.N., F.S., C.S., U.N. and T.P. All authors have read and agreed to the published version of the manuscript.

Funding: This research received no external funding.

Institutional Review Board Statement: The study was conducted according to the guidelines of the Declaration of Helsinki and approved by the Ethics Committee in Bern, Switzerland (decision number 2021-01822 and date of approval 6 September 2021).

Informed Consent Statement: Informed consent was obtained from all subjects involved in the study.

Data Availability Statement: No data supporting the reported results are deposited elsewhere. The data presented in this study are available on request from the corresponding author. The data are not publicly available due to institution-related patient identity restrictions.

Conflicts of Interest: The authors declare no conflict of interest.

References

1. Sermer, D.; Brentjens, R. CAR T-cell therapy: Full speed ahead. *Hematol. Oncol.* **2019**, *37*, 95–100. [CrossRef] [PubMed]
2. Mathys, A.; Bacher, U.; Banz, Y.; Legros, M.; Taleghani, B.M.; Novak, U.; Pabst, T. Outcome of patients with mantle cell lymphoma after autologous stem cell transplantation in the pre-CAR T-cell era. *Hematol. Oncol.* **2021**, *40*, 292–296. [CrossRef] [PubMed]
3. Brechbühl, S.; Bacher, U.; Jeker, B.; Pabst, T. Real-World Outcome in the pre-CAR-T Era of Myeloma Patients Qualifying for CAR-T Cell Therapy. *Mediterr. J. Hematol. Infect. Dis.* **2020**, *13*, e2021012. [CrossRef]
4. Heini, A.D.; Bacher, U.; Kronig, M.N.; Wiedemann, G.; Novak, U.; Zeerleder, S.; Mansouri Taleghani, B.; Daskalakis, M.; Pabst, T. Chimeric antigen receptor T-cell therapy for relapsed mantle cell lymphoma: Real-world experience from a single tertiary care center. *Bone Marrow Transplant.* **2022**, *57*, 1010–1012. [CrossRef] [PubMed]
5. Hill, J.A.; Giralt, S.; Torgerson, T.R.; Lazarus, H.M. CAR-T– and a side order of IgG, to go?—Immunoglobulin Replacement in Patients Receiving CAR-T Cell Therapy. *Blood Rev.* **2019**, *38*, 100596. [CrossRef] [PubMed]
6. Messmer, A.S.; Que, Y.A.; Schankin, C.; Banz, Y.; Bacher, U.; Novak, U.; Pabst, T. CAR T-cell therapy and critical care. *Wien. Klin. Wochenschr.* **2021**, *133*, 1318–1325. [CrossRef] [PubMed]
7. Nydegger, A.; Novak, U.; Kronig, M.N.; Legros, M.; Zeerleder, S.; Banz, Y.; Bacher, U.; Pabst, T. Transformed Lymphoma Is Associated with a Favorable Response to CAR-T-Cell Treatment in DLBCL Patients. *Cancers* **2021**, *13*, 6073. [CrossRef] [PubMed]
8. Pabst, T.; Joncourt, R.; Shumilov, E.; Heini, A.; Wiedemann, G.; Legros, M.; Seipel, K.; Schild, C.; Jalowiec, K.; Taleghani, B.M.; et al. Analysis of IL-6 serum levels and CAR T cell-specific digital PCR in the context of cytokine release syndrome. *Exp. Hematol.* **2020**, *88*, 7–14.e3. [CrossRef] [PubMed]
9. Bupha-Intr, O.; Haeusler, G.; Chee, L.; Thursky, K.; Slavin, M.; Teh, B. CAR-T cell therapy and infection: A review. *Expert Rev. Anti-Infect. Ther.* **2020**, *19*, 749–758. [CrossRef] [PubMed]
10. European Medicines Agency. Comirnaty; Spikevax (Previously COVID-19 Vaccine Moderna). Available online: https://www.ema.europa.eu/en/medicines/human (accessed on 15 January 2022).
11. European Society for Blood and Marrow Transplantation. COVID-19 Vaccines, Version 8, 3 January 2022. Available online: https://www.ebmt.org/covid-19-and-bmt (accessed on 13 March 2022).
12. Dhakal, B.; Abedin, S.; Fenske, T.; Chhabra, S.; Ledeboer, N.; Hari, P.; Hamadani, M. Response to SARS-CoV-2 vaccination in patients after hematopoietic cell transplantation and CAR T-cell therapy. *Blood* **2021**, *138*, 1278–1281. [CrossRef] [PubMed]
13. Ram, R.; Hagin, D.; Kikozashvilli, N.; Freund, T.; Amit, O.; Bar-On, Y.; Beyar-Katz, O.; Shefer, G.; Moshiashvili, M.M.; Karni, C.; et al. Safety and Immunogenicity of the BNT162b2 mRNA COVID-19 Vaccine in Patients after Allogeneic HCT or CD19-based CART therapy—A Single-Center Prospective Cohort Study. *Transplant. Cell. Ther.* **2021**, *27*, 788–794. [CrossRef] [PubMed]
14. Ram, R.; Freund, T.; Halperin, T.; Ben-Ami, R.; Amit, O.; Bar-On, Y.; Beyar-Katz, O.; Eilaty, N.; Gold, R.; Kay, S.; et al. Immunogenicity of a Third Dose of the BNT162b2 mRNA Covid-19 Vaccine in Patients with Impaired B Cell Reconstitution After Cellular Therapy—A Single Center Prospective Cohort Study. *Transplant. Cell. Ther.* **2022**, *28*, 278.e1–278.e4. [CrossRef] [PubMed]
15. Cordonnier, C.; Einarsdottir, S.; Cesaro, S.; Di Blasi, R.; Mikulska, M.; Rieger, C.; de Lavallade, H.; Gallo, G.; Lehrnbecher, T.; Engelhard, D.; et al. Vaccination of haemopoietic stem cell transplant recipients: Guidelines of the 2017 European Conference on Infections in Leukaemia (ECIL 7). *Lancet Infect. Dis.* **2019**, *19*, e200–e212. [CrossRef]
16. Alejo, J.L.; Mitchell, J.; Chiang, T.P.Y.; Abedon, A.T.; Boyarsky, B.J.; Avery, R.K.; Tobian, A.A.R.; Levan, M.L.; Massie, A.B.; Garonzik-Wang, J.M.; et al. Antibody Response to a Fourth Dose of a SARS-CoV-2 Vaccine in Solid Organ Transplant Recipients: A Case Series. *Transplantation* **2021**, *105*, e280–e281. [CrossRef] [PubMed]

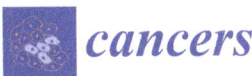

Review

T-Cell Engagers in Solid Cancers—Current Landscape and Future Directions

Mohamed Shanshal [1,*], Paolo F. Caimi [2], Alex A. Adjei [2] and Wen Wee Ma [2,*]

[1] Department of Oncology, Mayo Clinic, Rochester, MN 55902, USA
[2] Cleveland Clinic, Cleveland, OH 44195, USA
* Correspondence: shanshal.mohamed@mayo.edu (M.S.); maw4@ccf.org (W.W.M.)

Simple Summary: There are multiple strategies to target cancer cells, and among the rapidly evolving field is the use of bispecific antibodies and T-cell engagers in the treatment of cancers. These drugs work by recruiting and activating T-cells, a type of white blood cell, to recognize and attack cancer cells. These agents consist of two different antibody fragments: one that binds to a tumor antigen on cancer cells and another that binds to the CD3 receptor on T-cells. Once the T-cell engager binds to both the cancer cell and T-cell, it brings the T-cell into close proximity to the cancer cell, leading to the activation of T-cells and the release of cytokines and cytotoxic molecules that kill the cancer cell. T-cell engagers have shown promising results in the treatment of a variety of hematological malignancies. Research is ongoing to explore their use in the treatment of variety of solid cancers. Nevertheless, T-cell engagers can cause side effects like cytokine release syndrome and neurotoxicity. More research is ongoing to determine their long-term safety and effectiveness.

Abstract: Monoclonal antibody treatment initially heralded an era of molecularly targeted therapy in oncology and is now widely applied in modulating anti-cancer immunity by targeting programmed cell receptors (PD-1, PD-L1), cytotoxic T-lymphocyte-associated protein 4 (CTLA-4) and, more recently, lymphocyte-activation gene 3 (LAG3). Chimeric antigen receptor T-cell therapy (CAR-T) recently proved to be a valid approach to inducing anti-cancer immunity by directly modifying the host's immune cells. However, such cell-based therapy requires extensive resources such as leukapheresis, ex vivo modification and expansion of cytotoxic T-cells and current Good Manufacturing Practice (cGMP) laboratories and presents significant logistical challenges. Bi-/trispecific antibody technology is a novel pharmaceutical approach to facilitate the engagement of effector immune cells to potentially multiple cancer epitopes, e.g., the recently approved blinatumomab. This opens the opportunity to develop 'off-the-shelf' anti-cancer agents that achieve similar and/or complementary anti-cancer effects as those of modified immune cell therapy. The majority of bi-/trispecific antibodies target the tumor-associated antigens (TAA) located on the extracellular surface of cancer cells. The extracellular antigens represent just a small percentage of known TAAs and are often associated with higher toxicities because some of them are expressed on normal cells (off-target toxicity). In contrast, the targeting of intracellular TAAs such as mutant RAS and TP53 may lead to fewer off-target toxicities while still achieving the desired antitumor efficacy (on-target toxicity). Here, we provide a comprehensive review on the emerging field of bi-/tri-specific T-cell engagers and potential therapeutic opportunities.

Keywords: bi-/trispecific antibodies; T-cell engagers; solid tumors

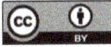

1. Introduction

The use of monoclonal antibody (mAb) technology in anti-cancer therapy has evolved rapidly since the Food and Drug Administration first approved the use of the anti-CD20 mAb rituximab in 1997 for treating relapsed CD20-positive B-cell lymphoma. Improvements in gene sequencing, proteomics and computational platforms resulted in the production of antibodies with increasing affinity to antigenic epitopes and efficacy [1]. Targeting tumor-associated antigens (TAA) continues to be a major focus in anti-cancer drug development and has become particularly relevant in the era of immunotherapeutics because these antigens may be targeted to elicit antitumor immune responses [2,3]. However, this approach can be hindered by several resistance mechanisms, including but not limited to downregulation of TAA expression by cancer cells, activation of signaling pathway granting cancer cells resistance to apoptosis as well as tumor microenvironmental factors impeding mAb activity [4]. Furthermore, inducing immune responses that alter antibody-dependent cellular cytotoxicity and complement-dependent cytotoxicity may impair the efficacy of these mAbs [5].

Bispecific antibodies (BsAbs) are a proven anti-cancer drug platform capable of simultaneously targeting multiple TAAs and potentially overcoming these resistance mechanisms, and, in the era of immuno-oncology, they modulate/induce immune cell responses by simultaneously targeting the TAA(s) and antigens/receptors on the effector cells [6]. The majority of BsAbs are designed based on IgG molecules (Figure 1). The antigen-binding site (ABS) is an area between the heavy variable (V_H) and light variable (V_L) chains and is designed via the re-arrangement of the complementarity-determining regions (CDRs) [7].

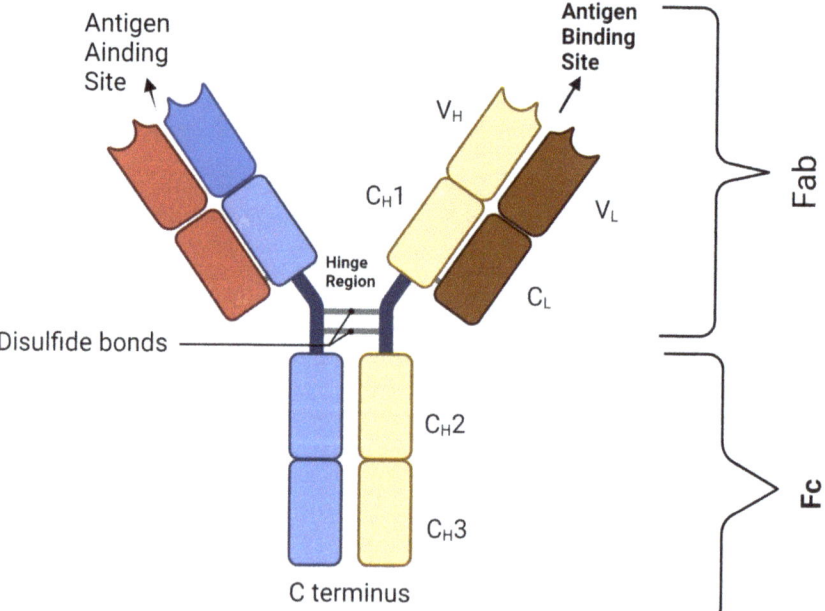

Figure 1. Basic BsAb structure showing the antigen-binding site that harbors the complementarity-determining region (CDR) segment, disulfide bond, light chains (L) and heavy chains (H); C: constant domain; V: variable domain, Fab: fragment antigen-binding domain; Fc: fragment-crystallizable domain. Figure created by BioRender.com (accessed on 14 May 2023).

Optimizing the CDRs is important for higher affinity (on-target efficacy) and avoidance of bystander cells (off-tumor toxicity) [8]. The design of an effective BsAbs involves multiple processes, and for the purposes of this review we will summarize it into four key steps: (A) lead identification, which is the detailed analysis/identification of the antibody-binding site for an antigen e.g., protein docking [9,10]; (B) predicting the antibody structure through proteomic computational methods, e.g., AlphaFold [11]; (C) lead optimization, which is the prediction of the binding affinity between the antibody (paratope) and the antigen (epitope), e.g., the PInet [12]; and finally (D): for the antibody to be effective, it does require good solubility to avoid overt immunogenicity. Lead identification, optimization and assessment of the relative positions of both parts of the paratope–epitope complex are crucial steps for the development of successful therapeutic antibodies [13].

BsAbs are designed in a way that one target is the neoepitope of cancer cells (TAA) and the other target site is dedicated to engaging with targets that can facilitate an antineoplastic effect. The antineoplastic activity can be achieved through several mechanisms: (1) direct engagement with surface antigens of immune effector cells, such as CD3 in T-cells, CD16 in NK cells or CD47 in macrophages; (2) engagement with receptors that modulate T-cell response; and (3) interaction with other signaling pathways.

The most common BsAbs are the bispecific T-cell engagers (BiTEs), which act through the simultaneous engagement of TAAs and CD3, resulting in the activation of T-cells irrespective of MHC, with the resultant release of perforins and granzymes [14]. In solid tumors, the success in targeting GP100 through construction of gp100/HLA*0201 fused to anti-CD3 single-chain variable fragments (scFv) led to tebentafusp's approval for the treatment of uveal melanoma.

BsAbs' T-cell-modulating targets include those that are immune-inhibitory such as PD-L1/CTLA-4 [15] and those that are immune-stimulatory such as the TNF receptors OX40, CD27 and CD137 (4-1BB) or the T-cell costimulatory receptor CD28. Engagement of one or more of these receptors may enhance the antitumor immune response or activate exhausted tumor-infiltrating lymphocytes in the tumor immune microenvironment [16].

Antibody–drug conjugates are another approach that utilize the mAb platform for targeted delivery of cytotoxic agents [17]. The use of trastuzumab deruxtecan in the treatment of HER2+ breast cancer is a successful example in which the BsAb binds to HER2/CD63 or HER2/PRLR and concurrently facilitates the internalization and lysosomal degradation essential for the action of the cytotoxic payload [18,19].

At the time of the writing of this review, there were a total of seven BsAbs approved for the treatment of different malignant diseases: amivantamab (EGFR/cMET), blinatumomab (CD3/CD19), catumaxomab (CD3/EpCAM), mosunetuzumab (CD3/CD20), tebentafusp (GP100/CD3), teclistamab (CD3/BCMA) and zenocutuzumab (HER2/HER3) [20,21].

Here, we focus on conditional T-cell engagers in solid tumors using the bi-/trispecific antibody platform and contrast this with immune effector cell therapies such as CAR-T therapy. We will also discuss the potential benefits of targeting intracellular TAAs and provide a summary of currently approved agents and those in development for the treatment of solid tumors.

2. Structural Mechanism of T-Cell Engagers

Bispecific antibodies (BsAbs) are divided into two major categories based on their structure and mechanism of action.

2.1. T-Cell Engagers without FC Fragment

Characterized by a lack of immune-mediated target cell killing (ADCC), as they lack the FC domain, these agents have lower stability and a short plasma half-life but have better tissue penetration given their lower molecular weight. These are particularly useful in targeting the central nervous system (CNS), and examples include nanobodies and svFC [22,23] (Figure 2A).

2.2. T-Cell Engagers with FC Fragment

These agents have the potential to exert actions related to their FC fragment, including ADCC. BsAbs with FC fragments are characterized by a longer half-life and higher stability. The design examples include the knob-in-hole technique in which the heavy chain is engineered with a knob, and the other heavy chain consists of a hole [24]. The disadvantages of including an FC fragment on a BsAb are both structural and functional. The structural disadvantage is that the large size of the molecule impedes tissue distribution and access to neoplastic cells. In addition, the non-covalent binding of the two variable domains via a hydrophobic interface is more challenging from the design and manufacturing aspects

(Figure 2B). From a functional standpoint, the presence of an intact FC domain decreases T-cell trafficking and limits the antineoplastic activity, though it can be improved by FC silencing via FC fragment modifications [25].

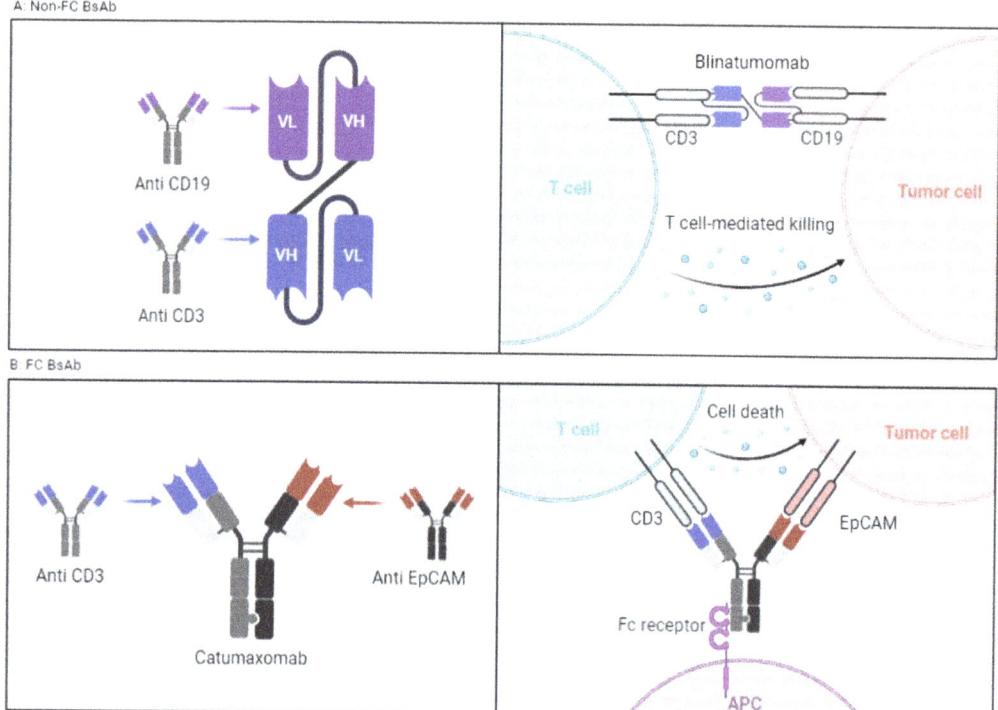

Figure 2. (**A**) BsAbs without FC portion connected via a linker. Example is blinatumomab. (**B**) Classic BsAbs with FC portion that requires antigen-presenting cells and activation of which results in ADCC. Example is catumaxomab. Figure created by BioRender.com (accessed on 14 May 2023).

3. T-Cell Engagers in Solid Tumors

Most approved BiTEs are used in the treatment of hematologic malignancies. While TAAs have been identified both in hematologic malignancies and solid tumors, most are also present in normal cellular counterparts, which results in "on-target" toxicities. These on-target toxicities in normal tissues are more manageable in hematologic malignancies than in solid tumors. For example, CD19 targeting results in B-cell aplasia and hypogammaglobulinemia and increases the risk of infection; such infections can be managed by being vigilant clinically and the prompt use of antibiotic(s). On the other hand, targeting epidermal growth factor (EGFR) in lung cancer leads to generalized cutaneous toxicity and cardiotoxicity in the treatment of HER2-positive breast cancer using trastuzumab [26,27].

These "on-target" toxicities can further be mitigated through the use of conditional T-cell engagers (cTCE), which are inactive precursors of TCEs activated by tumor-associated proteases. This induces TCEs to kill tumor cells expressing the target antigen in the tumor microenvironment without affecting distant tissues. The decreased toxicity of cTCEs potentially confers upon them a superior therapeutic index and may allow the administration of a higher dose. An example is ProTriTACs, where a half-life-extending albumin-binding domain masks the CD3-binding domain [28,29].

Intracellular TAA targeting may sidestep the challenges of mAb targeting of shared cell surface TAAs between tumor and normal tissues in solid tumors. This strategy may lead to higher tumor cell killing (on-target/on-tumor effect), decreased risk of damaging normal tissues (on-target/off-tumor toxicity) as well as lower bystander toxicity (off-target/off-tumor toxicity).

However, intracellular TAA targeting is currently challenged by a lack of effective tools to penetrate the cell surface and deliver the antibody arm of TCEs into neoplastic cells. This is an area of active research, and novel approaches include technologies that promote the expression of intracellular TAAs or enhance the delivery of BsAbs into tumor cells.

3.1. Targeting Tumor-Associated Peptides Presented by MHC

Aberrant intracellular proteins can be presented by MHC class 1 molecules on the cell surface (Figure 3E). One example is p53: a small fraction of intracellular p53 is degraded via proteosomes and can be presented by HLA on the cell surface. Specific peptides of mutated p53 (R175H) can bind to HLA-A*02:01 on the surface of cancer cells. Hsiue et al. developed CD3 engagers that bind specifically to the p53-R175H peptide–HLA complex with high affinity and resulted in tumor cell killing [30–32].

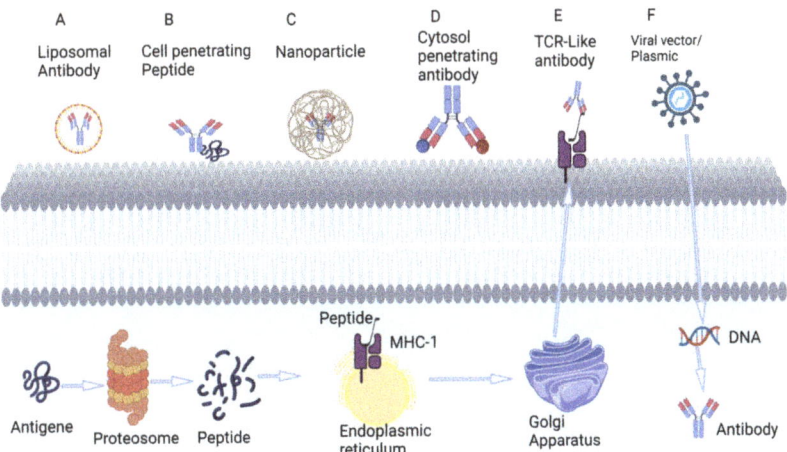

Figure 3. Techniques under investigation for targeting intracellular tumor antigens using antibodies. (**A**) Liposomal coating of antibodies. (**B**) Cell-penetrating peptides that adhere to the phospholipid bilayers. (**C**) Nanoparticles. (**D**) Cytosol-penetrating antibodies. (**E**) TCR-like antibodies that can target low-concentration intracellular peptide fragments that are presented to extracellular space via MHC. (**F**) Viral vectors that incorporate into the genome and produce intracellular antibodies. Figure created by BioRender.com (accessed on 14 May 2023).

A similar strategy is the use of oncolytic vaccines such as MAGE-1 and NY-ESO-1. These are incorporated into the tumor genome and are translated into antigens which, when degraded, are presented by MHC to the extracellular surface of tumor cells, making them recognizable by T-cell engagers. An example is melanoma-associated antigen A4 (MAGE-A4) solid cancers in patients with the HLA-A*02:01 genotype. MAGE-A4 is processed intracellularly, resulting in peptide fragments that are co-presented with HLA-A*02:01 (Figure 3E). Afamitresgene autoleucel is an HLA-restricted autologous T-cell therapy that targets MAGE-A4 that was evaluated in a phase 1 trial in solid tumor patients with HLA*02:01. The overall response rate was 24% (all partial response). All patients experienced grade 3 and above hematologic toxicity; 55% of patients experienced =< grade 2 cytokine release syndrome [33].

3.2. Intracellular Delivery of Antibodies

The delivery of larger antibodies to intracellular targets is an area of intense research, and approaches under investigation include the use of liposomes, cell-penetrating peptides, nanoparticles, cytosol-penetrating antibodies, TCR-Like antibody and the use of viral vectors (Figure 3A–F). The successful targeting of intracellular p53 and KRAS mutants had been demonstrated in preclinical studies [34].

3.3. Successful Examples of T-Cell Engagers in Solid Tumors

This section highlights the importance of T-cell engagers in the treatment of advanced solid tumors. Some of these example are FDA-approved, while others are in later stages of drug development. (Figure 4, summarize therapeutic targets in solid tumors).

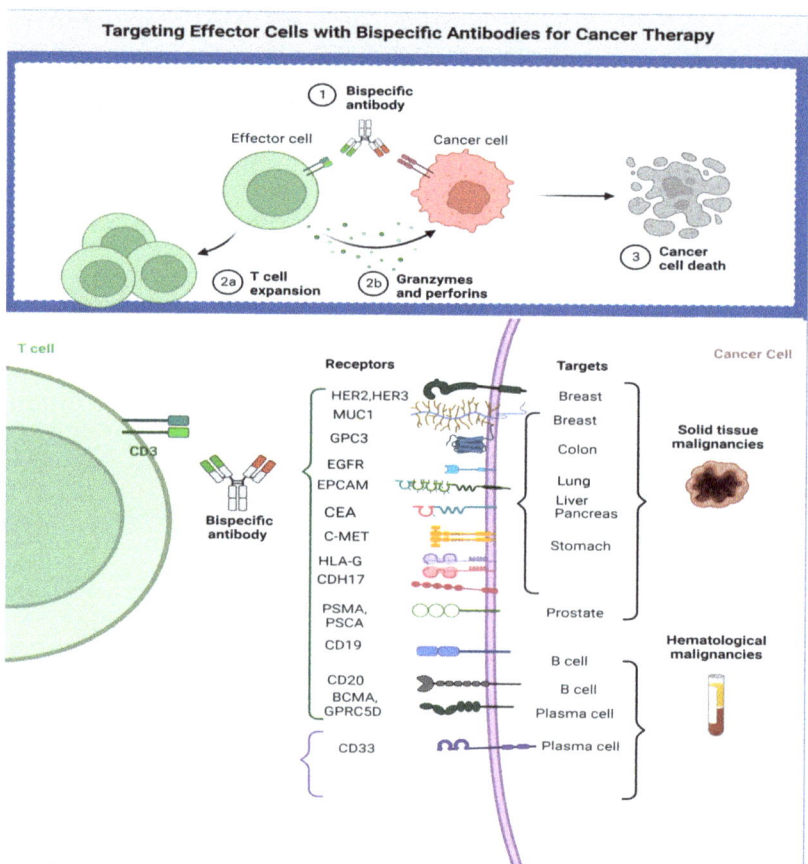

Figure 4. Therapeutic targets for bi- and trispecific antibodies. Figure created by BioRender.com (accessed on 14 May 2023).

- GP100

Melanoma-associated antigen (gp100) is a membrane-bound protein expressed on the surface of melanocytes and most malignant melanoma. T-lymphocytes recognize gp100 presented by HLA proteins such as HLA-A*02:01. Vaccination with gp100 peptide vaccine was evaluated in a phase II randomized trial in the treatment of metastatic melanoma in combination with IL2; the overall response rate (ORR) was 16%, and overall survival (OS) was 17 months [35]. This suggested gp100 as a potential TAA, which led to designer BiTEs' with a high-affinity TCR-binding domain and an anti-CD3 T-cell-engaging domain. Such a construct facilitates and redirects T-cells to attack gp100-expressing tumor cells. Tebentafusp is a gp100/CD3 BsAb and was evaluated in a phase 1 study of 42 patients with metastatic uveal melanoma. The study found that tebentafusp was generally well-tolerated, with the most common adverse events (AEs) being fever (91%), rash and pruritus (83%), fatigue (71%) and chills (69%). The overall response rate was 11.9% (95% CI, 4.0 to 25.6). The median overall survival was 25.5 months (range, 0.89–31.1 months), and the 1-year overall survival rate was 67% [36]. The subsequent phase 3 trial in HLA-A*02:01-expressing patients with treatment-naive metastatic uveal and cutaneous melanoma compared tebentafusp against the investigator's choice of treatment (pembrolizumab, ipilimumab or dacarbazine). At a median follow-up of 14 months, the tebentafusp-containing arm achieved superior survival compared to the investigator's choice (median OS 22 months versus 16 months; 6-month PFS 31% versus 19%, respectively). A 1-year overall survival rate of 65% was reported for both patient cohorts [37,38]. This pivotal trial led to Food and Drug Administration (FDA) approval of tebentafusp in April 2022. Cytokine release syndrome (CRS) occurred in 89% of patients, though the adverse events improved during subsequent dosing. Only 2% of patients discontinued treatment due to treatment-related side effects, and there were no treatment-related deaths.

- EPCAM

Catumaxomab is a T-cell engager with specificity for CD3 and epithelial cell adhesion molecule (EpCAM). Interestingly, this agent can be considered "trifunctional" because the mAb has a functional FC receptor capable of engaging FCγ receptors that induce immune reaction [39]. Catumaxomab was approved by the European Medical Agency in 2009 for treatment of EpCAM-positive carcinomas and malignant ascites. However, catumaxomab was withdrawn from the market in 2017 due to unacceptable CRS and high-grade liver toxicity which was fatal in some patients [40]. The severity of the toxicities was likely due to the high immunogenicity and wide expression of EpCAM in normal tissues such as the Kupffer cells of the liver.

- PSMA

Pasotuxizumab, a CD3/PSMA T-cell engager, was evaluated in a phase 1 trial of patients with metastatic castrate-resistant prostate cancer (mCRPC). The BsAb was administered as a continuous IV infusion over 12 weeks. Of the 16 patients treated, 13 (81%) experienced grade ≥ 3 adverse events (AEs). The most frequent all-grade AEs were flu-like illness and fatigue, whereas the most frequent grade ≥ 3 AEs were decreased lymphocytes and infections (44%). Three patients had a reduction of >50% in serum PSA levels, two of them had long-term responses, and one achieved a near CR as assessed by PSMA PET imaging [41]. The development of pasotuxizumab was halted after this study in favor of acapatamab.

Acapatamab is T-cell engager targeting CD3/PSMA but has a longer half-life than pasotuxizumab. Acapatamab was evaluated alone or in combination with pembrolizumab in a phase 1 trial involving patients with mCRPC. In the monotherapy cohort, a 'confirmed $\geq$ 30% PSA reduction' was achieved in 27.6% of patients, a partial response in 20% and stable disease in 53.3%. However, 60.5% had grade 2 CRS, and 25.6% had grade 3 CRS. [42,43]. The CD3/PSMA T-cell engager is being compared to enzalutamide and abiraterone in patients with mCRPC in a phase 2 trial (NCT04631601). The study has completed accrual, and the results are pending.

- CD33 (MDSC-targeting)

CD33 is a transmembrane receptor expressed on the surface of various myeloid cells, including myeloid-derived suppressor cells (MDSCs), and is known to promote tumor growth and suppress antitumor immune response in solid tumors [44]. AMV564 is a novel CD3/CD33 T-cell engager which induces antitumor immune response via T-cell-directed lysis of CD33 cells [45]. The agent was evaluated in a phase 1 trial which included 30 patients with advanced solid tumors. AMV564 was given via subcutaneous injections on days 1–5 and 8–12 of a 21-day cycle, either alone (20 patients) or in combination with pembrolizumab (10 patients) at a dose of 200 mg IV q3w. The monotherapy cohort dosing was 15, 50 and 75 mcg/day, while the combination therapy cohort dosing was 5, 15 and 50 mcg/day. Complete response was achieved in patients with ovarian cancer in the monotherapy cohort. The agent was well tolerated, with 2 cases of grade 2 CRS at 75 mcg/day and no dose-limiting toxicities. The most common side effects were injection site reactions, fever, fatigue, anemia, hypotension and nausea. Subcutaneous injection of AMV564 resulted in relevant plasma exposure [46].

3.4. Toxicity Profile and Management of Toxicity of T-Cell Engagers in Solid Tumors

The major advantages of T-cell-engaging immunotherapeutics such as BsAbs and T-cell engagers over cellular therapeutics, e.g., CAR-T, include their "off-the-shelf" availability and their requiring no lymphodepletion prior to administration. Both treatment modalities (T-cell engagers and CAR-T-cells) have similar toxicity profiles, including CRS and immune effector-associated neurotoxicity syndrome (ICANS). These toxicities are less severe or less frequent in T-cell engagers and may be related to their dosing (Table 1 and Table 3) [47,48]. While CAR-T-cell treatment is often administered in a single dose, T-cell engagers may be administered repeatedly. As such, T-cell engager administration includes a period of step-up dosing to mitigate the risk of these toxicities and is followed by the full doses about 1 to 2 weeks after.

Table 1. Unique toxicities based on therapeutic targets of T-cell engagers.

Target Antigen	Specific Toxicity
EPCAM	Immune-mediated hepatotoxicity
HER2	Hypotension, hypertension, tachycardia
PSMA	Hepatotoxicity
DLL3	Pneumonitis
Myeloid-derived suppressor cells (MDSC)	Anemia, hypotension, pruritis
EGFRvIII	Dermatologic toxicities, SJS, TEN
CEA	Hepatotoxicity

- Cytokine release syndrome

The immune-mediated toxicities associated with treatment using CAR-T-cells and T-cell engagers are significant challenges requiring close attention. The binding of the target antigen induces T-cell expansion and the release of proinflammatory cytokines, which then leads to the recruitment of other endogenous immune cells such as macrophages and further escalation of the immune response [49]. The overactive and uncontrolled immune response results in CRS, which is characterized by fever and multiple-end-organ dysfunction/damage. This systemic toxicity is experienced by approximately 15% of patients treated using blinatumomab. The incidence is dependent on the BiTEs' structure, affinity for CD3 engagement and TAA abundance, e.g., grade 3 and above CRS being reported in 2% of patients with MUC17/CD3 (AMG199) and 25% of patients with PSMA/CD3 (acapatamab) [42].

The risk can be mitigated by close monitoring and premedication with corticosteroids. Step-up dosing can also reduce CRS risk by starting at a lower dose and escalating during the first cycle of treatment. The use of a subcutaneous route has been proposed to decrease the risk of CRS [50]. A recent computational study showed that the co-administration of the interleukin (IL)-6 receptor-blocking mAb tocilizumab and/or anti-TNFα may reduce the incidence without compromising antitumor activity [51].

The management of low-grade CRS includes the use of antihistamines, antipyretics and intravenous fluids. CRS of grade 2 and above requires admission to the hospital and may require pressors for hypotension, as well as supplemental oxygen for respiratory distress [52,53]. Severe CRS will require intensive care unit care with early initiation of high-dose corticosteroids—for example, methylprednisone at 1 mg/kg/day and tocilizumab at 8 to 12 mg/kg based on body weight. Tocilizumab can be repeated after an interval of

8 h, and it should not exceed 4 doses in total [54]. Supportive therapies include the use of intravenous vasopressors or mechanical ventilation to assist with respiratory distress.

- Neurotoxicity

Immune effector-associated neurotoxicity syndrome (ICANS) with T-cell engager treatment may manifest as mild confusion, headache, dysgraphia and, in more severe cases, encephalopathy. The pathophysiology of ICANS is not yet fully understood. Cerebral microvasculature damage from activated immune cells, endothelial damage, blood–brain barrier disruption and direct effects of cytokines have been hypothesized as underlying mechanisms [55].

The neurotoxicity risk from T-cell engagers may be mitigated by step-up dosing and pre-treatment with corticosteroids. Once it has occurred, management consists primarily of aggressive supportive care and corticosteroids. Tocilizumab, however, is not recommended for neurotoxicity, as it can increase IL-6 plasma concentration and exacerbate ICANS.

The management of ICANS often involves supportive care measures such as hydration, electrolyte balancing, the use of steroids and seizure management. For patients with more severe symptoms, more aggressive interventions may be indicated including mechanical ventilation or intracranial pressure monitoring. A neurologist or other specialist with experience in managing neurological complications of immunotherapy should be consulted if one has not been already.

The prophylactic use of corticosteroids has been shown to be effective in ameliorating the side effects of CRS and ICANS. The ZUMA-1 study showed the superiority of prophylactic use of dexamethasone at 10 mg for 3 days before axicabtagene ciloleucel (no grade 3 CRS) compared to the 13% incidence of CRS among patients who received steroids after an infusion of axicabtagene ciloleucel. The efficacy was not compromised in this approach, though there was a higher rate of ICANS [56].

Based on the above information, clinicians should be aware of the potential side effects of CRS and ICANS when using T-cell engagers. Early identification and prompt management are key to preventing the development of severe side effects. A multidisciplinary team with experience in immunotoxicity provides the best outcome.

- TAA-specific toxicities

Other less common but important side effects include hepatotoxicity and cardiac toxicity, which are mostly managed with supportive care and interventions described above. Table 1 lists toxicities described for solid tumor T-cell engagers.

- T-cell engagers undergoing clinical evaluation in solid tumors

Publicly available databases including PubMed, meeting abstracts of major scientific meetings and ClinicalTrials.gov were searched for T-cell engagers that are in the early phases clinical testing (summarized in Table 2).

Table 2. Summary of T-cell engagers in development against solid tumors.

	Target Population	Phase of Study/References	Number of Patients	Results	Clinical Trial Number
CD3/HER2	Advanced HER2-positive breast cancer	Phase 2 [57]	32 patients, 8 patients had stable disease.	The median OS was 13.1, 15.2 and 12.3 months for the entire group, HER2-HR+ and TNBC patients, respectively. Plan for phase 3.	NCT03272334
EGFRvIII/CD3 (AMG596), (CX-904) EGFR/CD3.	EGFRvIII-positive GBM or malignant glioma	Phase 1/1b [58]	Total 14 patients.	1 partial response, 2 stable disease.	NCT03296696
	Tumor expression EGFR	Early phase 1	Plan for 100 patients	Not published	NCT05387265

Table 2. Cont.

	Target Population	Phase of Study/References	Number of Patients	Results	Clinical Trial Number
Tyrosinase Related Protein 1 (TYRP1) (RO7293583)	Melanoma	Phase 1	20 patients	Not published	NCT04551352
MUC17/CD3	Advanced gastric, GE junction, CRC and pancreatic (AMG199)	Phase 1 [59]	Total 64 patients.	13 had PR, 17 SD. CRS > grade 3 occurred in 2%	NCT04117958
	Advanced liver cancer	Phase 2 [60]	11 Patients	Median PFS 4 months, median OS 13.2 months; 5 discontinued treatments due to severe side effects	NCT03146637
DLL3/CD3	Small cell lung cancer	Phase 1 [61]	Confirmed partial responses in 20% of patients and duration of response of 8.7 months	Phase 2 ongoing	NCT05060016
CEA (MEDI-565)	Advanced GI cancers	Phase 1	Total 39 patients,	11 patients have stable disease as best response.	NCT01284231
PSMA	Prostate cancer	Phase 1/2	LAVA-1207	Not published	NCT05369000
		Phase 1 [62]	AMG 509	Not published	NCT04221542
		Phase 1	BAY 2010112	47 patients, 12 patients had >50% decrease in PSA	NCT01723475
EpCAM	Advanced solid tumors	Solitomab: Phase 1 Catumoximab: Phase 2 [63]	Catumoximab and Solitomab: for malignant ascites both associated with sever toxicities precluding development of Solitomab.	Solitomab DLT in phase-limiting escalation. Catumoximab, withdrawn from market due to toxicities.	NCT00635596 NCT00836654
Myeloid-derived suppressor cells (MDSC)	Advanced solid tumors. with and without pembrolizumab	Phase 1	20 patients in monotherapy arm. 10 in combination arm.	Not fully published, study mentioned One CR. Study is going to phase 2.	NCT04128423
CLDN18.2 (AMG 910)	Gastric and gastroesophageal junction (G/GEJ) adenocarcinoma	Phase 1 [64]	Plan recruitment 34 patients	Not finished	(NCT04260191)
HLA-G	Advanced solid tumors	Phase 1	Actively recruiting	Not finished	NCT04991740

4. Conclusions

Bispecific T-cell engagers have emerged as a valid and clinically relevant anti-cancer therapeutic. The practical advantages of T-cell engagers over immune effector cell therapies, such as off-the-shelf availability and avoidance of complex cell handling facilities, broaden the applications of this class of immune therapeutics in cancer care (Table 3).

The majority of bispecific antibodies can be given on an outpatient basis; however, this can vary based on the drug toxicity profile and the clinical condition of the patient. Therefore, there are no standards of care of management, and many clinicians prefer to admit patients to inpatient care for cycle 1 to monitor for side effects before continuing via outpatient care.

Table 3. Comparison of T-cell engagers and CAR-T therapies.

	T-Cell Engagers	CAR-T
Basic Structure	Bispecific antibody that binds TAA and CD3 on T-cells	Engineered T-cell that express engineered scFV fused to linker and activation domain
Source of T-cells	Endogenous T-cell activation	Requires ex vivo expansion of engineered T-cells
Availability	Outpatient	Inpatient and only at high-volume medical centers
Drug properties	Off the shelf	Must be engineered (2–4 weeks)
Dosing	Requires multiple doses, sometimes requires pump	One dose, sometimes multiple dosing if HLA is eliminated
Toxicity	Less CRS	Higher CRS and neurotoxicity
Lymphodepletion prior to treatment	Not required	Required
Operational Cost	High (USD 90,000) per course	Very high (USD 450,000 to 750,000)

CAR-T, chimeric antigen receptor-T-cells; CRS, cytokine release syndrome; scFV, single-chain, fragment variable antibody; TAA, tumor-associated antigen.

Significant efforts are now underway in search of clinically relevant TAAs, optimizing molecular structures and identifying their roles in the treatment of hematologic and solid cancers. The majority of BiTEs in clinical development are directed towards extracellular proteins that represent 10% of the known targetable proteome [65]. Intracellular TAAs are the next frontier for T-cell engagers, and research to direct CD3 cells towards targets such as $p53^{R175H}$ and RAS proteins on MHC molecules of tumor cells are underway [32,66]. Conditional activation of T-cell engagers is another approach to enhance tumor selectivity and on-target/on-tumor efficacy while lessening off-tumor toxicity. Here, inactive T-cell engagers become activated upon entering a tumor by either leveraging tumor proteases or modulating the pH of the microenvironment [67]. In summary, this class of immune therapeutics holds great promise, especially in highly heterogeneous solid tumors, and commands the attention of anti-cancer drug developers.

Author Contributions: M.S.: writing—original draft preparation. W.W.M.: writing—review and editing and supervision. P.F.C. and A.A.A.: writing—review and editing. All authors have read and agreed to the published version of the manuscript.

Funding: This research received no external funding.

Conflicts of Interest: The authors declare no conflict of interest.

References

1. Oostindie, S.C.; Lazar, G.A.; Schuurman, J.; Parren, P. Avidity in antibody effector functions and biotherapeutic drug design. *Nat. Rev. Drug. Discov.* **2022**, *21*, 715–735. [CrossRef] [PubMed]
2. Tran, E.; Robbins, P.F.; Rosenberg, S.A. 'Final common pathway' of human cancer immunotherapy: Targeting random somatic mutations. *Nat. Immunol.* **2017**, *18*, 255–262. [CrossRef] [PubMed]
3. Schumacher, T.N.; Schreiber, R.D. Neoantigens in cancer immunotherapy. *Science* **2015**, *348*, 69–74. [CrossRef] [PubMed]
4. Torka, P.; Barth, M.; Ferdman, R.; Hernandez-Ilizaliturri, F.J. Mechanisms of Resistance to Monoclonal Antibodies (mAbs) in Lymphoid Malignancies. *Curr. Hematol. Malig. Rep.* **2019**, *14*, 426–438. [CrossRef] [PubMed]
5. Pierpont, T.M.; Limper, C.B.; Richards, K.L. Past, Present, and Future of Rituximab-The World's First Oncology Monoclonal Antibody Therapy. *Front. Oncol.* **2018**, *8*, 163. [CrossRef]
6. Ma, J.; Mo, Y.; Tang, M.; Shen, J.; Qi, Y.; Zhao, W.; Huang, Y.; Xu, Y.; Qian, C. Bispecific Antibodies: From Research to Clinical Application. *Front. Immunol.* **2021**, *12*, 626616. [CrossRef]
7. Abanades, B.; Georges, G.; Bujotzek, A.; Deane, C.M. ABlooper: Fast accurate antibody CDR loop structure prediction with accuracy estimation. *Bioinformatics* **2022**, *38*, 1877–1880. [CrossRef]
8. Pantazes, R.J.; Maranas, C.D. OptCDR: A general computational method for the design of antibody complementarity determining regions for targeted epitope binding. *Protein Eng. Des. Sel.* **2010**, *23*, 849–858. [CrossRef]

9. Guest, J.D.; Vreven, T.; Zhou, J.; Moal, I.; Jeliazkov, J.R.; Gray, J.J.; Weng, Z.; Pierce, B.G. An expanded benchmark for antibody-antigen docking and affinity prediction reveals insights into antibody recognition determinants. *Structure* **2021**, *29*, 606–621.e5. [CrossRef]
10. Ambrosetti, F.; Jiménez-García, B.; Roel-Touris, J.; Bonvin, A.M.J.J. Modeling Antibody-Antigen Complexes by Information-Driven Docking. *Structure* **2019**, *28*, 119–129. [CrossRef]
11. Tunyasuvunakool, K.; Adler, J.; Wu, Z.; Green, T.; Zielinski, M.; Žídek, A.; Bridgland, A.; Cowie, A.; Meyer, C.; Laydon, A.; et al. Highly accurate protein structure prediction for the human proteome. *Nature* **2021**, *596*, 590–596. [CrossRef]
12. Dai, B.; Bailey-Kellogg, C. Protein Interaction Interface Region Prediction by Geometric Deep Learning. *Bioinformatics* **2021**, *37*, 2580–2588. [CrossRef] [PubMed]
13. Kuroda, D.; Tsumoto, K. Antibody Affinity Maturation by Computational Design. *Methods Mol. Biol.* **2018**, *1827*, 15–34. [PubMed]
14. Garrido, F. HLA class-I expression and cancer immunotherapy. In *MHC Class-I Loss and Cancer Immune Escape*; Springer: Berlin/Heidelberg, Germany, 2019; pp. 79–90.
15. Dovedi, S.; Mazor, Y.; Elder, M.; Hasani, S.; Wang, B.; Mosely, S.; Jones, D.; Hansen, A.; Yang, C.; Wu, Y.; et al. Abstract 2776: MEDI5752: A novel bispecific antibody that preferentially targets CTLA-4 on PD-1 expressing T-cells. *Cancer Res.* **2018**, *78*, 2776. [CrossRef]
16. Halim, L.; Das, K.K.; Larcombe-Young, D.; Ajina, A.; Candelli, A.; Benjamin, R.; Dillon, R.; Davies, D.M.; Maher, J. Engineering of an Avidity-Optimized CD19-Specific Parallel Chimeric Antigen Receptor That Delivers Dual CD28 and 4-1BB Co-Stimulation. *Front. Immunol.* **2022**, *13*, 836549. [CrossRef]
17. Marei, H.E.; Cenciarelli, C.; Hasan, A. Potential of antibody-drug conjugates (ADCs) for cancer therapy. *Cancer Cell. Int.* **2022**, *22*, 255. [CrossRef]
18. de Goeij, B.E.; Vink, T.; Ten Napel, H.; Breij, E.C.; Satijn, D.; Wubbolts, R.; Miao, D.; Parren, P.W. Efficient Payload Delivery by a Bispecific Antibody-Drug Conjugate Targeting HER2 and CD63. *Mol. Cancer Ther.* **2016**, *15*, 2688–2697. [CrossRef]
19. Andreev, J.; Thambi, N.; Perez Bay, A.E.; Delfino, F.; Martin, J.; Kelly, M.P.; Kirshner, J.R.; Rafique, A.; Kunz, A.; Nittoli, T.; et al. Bispecific Antibodies and Antibody-Drug Conjugates (ADCs) Bridging HER2 and Prolactin Receptor Improve Efficacy of HER2 ADCs. *Mol. Cancer Ther.* **2017**, *16*, 681–693. [CrossRef]
20. Esfandiari, A.; Cassidy, S.; Webster, R.M. Bispecific antibodies in oncology. *Nat. Rev. Drug. Discov.* **2022**, *21*, 411–412. [CrossRef]
21. Schram, A.M.; Goto, K.; Kim, D.-W.; Martin-Romano, P.; Ou, S.-H.I.; O'Kane, G.M.; O'Reilly, E.M.; Umemoto, K.; Duruisseaux, M.; Neuzillet, C.; et al. Efficacy and safety of zenocutuzumab, a HER2 x HER3 bispecific antibody, across advanced NRG1 fusion (NRG1+) cancers. *J. Clin. Oncol.* **2022**, *40*, 105. [CrossRef]
22. Kariolis, M.S.; Wells, R.C.; Getz, J.A.; Kwan, W.; Mahon, C.S.; Tong, R.; Kim, D.J.; Srivastava, A.; Bedard, C.; Henne, K.R.; et al. Brain delivery of therapeutic proteins using an Fc fragment blood-brain barrier transport vehicle in mice and monkeys. *Sci. Transl. Med.* **2020**, *12*, eaay1359. [CrossRef] [PubMed]
23. Yin, W.; Zhao, Y.; Kang, X.; Zhao, P.; Fu, X.; Mo, X.; Wang, Y.; Huang, Y. BBB-penetrating codelivery liposomes treat brain metastasis of non-small cell lung cancer with EGFR(T790M) mutation. *Theranostics* **2020**, *10*, 6122–6135. [CrossRef] [PubMed]
24. Wang, Q.; Chen, Y.; Park, J.; Liu, X.; Hu, Y.; Wang, T.; McFarland, K.; Betenbaugh, M.J. Design and Production of Bispecific Antibodies. *Antibodies* **2019**, *8*, 43. [CrossRef]
25. Wang, L.; Hoseini, S.S.; Xu, H.; Ponomarev, V.; Cheung, N.K. Silencing Fc Domains in T cell-Engaging Bispecific Antibodies Improves T-cell Trafficking and Antitumor Potency. *Cancer Immunol. Res.* **2019**, *7*, 2013–2024. [CrossRef] [PubMed]
26. Ellerman, D. Bispecific T-cell engagers: Towards understanding variables influencing the in vitro potency and tumor selectivity and their modulation to enhance their efficacy and safety. *Methods* **2019**, *154*, 102–117. [CrossRef]
27. Middelburg, J.; Kemper, K.; Engelberts, P.J.; Labrijn, A.F.; Schuurman, J.; van Hall, T. Overcoming Challenges for CD3-Bispecific Antibody Therapy in Solid Tumors. *Cancers* **2021**, *13*, 287. [CrossRef] [PubMed]
28. Baeuerle, P.A. Abstract IAP0301: Bispecific T cell engagers (TCEs) for treatment of solid tumors: Challenges and opportunities. *Mol. Cancer Ther.* **2021**, *20*, IAP0301. [CrossRef]
29. Lin, S.J.; Rocha, S.S.; Kwant, K.; Dayao, M.R.; Ng, T.M.; Banzon, R.R.; Thothathri, S.; Aaron, W.; Callihan, E.; Hemmati, G.; et al. Abstract 933: ProTriTAC is a modular and robust T cell engager prodrug platform with therapeutic index expansion observed across multiple tumor targets. *Cancer Res.* **2021**, *81*, 933. [CrossRef]
30. Weidle, U.H.; Maisel, D.; Klostermann, S.; Schiller, C.; Weiss, E.H. Intracellular proteins displayed on the surface of tumor cells as targets for therapeutic intervention with antibody-related agents. *Cancer Genom. Proteom.* **2011**, *8*, 49–63.
31. Thura, M.; Al-Aidaroos, A.Q.O.; Yong, W.P.; Kono, K.; Gupta, A.; Lin, Y.B.; Mimura, K.; Thiery, J.P.; Goh, B.C.; Tan, P.; et al. PRL3-zumab, a first-in-class humanized antibody for cancer therapy. *JCI Insight* **2016**, *1*, e87607. [CrossRef]
32. Hsiue, E.H.; Wright, K.M.; Douglass, J.; Hwang, M.S.; Mog, B.J.; Pearlman, A.H.; Paul, S.; DiNapoli, S.R.; Konig, M.F.; Wang, Q.; et al. Targeting a neoantigen derived from a common TP53 mutation. *Science* **2021**, *371*, eabc8697. [CrossRef] [PubMed]
33. Hong, D.S.; Van Tine, B.A.; Biswas, S.; McAlpine, C.; Johnson, M.L.; Olszanski, A.J.; Clarke, J.M.; Araujo, D.; Blumenschein, G.R., Jr.; Kebriaei, P.; et al. Autologous T cell therapy for MAGE-A4(+) solid cancers in HLA-A*02(+) patients: A phase 1 trial. *Nat. Med.* **2023**, *29*, 104–114. [CrossRef] [PubMed]
34. Shin, S.-M.; Kim, J.-S.; Park, S.-W.; Jun, S.-Y.; Kweon, H.-J.; Choi, D.-K.; Lee, D.; Cho, Y.B.; Kim, Y.-S. Direct targeting of oncogenic RAS mutants with a tumor-specific cytosol-penetrating antibody inhibits RAS mutant–driven tumor growth. *Sci. Adv.* **2020**, *6*, eaay2174. [CrossRef] [PubMed]

35. Sosman, J.A.; Carrillo, C.; Urba, W.J.; Flaherty, L.; Atkins, M.B.; Clark, J.I.; Dutcher, J.; Margolin, K.A.; Mier, J.; Gollob, J.; et al. Three phase II cytokine working group trials of gp100 (210M) peptide plus high-dose interleukin-2 in patients with HLA-A2-positive advanced melanoma. *J. Clin. Oncol.* **2008**, *26*, 2292–2298. [CrossRef]
36. Carvajal, R.D.; Nathan, P.; Sacco, J.J.; Orloff, M.; Hernandez-Aya, L.F.; Yang, J.; Luke, J.J.; Butler, M.O.; Stanhope, S.; Collins, L.; et al. Phase I Study of Safety, Tolerability, and Efficacy of Tebentafusp Using a Step-Up Dosing Regimen and Expansion in Patients With Metastatic Uveal Melanoma. *J. Clin. Oncol.* **2022**, *40*, 1939–1948. [CrossRef]
37. Middleton, M.R.; McAlpine, C.; Woodcock, V.K.; Corrie, P.; Infante, J.R.; Steven, N.M.; Evans, T.R.J.; Anthoney, A.; Shoushtari, A.N.; Hamid, O.; et al. Tebentafusp, A TCR/Anti-CD3 Bispecific Fusion Protein Targeting gp100, Potently Activated Antitumor Immune Responses in Patients with Metastatic Melanoma. *Clin. Cancer Res.* **2020**, *26*, 5869–5878. [CrossRef]
38. Nathan, P.; Hassel, J.C.; Rutkowski, P.; Baurain, J.F.; Butler, M.O.; Schlaak, M.; Sullivan, R.J.; Ochsenreither, S.; Dummer, R.; Kirkwood, J.M.; et al. Overall Survival Benefit with Tebentafusp in Metastatic Uveal Melanoma. *N. Engl. J. Med.* **2021**, *385*, 1196–1206. [CrossRef]
39. Linke, R.; Klein, A.; Seimetz, D. Catumaxomab: Clinical development and future directions. *mAbs* **2010**, *2*, 129–136. [CrossRef]
40. Borlak, J.; Länger, F.; Spanel, R.; Schöndorfer, G.; Dittrich, C. Immune-mediated liver injury of the cancer therapeutic antibody catumaxomab targeting EpCAM, CD3 and Fcγ receptors. *Oncotarget* **2016**, *7*, 28059–28074. [CrossRef]
41. Hummel, H.-D.; Kufer, P.; Grüllich, C.; Deschler-Baier, B.; Chatterjee, M.; Goebeler, M.-E.; Miller, K.; Santis, M.D.; Loidl, W.C.; Buck, A.; et al. Phase 1 study of pasotuxizumab (BAY 2010112), a PSMA-targeting Bispecific T cell Engager (BiTE) immunotherapy for metastatic castration-resistant prostate cancer (mCRPC). *J. Clin. Oncol.* **2019**, *37*, 5034. [CrossRef]
42. Tran, B.; Horvath, L.G.; Dorff, T.B.; Greil, R.; Machiels, J.-P.H.; Roncolato, F.T.; Autio, K.A.; Rettig, M.B.; Fizazi, K.; Lolkema, M.P.; et al. Phase I study of AMG 160, a half-life extended bispecific T-cell engager (HLE BiTE) immune therapy targeting prostate-specific membrane antigen (PSMA), in patients with metastatic castration-resistant prostate cancer (mCRPC). *J. Clin. Oncol.* **2020**, *38*, TPS5590. [CrossRef]
43. ESMO Virtual Congress 2020: Novel Immunotherapy for Prostate Cancer—AMG 160—PSMA-Targeted, Bispecific T-Cell Engager (BiTE®) Immune Therapy for Metastatic Castration-Resistant Prostate Cancer—Invited Discussan. Available online: https://www.urotoday.com/conference-highlights/esmo-2020/prostate-cancer/124635-esmo-virtual-congress-2020-novel-immunotherapy-for-prostate-cancer-amg-160-psma-targeted-bispecific-t-cell-engager-bite-immune-therapy-for-metastatic-castration-resistant-prostate-cancer-invited-discussant.html (accessed on 14 May 2023).
44. Tolcher, A.W.; Gordon, M.; Mahoney, K.M.; Seto, A.; Zavodovskaya, M.; Hsueh, C.H.; Zhai, S.; Tarnowski, T.; Jürgensmeier, J.M.; Stinson, S.; et al. Phase 1 first-in-human study of dalutrafusp alfa, an anti-CD73-TGF-β-trap bifunctional antibody, in patients with advanced solid tumors. *J. Immunother. Cancer* **2023**, *11*, e005267. [CrossRef] [PubMed]
45. Cheng, P.; Chen, X.; Dalton, R.; Calescibetta, A.; So, T.; Gilvary, D.; Ward, G.; Smith, V.; Eckard, S.; Fox, J.A.; et al. Immunodepletion of MDSC by AMV564, a novel bivalent, bispecific CD33/CD3 T cell engager, ex vivo in MDS and melanoma. *Mol. Ther.* **2022**, *30*, 2315–2326. [CrossRef] [PubMed]
46. Mettu, N.B.; Starodub, A.; Piha-Paul, S.A.A.; Abdul-Karim, R.M.; Tinoco, G.; Shafique, M.R.; Smith, V.; Baccei, C.; Chun, P.Y. Results of a phase 1 dose-escalation study of AMV564, a novel T-cell engager, alone and in combination with pembrolizumab in patients with relapsed/refractory solid tumors. *J. Clin. Oncol.* **2021**, *39*, 2555. [CrossRef]
47. Yan, Z.; Zhang, H.; Cao, J.; Zhang, C.; Liu, H.; Huang, H.; Cheng, H.; Qiao, J.; Wang, Y.; Wang, Y.; et al. Characteristics and Risk Factors of Cytokine Release Syndrome in Chimeric Antigen Receptor T Cell Treatment. *Front. Immunol.* **2021**, *12*, 611366. [CrossRef]
48. Weddell, J. Mechanistically modeling peripheral cytokine dynamics following bispecific dosing in solid tumors. *CPT Pharmacomet. Syst. Pharmacol.* **2023**. Online ahead of print. [CrossRef]
49. Morris, E.C.; Neelapu, S.S.; Giavridis, T.; Sadelain, M. Cytokine release syndrome and associated neurotoxicity in cancer immunotherapy. *Nat. Rev. Immunol.* **2022**, *22*, 85–96. [CrossRef]
50. Lesokhin, A.M.; Levy, M.Y.; Dalovisio, A.P.; Bahlis, N.J.; Solh, M.; Sebag, M.; Jakubowiak, A.; Jethava, Y.S.; Costello, C.L.; Chu, M.P.; et al. Preliminary Safety, Efficacy, Pharmacokinetics, and Pharmacodynamics of Subcutaneously (SC) Administered PF-06863135, a B-Cell Maturation Antigen (BCMA)-CD3 Bispecific Antibody, in Patients with Relapsed/Refractory Multiple Myeloma (RRMM). *Blood* **2020**, *136*, 8–9. [CrossRef]
51. Selvaggio, G.; Parolo, S.; Bora, P.; Leonardelli, L.; Harrold, J.; Mehta, K.; Rock, D.A.; Marchetti, L. Computational Analysis of Cytokine Release Following Bispecific T-Cell Engager Therapy: Applications of a Logic-Based Model. *Front. Oncol.* **2022**, *12*, 818641. [CrossRef]
52. Neelapu, S.S.; Tummala, S.; Kebriaei, P.; Wierda, W.; Gutierrez, C.; Locke, F.L.; Komanduri, K.V.; Lin, Y.; Jain, N.; Daver, N.; et al. Chimeric antigen receptor T-cell therapy—Assessment and management of toxicities. *Nat. Rev. Clin. Oncol.* **2018**, *15*, 47–62. [CrossRef]
53. Lee, D.W.; Santomasso, B.D.; Locke, F.L.; Ghobadi, A.; Turtle, C.J.; Brudno, J.N.; Maus, M.V.; Park, J.H.; Mead, E.; Pavletic, S.; et al. ASTCT Consensus Grading for Cytokine Release Syndrome and Neurologic Toxicity Associated with Immune Effector Cells. *Biol. Blood Marrow Transplant.* **2019**, *25*, 625–638. [CrossRef] [PubMed]
54. Si, S.; Teachey, D.T. Spotlight on Tocilizumab in the Treatment of CAR-T-Cell-Induced Cytokine Release Syndrome: Clinical Evidence to Date. *Ther. Clin. Risk Manag.* **2020**, *16*, 705–714. [PubMed]

55. Gust, J.; Hay, K.A.; Hanafi, L.A.; Li, D.; Myerson, D.; Gonzalez-Cuyar, L.F.; Yeung, C.; Liles, W.C.; Wurfel, M.; Lopez, J.A.; et al. Endothelial Activation and Blood-Brain Barrier Disruption in Neurotoxicity after Adoptive Immunotherapy with CD19 CAR-T Cells. *Cancer Discov.* **2017**, *7*, 1404–1419. [CrossRef] [PubMed]
56. Oluwole, O.O.; Bouabdallah, K.; Muñoz, J.; De Guibert, S.; Vose, J.M.; Bartlett, N.L.; Lin, Y.; Deol, A.; McSweeney, P.A.; Goy, A.H.; et al. Prophylactic corticosteroid use in patients receiving axicabtagene ciloleucel for large B-cell lymphoma. *Br. J. Haematol.* **2021**, *194*, 690–700. [CrossRef] [PubMed]
57. Lum, L.G.; Al-Kadhimi, Z.; Deol, A.; Kondadasula, V.; Schalk, D.; Tomashewski, E.; Steele, P.; Fields, K.; Giroux, M.; Liu, Q.; et al. Phase II clinical trial using anti-CD3 × anti-HER2 bispecific antibody armed activated T cells (HER2 BATs) consolidation therapy for HER2 negative (0-2+) metastatic breast cancer. *J. Immunother. Cancer* **2021**, *9*, e002194. [CrossRef] [PubMed]
58. Sternjak, A.; Lee, F.; Thomas, O.; Balazs, M.; Wahl, J.; Lorenczewski, G.; Ullrich, I.; Muenz, M.; Rattel, B.; Bailis, J.M.; et al. Preclinical Assessment of AMG 596, a Bispecific T-cell Engager (BiTE) Immunotherapy Targeting the Tumor-specific Antigen EGFRvIII. *Mol. Cancer Ther.* **2021**, *20*, 925–933. [CrossRef]
59. Chao, J.; Buxó, E.; Cervantes, A.; Dayyani, F.; Lima, C.M.S.P.R.; Greil, R.; Laarhoven, H.W.M.V.; Lorenzen, S.; Heinemann, V.; Kischel, R.; et al. Trial in progress: A phase I study of AMG 199, a half-life extended bispecific T-cell engager (HLE BiTE) immune therapy, targeting MUC17 in patients with gastric and gastroesophageal junction (G/GEJ) cancer. *J. Clin. Oncol.* **2020**, *38*, TPS4649. [CrossRef]
60. Lu, Y.Y.; Yu, H.; Tang, Y. Efficacy and safety of MUC1 targeted CIK cells for the treatment of advanced liver cancer. *J. Clin. Oncol.* **2021**, *39*, e16278. [CrossRef]
61. Wermke, M.; Felip, E.; Gambardella, V.; Kuboki, Y.; Morgensztern, D.; Oum'Hamed, Z.; Geng, J.; Studeny, M.; Owonikoko, T.K. A phase I, open-label, dose-escalation trial of BI 764532, a DLL3/CD3 bispecific antibody, in patients (pts) with small cell lung carcinoma (SCLC) or other neuroendocrine neoplasms expressing DLL3. *J. Clin. Oncol.* **2021**, *39*, TPS8588. [CrossRef]
62. Danila, D.C.; Waterhouse, D.M.; Appleman, L.J.; Pook, D.W.; Matsubara, N.; Dorff, T.B.; Lee, J.-L.; Armstrong, A.J.; Kim, M.; Horvath, L.; et al. A phase 1 study of AMG 509 in patients (pts) with metastatic castration-resistant prostate cancer (mCRPC). *J. Clin. Oncol.* **2022**, *40*, TPS5101. [CrossRef]
63. Heiss, M.M.; Murawa, P.; Koralewski, P.; Kutarska, E.; Kolesnik, O.O.; Ivanchenko, V.V.; Dudnichenko, A.S.; Aleknaviciene, B.; Razbadauskas, A.; Gore, M.; et al. The trifunctional antibody catumaxomab for the treatment of malignant ascites due to epithelial cancer: Results of a prospective randomized phase II/III trial. *Int. J. Cancer* **2010**, *127*, 2209–2221. [CrossRef] [PubMed]
64. Lordick, F.; Chao, J.; Buxò, E.; van Laarhoven, H.; Lima, C.; Lorenzen, S.; Dayyani, F.; Heinemann, V.; Greil, R.; Stienen, S. 1496TiP Phase I study evaluating safety and tolerability of AMG 910, a half-life extended bispecific T cell engager targeting claudin-18.2 (CLDN18. 2) in gastric and gastroesophageal junction (G/GEJ) adenocarcinoma. *Ann. Oncol.* **2020**, *31*, S928–S929. [CrossRef]
65. de Souza, J.E.; Galante, P.A.; de Almeida, R.V.; da Cunha, J.P.; Ohara, D.T.; Ohno-Machado, L.; Old, L.J.; de Souza, S.J. SurfaceomeDB: A cancer-orientated database for genes encoding cell surface proteins. *Cancer Immun.* **2012**, *12*, 15. [PubMed]
66. Malekzadeh, P.; Pasetto, A.; Robbins, P.F.; Parkhurst, M.R.; Paria, B.C.; Jia, L.; Gartner, J.J.; Hill, V.; Yu, Z.; Restifo, N.P.; et al. Neoantigen screening identifies broad TP53 mutant immunogenicity in patients with epithelial cancers. *J. Clin. Investig.* **2019**, *129*, 1109–1114. [CrossRef]
67. Cattaruzza, F.; Nazeer, A.; Lange, Z.; Hammond, M.; Koski, C.; Henkensiefken, A.; Derynck, M.K.; Irving, B.; Schellenberger, V. Abstract 3376: HER2-XPAT and EGFR-XPAT: Pro-drug T-cell engagers (TCEs) engineered to address on-target, off-tumor toxicity with potent efficacy in vitro and in vivo and large safety margins in NHP. *Cancer Res.* **2020**, *80*, 3376. [CrossRef]

Disclaimer/Publisher's Note: The statements, opinions and data contained in all publications are solely those of the individual author(s) and contributor(s) and not of MDPI and/or the editor(s). MDPI and/or the editor(s) disclaim responsibility for any injury to people or property resulting from any ideas, methods, instructions or products referred to in the content.

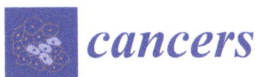

Article

mRNA-Lipid Nanoparticle (LNP) Delivery of Humanized EpCAM-CD3 Bispecific Antibody Significantly Blocks Colorectal Cancer Tumor Growth

Vita Golubovskaya [1,*], John Sienkiewicz [1], Jinying Sun [1], Yanwei Huang [1], Liang Hu [1], Hua Zhou [1], Hizkia Harto [1], Shirley Xu [1], Robert Berahovich [1], Walter Bodmer [2] and Lijun Wu [1,3,*]

1. Promab Biotechnologies, 2600 Hilltop Drive, Richmond, CA 94806, USA; liang.hu@promab.com (L.H.)
2. Cancer & Immunogenetics Laboratory, Weatherall Institute of Molecular Medicine, John Radcliffe Hospital, Oxford OX3 9DS, UK
3. Forevertek Biotechnology, Janshan Road, Changsha Hi-Tech Industrial Development Zone, Changsha 410205, China
* Correspondence: vita.gol@promab.com (V.G.); john@promab.com (L.W.); Tel.: +1-510-974-0697 (V.G.); +1-510-529-3021 (L.W.)

Simple Summary: Colorectal cancer is one of the most common cancers worldwide, and novel treatments are urgently needed to improve treatment for cancer patients. In this report, three different designs of humanized EpCAM-CD3 antibodies were engineered and tested against colorectal tumors. The antibodies demonstrated high efficacy and specificity. In addition, the study demonstrates a novel method of delivering bispecific antibodies using mRNA-lipid nanoparticle (LNP) technology. The delivery of EpCAM-CD3 human Fc (hFc) mRNA-LNPs into mice tumors with intravenous T cell injection significantly blocked OVCAR-5 xenograft tumor growth in vivo. The data provide a basis for future clinical studies.

Citation: Golubovskaya, V.; Sienkiewicz, J.; Sun, J.; Huang, Y.; Hu, L.; Zhou, H.; Harto, H.; Xu, S.; Berahovich, R.; Bodmer, W.; et al. mRNA-Lipid Nanoparticle (LNP) Delivery of Humanized EpCAM-CD3 Bispecific Antibody Significantly Blocks Colorectal Cancer Tumor Growth. *Cancers* **2023**, *15*, 2860. https://doi.org/10.3390/cancers15102860

Academic Editor: Alfons Navarro

Received: 18 March 2023
Revised: 19 May 2023
Accepted: 20 May 2023
Published: 22 May 2023

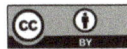

Copyright: © 2023 by the authors. Licensee MDPI, Basel, Switzerland. This article is an open access article distributed under the terms and conditions of the Creative Commons Attribution (CC BY) license (https://creativecommons.org/licenses/by/4.0/).

Abstract: The epithelial cell adhesion molecule (EpCAM) is often overexpressed in many types of tumors, including colorectal cancer. We sequenced and humanized an EpCAM mouse antibody and used it to develop bispecific EpCAM-CD3 antibodies. Three different designs were used to generate bispecific antibodies such as EpCAM-CD3 CrossMab knob-in-hole, EpCAM ScFv-CD3 ScFv (BITE), and EpCAM ScFv-CD3 ScFv-human Fc designs. These antibody designs showed strong and specific binding to the EpCAM-positive Lovo cell line and T cells, specifically killed EpCAM-positive Lovo cells and not EpCAM-negative Colo741 cells in the presence of T cells, and increased T cells' IFN-gamma secretion in a dose-dependent manner. In addition, transfection of HEK-293 cells with EpCAM ScFv-CD3 ScFv human Fc mRNA-LNPs resulted in antibody secretion that killed Lovo cells and did not kill EpCAM-negative Colo741 cells. The antibody increased IFN-gamma secretion against Lovo target cells and did not increase it against Colo741 target cells. EpCAM-CD3 hFc mRNA-LNP transfection of several cancer cell lines (A1847, C30, OVCAR-5) also demonstrated functional bispecific antibody secretion. In addition, intratumoral delivery of the EpCAM-CD3 human Fc mRNA-LNPs into OVCAR-5 tumor xenografts combined with intravenous injection of T cells significantly blocked xenograft tumor growth. Thus, EpCAM-CD3 hFc mRNA-LNP delivery to tumor cells shows strong potential for future clinical studies.

Keywords: colorectal cancer; EpCAM; CD3; bispecific antibody

1. Introduction

Colorectal cancer is one of the most common cancers worldwide [1,2]. Patients with metastatic colorectal cancer will typically have a poor prognosis and a low survival rate. Recently, different approaches for colorectal cancer therapy have been developed such as monoclonal antibodies, vaccines, checkpoint inhibitors, oncolytic viruses, and CAR-T cell therapy [3,4]. Novel therapeutic approaches are urgently needed to improve treatment for patients with colorectal cancer.

One of the attractive targets for immunotherapy is EpCAM (CD326), a 39–40 kDa human cell surface glycoprotein, which is highly expressed in many cancer cells such as ovarian, breast, colorectal, prostate, lung, pancreatic, and others [5]. EpCAM was discovered over 40 years ago as an epithelial antigen and was later classified as a cell adhesion molecule [6]. EpCAM plays an important role in colorectal cancer biology and is also involved in survival signaling, motility, differentiation, cell proliferation, adhesion, and metastasis [6–8]. EpCAM can be expressed not only in epithelial cells but also in the stem cells of different tissues and in embryonic stem cells [9]. Recently, the EpCAM AUA1 antibody was used to detect circulating tumor cells, which can be used for the early detection of many carcinomas [10].

EpCAM shows high potential as a target for developing anticancer therapies and immunotherapies with monoclonal antibodies or bispecific antibodies. Recent studies have targeted EpCAM with monoclonal antibodies [11], bispecific antibodies, immunotherapy [12], siRNA, and CAR-T cells [5,13–16].

Recently, lipid nanoparticles (LNPs) were used for the delivery of the COVID-19 mRNA vaccine by the biopharmaceutical companies Moderna and Pfizer [17–19]. The nanoparticle-based drug delivery demonstrated many advantages, such as high bioavailability, solubility, stability, passage through the blood–brain barrier, and low toxicity and minimal side effects [20].

In this study, mRNA-LNPs were used to deliver EpCAM-CD3 bispecific antibodies to tumor sites, stimulating T cells to kill colorectal tumors. Three different formats of novel bispecific antibodies based on the humanized AUA1 antibody [10] were engineered for this study. All bispecific antibodies demonstrated high efficacy and specificity with the EpCAM-positive Lovo cell line but not with the EpCAM-negative Colo741 cell line. In addition, we designed EpCAM-CD3 hFc mRNA, which was embedded into an LNP complex, and showed that the secreted antibodies had highly specific and effective killing activity when combined with T cells and induced the secretion of IFN-gamma in a dose-dependent manner against the EpCAM-positive target colorectal cell line. We also showed that OVCAR-5, A1847, and C30 cancer cells transfected with EpCAM-CD3 mRNA-LNPs secreted EpCAM-CD3 antibodies with high cytotoxic activity. In addition, EpCAM-CD3 hFc mRNA-LNP delivery to OVCAR-5 xenograft tumors with the intravenous injection of T cells demonstrated a significant decrease in tumor growth in vivo. These data provide a basis for the generation of EpCAM-CD3 antibodies in vivo through the mRNA-LNP delivery platform. The produced EpCAM-CD3 hFc antibody shows high antitumor efficacy and potential for use in clinical studies.

2. Materials and Methods

2.1. Cell Lines

The HEK-293, A1847, C30, OVCAR-5, HeLa, Hep3B, SKOV-3, and PC3 cell lines were obtained from ATCC. The A1847, C30, HeLa, Hep3B, and OVCAR-5 cells were cultured in Dulbecco's modified Eagle's medium (DMEM) medium with 10% FBS and penicillin/streptomycin. The PC3 cell line was cultured in an F-12K medium with 10% FBS and penicillin/streptomycin. The SKOV-3 cell line was cultured in a McCoy's 5A medium with 10% FBS and penicillin/streptomycin. Lovo and Colo741 cell lines were obtained from Dr. Walter Bodmer (Oxford University, Oxford, UK), whose laboratory authenticated the cell lines using SNPs, Sequenom MassARRAY iPLEX, and HumanOmniExpress-24 BeadChip arrays, and tested for the absence of Mycoplasma [21]. The Lovo cell line was cultured in Ham's F-12 K Medium with 10% FBS and penicillin/streptomycin. The Colo741 cell line was cultured in an RPMI-1640 medium with 10% FBS and penicillin/streptomycin. The Lovo cell line with knockout of EpCAM (Lovo EpCAM KO) was generated using electroporation of the EpCAM sgRNA kit from Synthego and caspase-9 protein following the manufacturer's protocol. The HEK-293 suspension cells were cultured in a FreeStyle™

F17 expression medium and supplemented with Gibco™ GlutaMAX™ and Pluronic™ F-68 nonionic surfactant (100×). The cell lines were authenticated by FACS using specific cell surface marker detection antibodies. Human peripheral blood mononuclear cells (PBMCs) were isolated from whole blood from the Stanford Hospital Blood Center according to the IRB-approved protocol (#13942). PBMCs were isolated using density sedimentation over Ficoll-Paque (GE Healthcare, Chicago, IL, USA) [22–25]. PBMCs were suspended at 1×10^6 cells/mL in an AIM-V medium (ThermoFisher, Waltham, MA, USA) containing 10% FBS and 10 ng/mL IL-2 (ThermoFisher), mixed with CD3/CD28 Dynabeads (ThermoFisher) at a 1:1 ratio, and cultured for 10–12 days in 24-well plates. Fresh medium with 10 ng/mL IL-2 was added every 2–3 days to maintain the PBMC cell number at $1-2 \times 10^6$ cells/mL. All cell lines and PBMCs were cultured in a humidified 5% CO_2 incubator.

2.2. Antibodies

APC antihuman CD326 (EpCAM) antibody was obtained from Biolegend (Cat No.: 324207). PE-conjugated anti-His tag antibody was from Biolegend (Cat. No.: 362603). APC antihuman CD3 antibody was obtained from Biolegend (Cat No.: 317318). Antihuman IgG was from Jackson ImmunoResearch (109-605-190). PE streptavidin was obtained from Biolegend (Cat. No.: 405204) and 7-AAD viability staining solution was obtained from Biolegend (Cat. No.: 420404).

2.3. Design and Cloning of Bispecific Antibody DNA Constructs

The AUA1 antibody was produced conventionally by immunizing BALB/c mice with the colon adenocarcinoma cell line Lovo. The mouse AUA1 EpCAM antibody was characterized by Dr. Walter Bodmer's Lab and described in [26]. Humanization of the mouse AUA1 antibody [27] was performed as described in [28,29]. The humanized antibody was first checked for functional activity in the chimeric antigen receptor (CAR) format as described in [29,30]. The humanized variable fragment heavy chain (VH) and light fragment chain (VL) of the AUA1 antibody were used for the engineering of CrossMab knob-in-hole design bivalent antibody constructs as described in [21]. Human Fc (IgG1) contained P329G and L234AL235A (LALA) mutations to silence the Fc region by preventing the binding of gamma receptors and activating innate immune cells [21]. Another design contained an EpCAM ScFv-CD3 ScFv-His tag (BITE) format. The third design was an EpCAM ScFv-CD3 ScFv-human Fc construct. All constructs were cloned into the pYD11 vector and confirmed by sequencing. For the design of DNA templates for RNA-based expression, the EpCAM ScFv-CD3 ScFv-human Fc sequence was cloned into a DNA vector with a T7AG promoter, 5′UTR, 3′UTR, and a 150 poly A tail as described [31]. The DNA template sequence for in vitro transcription was verified by sequencing.

2.4. In Vitro Transcription

The mRNA was in vitro transcribed from a DNA template using the HiScribe T7 mRNA Kit with CleanCap Reagent AG (NEB #E2080). In brief, a DNA template, $0.5 \times$ T7 CleanCap Reagent AG Reaction Buffer, 5 mM of ATP, CTP, pseudo-UTP, and GTP were added to 4 mM of CleanCapAG and T7 polymerase mix for 2 h at 37 °C. Then, DNAse I treatment was performed for 15 min at 37 °C. The mRNA was purified with the Monarch RNA Cleanup Kit (T2050) according to the manufacturer's protocol.

2.5. Embedding of mRNA into LNP and Transfection of mRNA-LNP into Cells

To generate an mRNA–LNP complex, an aqueous solution of mRNA in 100 mM sodium acetate (pH 4.0) was combined with a lipid mix containing the ethanol phase of SM-102 (Cayman), DSPC (Avanti), cholesterol (Sigma), and DMG-PEG2000 (Cayman) (at a molar % ratio of 50:10:38.5:1.5, respectively) at a flow rate ratio of 3:1 (aqueous:organic) using the PreciGenome Flex S System (San Jose, CA, USA). The mRNA-LNPs were purified and concentrated using Amicon® Ultra-15 centrifugal filter units (30–100 kDa). The size, zeta-potential, and polydispersity index (PDI) of the mRNA-LNPs were detected using an Anton Paar Litesizer 500 System, and the encapsulation efficiency was checked with the Quant-it™ RiboGreen RNA assay Kit. The mean mRNA-LNP size was 104 nm; the zeta-potential was −4.8 mV; the PDI was 0.14; and the encapsulation efficiency was 91.8 ± 4.5%.

In brief, 1 µg of mRNA-LNPs was used to transfect $0.5–1 \times 10^6$ HEK-293 cells or other cancer cell lines. The supernatant with secreted EpCAM-CD3 hFc bispecific antibody was collected 48–72 h after transfection, and the correct size was confirmed through Western blotting. The binding with target cells was performed using FACS.

2.6. Transfection of HEK-293 Cells with DNA Encoding Bispecific Antibodies

HEK293S cells were transfected using DNA constructs of the bispecific antibodies with the ALSTEM NanoFect Transfection Reagent. The cells were cultured in Freestyle F17 medium with 8 mM glutamine and 0.1% Pluronic F68 surfactant in suspension bottles using a shaker at 37 °C and 5% CO_2. Supernatants containing antibodies were collected on days 3–7 posttransfection. The supernatants containing antibodies with human Fc were purified using protein A or protein G columns. The supernatant containing EpCAM-CD3-His tag antibody was purified using Ni-NTA columns. The purified antibodies were checked for size on SDS gel and then used for functional analyses.

2.7. Flow Cytometry (FACS)

To measure the binding of the bispecific antibodies, 0.25×10^6 cells were suspended in 0.1 mL of 1 × PBS buffer containing 2 mM EDTA and 0.5% BSA and incubated on ice with 1 µL of human serum (Jackson ImmunoResearch, West Grove, PA, USA) for 10 min. The bispecific antibodies were added to the cells, which were then incubated on ice for 30 min. The cells were washed 3 times with FACS buffer and resuspended in 0.1 mL of buffer. Then, 1 µL of phycoerythrin (PE)-conjugated or APC-conjugated secondary antibody (BD Biosciences, San Jose, CA, USA) was added, and the cells were incubated on ice for 30 min. The antibodies containing human Fc or His Tag were stained with an antihuman-IgG antibody or anti-His tag antibody, respectively, and incubated on ice for 30 min, washed with FACS buffer three times, and stained with PE-streptavidin antibody on ice for 30 min. The cells were washed three times and resuspended in buffer for analysis on an FACSCalibur (BD Biosciences).

Supernatants containing EpCAM-CD3-hFc antibody (resulting from mRNA-LNP transfection to cancer cells) were collected 48–72 h posttransfection and incubated with the target cells on ice for 30 min. Cells were washed three times with FACS buffer, stained with antihuman-IgG (Fc fragment specific) (Jackson ImmunoResearch), and incubated on ice for 30 min. Cells were washed three times with FACS buffer and resuspended in the buffer for analysis on an FACSCalibur (BD Biosciences).

2.8. Real-Time Cytotoxicity Assay (RTCA)

Adherent Lovo ($EpCAM^+$) and Colo741 ($EpCAM^−$) target cells were seeded in triplicate into 96-well E-plates (Acea Biosciences/Agilent, San Diego, CA, USA) at $1–4 \times 10^4$ cells per well overnight using the impedance-based real-time cell analysis (RTCA) xCELLigence system (Acea Biosciences/Agilent). The next day, the medium was removed and replaced with AIM-V medium containing 10% FBS. Effector T cells were added to the target cells at a 10:1 ratio either alone or with different dilutions of antibodies, in triplicate. The cells in the E-plates were monitored for 24 h with the RTCA system, and the impedance was plotted over time. The supernatant was collected after RTCA and used in an ELISA to detect IFN-gamma secretion.

2.9. ELISA (Enzyme-Linked Immunoassay)

Target cells were cultured with different dilutions of bispecific antibodies in U-bottom 96-well plates in 200 µL of AIM-V medium containing 10% FBS, in triplicate, and then analyzed with the ELISA to determine human IFN-gamma secretion levels using the R&D

Systems Human IFN-gamma Quantikine Kit (Minneapolis, MN, USA) according to the manufacturer's protocol.

2.10. Mouse Xenograft Tumor Model

Six-week-old NSG mice (Jackson Laboratories, Bar Harbor, ME, USA) were housed and handled in strict accordance with the Institutional Animal Care and Use Committee (#LUM-001) (IACUC) guidelines. Each mouse was injected subcutaneously on day 0 with 100 µL of 2×10^6 OVCAR-5 cells. EpCAM-CD3 hFc mRNA-LNPs were injected intratumorally (1 µg/mice) on certain days, and 1×10^7 T cells were injected either 1 or 3 times intravenously 24–48 h after the injection of mRNA-LNPs. The tumors were measured twice a week with calipers, and the tumor volume was calculated using the following formula: $1/2$ (Length $\times$ Width^2). Tumor growth curves were generated for each group.

2.11. Statistical Analysis

Comparison between two groups was performed using the unpaired Student's *t*-test. Differences with $p < 0.05$ were considered significant.

3. Results

3.1. The AUA1 Mouse Antibody Was Humanized and Used to Engineer Three Designs of Humanized AUA1-CD3 Bispecific Antibodies

We used the mouse AUA1 antibody [26] for FACS with several different cancer cell lines and detected high binding to different types of cancer cell lines such as cervical cancer HeLa, hepatocellular carcinoma Hep3B, colorectal Lovo, ovarian SKOV-3, and prostate PC3 cancer cell lines (Figure 1A). We humanized the AUA1 antibody and tested binding by FACS using the EpCAM-positive Lovo cancer cell line and the EpCAM knockout (KO) Lovo cell line generated with CRISPR/Cas-9. The humanized EpCAM antibody showed binding to Lovo cells and did not show binding to the Lovo EpCAM-KO cell line (Figure 1B). This demonstrates the high specificity of the humanized AUA1 antibody.

We used this humanized antibody to generate bispecific antibodies using three different designs: bivalent EpCAM-CD3 CrossMab knob-in-hole with silenced Fc, EpCAM-CD3 KIH Fc (Figure 1C); EpCAM ScFv-CD3 ScFv-His tag (BITE) (Figure 1D); and EpCAM ScFv-CD3 ScFv human Fc (Figure 1E). All antibodies were purified, checked for correct size on SDS gel, and used for functional analysis with FACS, real-time cytotoxicity assay (RTCA), and IFN-gamma secretion.

3.2. EpCAM-CD3 Bispecific Antibodies Caused High Binding, Killing, and IFN-Gamma Secretion with EpCAM-Positive Target Cancer Cells

We tested bivalent EpCAM-CD3 CrossMab KIH Fc for binding to EpCAM-positive Lovo cells and CD3-positive T cells (Figure 2A) using FACS. The antibody showed binding to Lovo cells and T cells (Figure 2A) and did not show binding to EpCAM-negative Colo741 cells (not shown). The EpCAM-CD3 CrossMab KIH Fc killed Lovo cells when combined with T cells in a dose-dependent manner using the Agilent RTCA system (Figure 2B). The supernatant was collected and tested for the secretion of IFN-gamma by T cells, which showed high levels of secretion with Lovo target cells and did not show any increase in IFN-gamma secretion with Colo741 target cells (Figure 2C). Thus, EpCAM-CD3 CrossMab KIH Fc has high dose-dependent efficacy against EpCAM-positive Lovo cells.

Next, we tested the EpCAM-CD3 (BITE) antibody for binding to Lovo and T cells using FACS (Figure 3A). The antibody showed high binding to Lovo and T cells (Figure 3A). The antibody combined with T cells killed Lovo target cells (Figure 3B) and did not kill Colo741 cells (not shown). The EpCAM-CD3 antibody combined with T cells showed a high level of secreted IFN-gamma with Lovo target cells and did not show it with EpCAM-negative Colo741 target cells (Figure 3C).

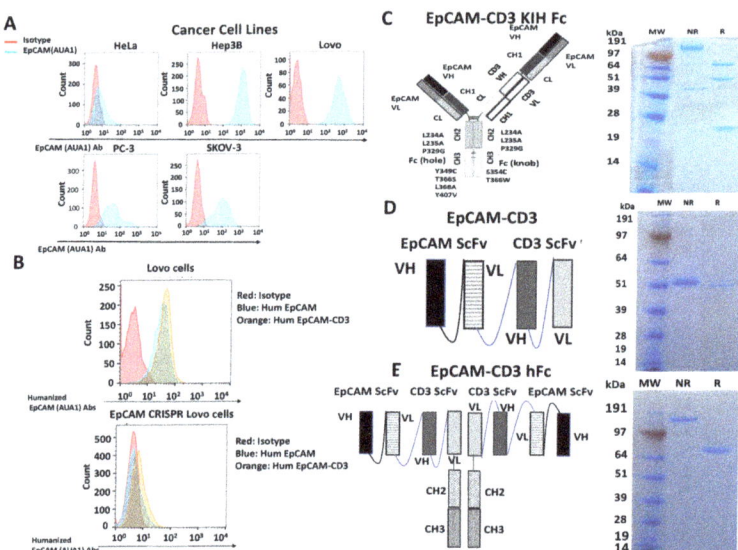

Figure 1. Different designs of humanized EpCAM(AUA-1)-CD3 bispecific antibodies. (**A**) The mouse AUA1 antibody detects EpCAM on different cancer cell surfaces by FACS analysis. This antibody was used for FACS staining with HeLa, Hep3B, Lovo, PC3, and SKOV-3 cells. (**B**) Humanized regular and bispecific humanized EpCAM ScFv-CD3 Scfv antibodies specifically bound to the EpCAM antigen in Lovo cells and did not bind in Lovo cells with CRISPR/Cas-9 knockout of EpCAM (EpCAM KO). (**C**) EpCAM-CD3 CrossMab KIH design and SDS gel for reduced (R) and nonreduced (NR) conditions are shown. (**D**) EpCAM-CD3 (BITE) format design and SDS gel for R and NR conditions are shown. (**E**) EpCAM-CD3 hFc format design and SDS gel for R and NR conditions are shown.

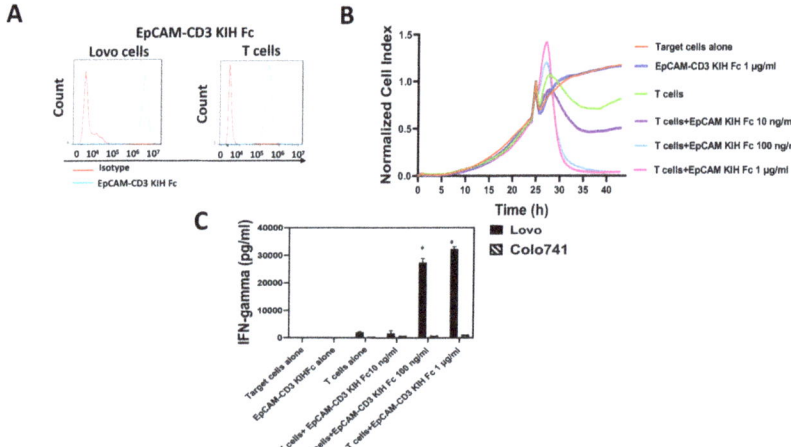

Figure 2. EpCAM-CD3 CrossMab KIH antibody specifically binds to EpCAM-positive cells and T cells, kills EpCAM-positive target cells, and induces IFN-gamma secretion with T cells. (**A**) FACS shows binding of bispecific antibody to EpCAM-positive Lovo cells and to T cells. (**B**) Real-time cytotoxicity (RTCA) assay demonstrates killing of EpCAM-positive Lovo cells by EpCAM CrossMab KIH-CD3 antibody with T cells, in a dose-dependent manner. (**C**) EpCAM CrossMab KIH-CD3 antibody induces IFN-gamma secretion by T cells against EpCAM-positive cells. There was no induction of IFN-gamma secretion against EpCAM-negative Colo741 cells. * $p < 0.05$, Student's *t*-test IFN-gamma secretion against Lovo cells versus Colo741 cells.

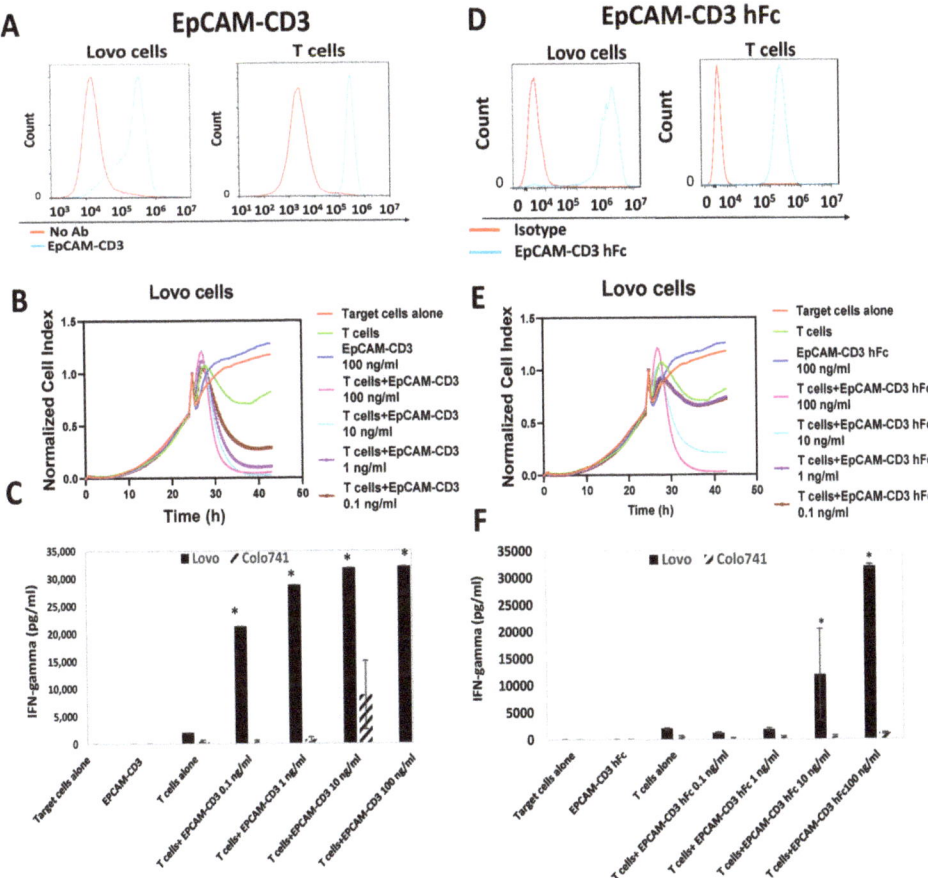

Figure 3. EpCAM-CD3 and EpCAM-CD3 human Fc antibodies bind to EpCAM-positive cells and T cells, kill EpCAM-positive target cells, and induce IFN-gamma secretion with T cells. (**A**) FACS shows binding of EpCAM-CD3 antibody to EpCAM-positive Lovo cells, as well as T cells. (**B**) RTCA assay demonstrates dose-dependent killing of Lovo target cells by antibody when incubated with T cells. (**C**) EpCAM-CD3 antibody with T cells induces IFN-gamma secretion against Lovo cells but not against Colo741 cells. (**D**) FACS shows binding of EpCAM-CD3 human Fc antibody to Lovo and T cells. (**E**) RTCA assay demonstrates the dose-dependent killing of EpCAM-positive target cells by antibody when incubated with T cells. (**F**) EpCAM-CD3 hFc antibody with T cells induces IFN-gamma secretion against Lovo cells and not against Colo741 cells. * $p < 0.05$, Student's t-test. IFN-gamma secretion increased when the antibody was incubated with T cells against Lovo cells and not against Colo741 cells.

Next, we tested the EpCAM-CD3 hFc antibody for binding to Lovo and T cells using FACS, killing activity, and IFN-gamma secretion. This antibody showed high binding to EpCAM-positive Lovo cells and T cells (Figure 3D), effectively killed Lovo cells (Figure 3E), and did not kill Colo741 cells (not shown). The EpCAM-CD3 hFc incubated with T cells caused the secretion of IFN-gamma against Lovo cells and not against Colo741 cells (Figure 3F). The antibody alone without T cells did not cause the secretion of IFN-gamma (Figure 3F). Thus, all three bispecific antibody designs had high and specific in vitro activity against EpCAM-positive cells.

3.3. EpCAM-CD3 hFc mRNA-LNPs Transfected in HEK293 Cells Produce EpCAM-CD3 hFc Antibody with Highly Specific Functional Activity against EpCAM-Positive Cells

To test the production of antibodies using mRNA, we used an EpCAM-CD3 hFc DNA design and subcloned this antibody-encoding sequence into a DNA template for in vitro transcription with a T7AG promoter, 5′UTR, 3′UTR, and a 150 poly A tail. This template was used for in vitro transcription to generate mRNA for this antibody. The mRNA was embedded into LNPs using the PreciGenome Flex S microfluidic system. EpCAM-CD3 hFc mRNA-LNPs were transfected into HEK-293 cells, and 48–72 h later, the supernatant containing antibodies was collected and used for functional assays. The supernatant showed binding to Lovo and T cells but did not bind to EpCAM-negative Colo741 cells (Figure 4A). Dose-dependent killing of Lovo cells but not Colo741 cells was observed with the collected supernatant (Figure 4B). This was also accompanied by T cell secretion of IFN-gamma with Lovo target cells and not with Colo741 target cells (Figure 4C).

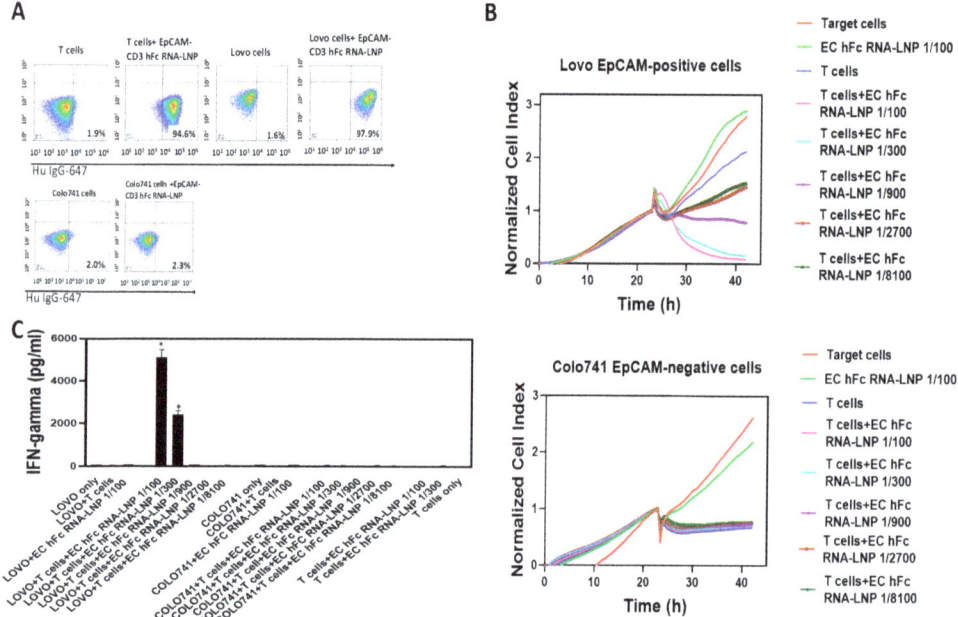

Figure 4. EpCAM-CD3 hFc mRNA-LNP transfection to HEK-293 cells generates antibodies that bind to Lovo and T cells and demonstrates specific killing. (**A**) FACS of Lovo, Colo741, and T cells is shown with supernatant collected from HEK-293 cells transfected with mRNA-LNPs. (**B**) RTCA assay of Lovo and Colo741 cells using supernatant at different dilutions collected from mRNA-LNP-transfected HEK-293 cells. RTCA demonstrates dose-dependent killing of target cells by antibody and T cells. As a negative control, supernatant from untransfected HEK-293 cells was used and tested in an RTCA assay at the same dilutions as the supernatant from transfected HEK-293 cells. (**C**) IFN-gamma secretion by T cells with EpCAM-CD3 hFc supernatant collected after RTCA against Lovo and Colo741 target cells. The secretion of IFN-gamma was significantly higher for Lovo target cells than for Colo741 target cells. * $p < 0.05$, Student's t-test, EpCAM-CD3 hFc with T cells against Lovo cells versus the same conditions against Colo741 cells.

Thus, transfection of the EpCAM-CD3 hFc mRNA-LNPs to HEK293 cells produced functional antibodies that showed binding to EpCAM-positive target cells and demonstrated highly specific killing activity and secretion of IFN-gamma when combined with T cells against EpCAM-positive target cells.

3.4. EpCAM-CD3 hFc mRNA-LNPs Transfected to Cancer Cells Produced Bispecific Antibody with Specific Functional Activity against EpCAM-Positive Cells

Next, we wanted to check whether cancer cells transfected with EpCAM-CD3 hFc mRNA-LNPs would produce functional antibodies. We transfected ovarian and colorectal cancer cell lines and detected that OVCAR-5 colorectal and ovarian A1847 and C30 cancer cell lines produced antibodies that showed binding to Lovo cells and T cells and did not show binding to Colo741 cells (Figure 5A). The antibodies generated from the OVCAR-5 cells killed Lovo cells with added T cells in a dose-dependent manner (Figure 5B) and induced the secretion of IFN-gamma by T cells (Figure 5C).

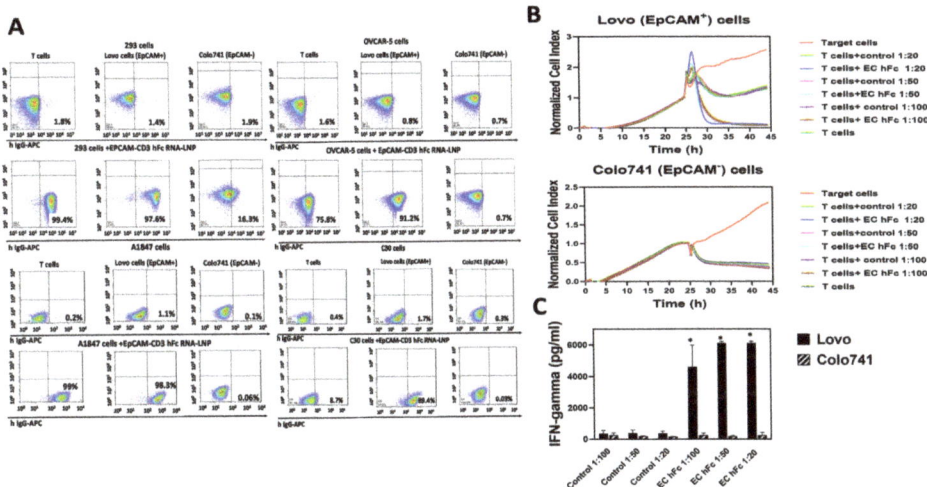

Figure 5. OVCAR-5, A1847, and C30 cancer cell lines secrete functional EpCAM-CD3-hFc antibody after mRNA-LNP transfection. (**A**) FACS with supernatant collected from EpCAM-CD3 hFc mRNA-LNP transfected OVCAR-5, A1847, and C30 cells shows high binding of secreted antibodies to EpCAM-positive Lovo and T cells and shows no binding to Colo741 cells. (**B**) RTCA assay shows that supernatant collected 48 h after EpCAM-CD3 hFc mRNA-LNP transfection of OVCAR-5 cells kills target Lovo cells in the presence of T cells and does not kill Colo741 cells under the same conditions. No killing was observed for the supernatant containing the EpCAM-CD3 hFc antibody alone against target cells without T cells. (**C**) Induction of IFN-gamma secretion by T cells detected in the supernatant collected after RTCA assay (**B**) for Lovo target cells and not for Colo741 target cells. * $p < 0.05$, Student's *t*-test, IFN-gamma secretion against Lovo cells versus Colo741 cells.

Thus, cancer cell lines can be transfected with EpCAM-CD3 hFc mRNA-LNPs and produce functional antibodies with specific EpCAM-dependent activity against cancer cells.

3.5. EpCAM-CD3 hFc mRNA-LNPs with T Cells Significantly Blocked OVCAR-5 Xenograft Tumor Growth

OVCAR-5 cells were injected subcutaneously into NSG mice, and then, one group of mice were injected at days 1, 8, and 15 intratumorally (i.t. group) with EpCAM-CD3 hFc mRNA-LNPs and then with T cells injected intravenously on days 3, 10, and 17 (Figure 6A). Another group (c, i.t. group) of mice were injected with OVCAR-5 cells pre-mixed together with EpCAM-CD3 hFc mRNA-LNPs (cellular injection, c.), and then, for a second time they were injected with EpCAM-CD3 hFc mRNA-LNPs on day 16 intratumorally (i.t.), and T cells were injected intravenously on the same days as above (Figure 6A). Both treatments of EpCAM-CD3 hFc mRNA-LNPs delivered to mice combined with T cells significantly decreased OVCAR-5 tumor growth (Figure 6B). The inhibition of tumor growth was significantly higher ($p < 0.05$) with EpCAM-CD3 mRNA-LNPs and T cell delivery than with T cells alone. EpCAM-CD3 hFc mRNA-LNPs alone without T cells did not block tumor growth (Figure 6B). Thus, the high antitumor activity of EpCAM-CD3 hFc mRNA-LNPs combined with T cells was demonstrated in vivo.

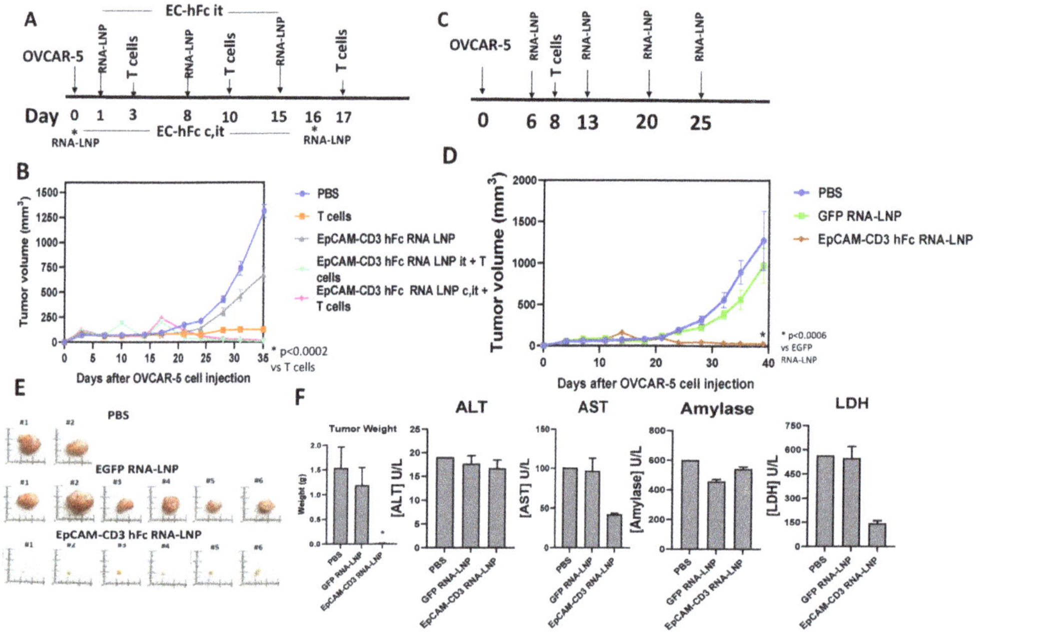

Figure 6. EpCAM-CD3 hFc mRNA-LNPs delivered to OVCAR-5 tumors with intravenous injection of T cells significantly decreased OVCAR-5 xenograft tumor growth. (**A**) The schedule for mRNA-LNP intratumoral (i.t.) injections and three T cell intravenous (i.v.) injections to OVCAR-5 tumor groups. Note: c. marks cellular delivery of EpCAM-CD3-hFc mRNA-LNP pre-mixed with OVCAR-5 cancer cells; i.t. marks intratumoral delivery; i.v. marks intravenous delivery of T cells. (**B**) EpCAM-CD3 hFc mRNA-LNPs combined with T cells significantly decreased OVCAR-5 xenograft tumor growth. (**C**) The schedule for mRNA-LNP intratumoral injection and a single injection of T cells i.v. delivered to OVCAR-5 xenograft tumor model. (**D**) EpCAM-CD3 hFc mRNA-LNPs significantly decreased OVCAR-5 tumor growth combined with a single injection of T cells. (**E**) Tumor size and weight significantly decreased with EpCAM-CD3-hFc mRNA-LNP and T cell treatment. Images of tumors (left panel) are shown at the end of experiment. Bars with averages of tumor weight are shown in the right panel. For tumor weights: * $p < 0.05$, EpCAM-CD3 hFc mRNA-LNP group versus PBS and GFP mRNA-LNP groups, Student's t-test. (**F**) There was no increase in ALT, AST, amylase, or LDH levels in mouse serum collected at the end of treatment for the EpCAM-CD3-hFc mRNA-LNP group versus the GFP mRNA-LNP group for the OVCAR-5 xenograft tumor model.

Next, we tested EpCAM-CD3 hFc mRNA-LNPs delivered intratumorally on days 6, 13, 20, and 25 with only a single injection of T cells i.v. on day 8 (Figure 6C). As a negative control, we used GFP mRNA-LNPs. The EpCAM-CD3 mRNA-LNPs significantly blocked OVCAR-5 xenograft tumor growth while the GFP mRNA-LNPs did not (Figure 6D). The images of tumors at the end of treatment are shown in Figure 6E. There was significant reduction in tumor size and weight in the EpCAM-CD3 hFc mRNA-LNP and T cell–treated group versus the PBS and GFP mRNA-LNP–treated group. In addition, we collected serum from the treated mice and showed that there was no increase in blood toxicology markers (AST, ALT, amylase, and LDH) caused by EpCAM-CD3 hFc mRNA-LNP treatment versus GFP mRNA-LNP treatment suggesting no toxicity of the EpCAM-CD3 mRNA-LNPs (Figure 6F). AST and LDH levels were significantly decreased by EpCAM-CD3 hFc mRNA-LNP versus GFP mRNA-LNP treatment (Figure 6F).

Thus, EpCAM-CD3 hFc mRNA-LNPs can produce antibodies inside cancer cells with high antitumor efficacy in vivo.

4. Discussion

We tested three different designs of humanized EpCAM-CD3 antibodies such as bivalent CrossMAB knob-in-hole KIH Fc, EpCAM-CD3 (BITE), and EpCAM-CD3-hFc. All the antibodies demonstrated highly specific binding and killing activity against EpCAM-positive target cells and not against EpCAM-negative cells. In addition, we developed mRNA-LNP technology to produce EpCAM-CD3 hFc antibodies that showed highly specific anticancer efficacy in vitro in HEK-293 cells and in various cancer cells. The delivery of mRNA-LNPs into mice tumors with intravenous T cell significantly blocked OVCAR-5 xenograft tumor growth in vivo.

This study demonstrates a novel method of delivering bispecific antibodies using mRNA-LNP technology. The mRNA-LNP technology platform was recently used for COVID-19 vaccines by Moderna and Pfizer and was proven to be safe, which provides a solid basis for future anticancer vaccine, antibody production, and novel therapeutics development.

The production of efficacious antibodies was shown by the intratumoral delivery of EpCAM-CD3 hFc mRNA-LNPs. This delivery was shown to be safe as there was no increase in toxicology blood markers such as ALT, AST, amylase, and LDH in the collected serum of treated mice. The encoding of antibodies and drugs through mRNA has been discussed using nanotechnology and oncolytic viruses [20,32]. This study shows nonviral delivery of mRNA-LNP to tumors.

We also tested the same EpCAM-CD3 antibody with mutant, silenced Fc as was shown for the CrossMab KIH design to decrease potential immune activation through NK receptors. The EpCAM-CD3 mutant Fc antibody generated with mRNA-LNP technology demonstrated the same high efficacy as the wild-type Fc antibody (not shown).

The production of bispecific antibodies through mRNA-LNP injection in vivo has many advantages versus RNA or antibody proteins. The mRNA–LNP complexes are more stable than regular mRNA, and the production of antibodies through mRNA-LNPs is less costly than antibody protein manufacturing and shows potential for further optimizations in future studies.

This novel approach included bispecific antibody generation using safe and local intratumoral delivery using mRNA-LNP technology. Moreover, it combined a cell therapy approach by using T cells to kill tumors. This approach can be used similarly to attract NK cells or gamma–delta T cells to tumors using specific immune cell receptors. In addition, different stimulators of immune cells can be used to increase the efficacy of this therapy such as checkpoint inhibitor players, chemokines, cytokines, growth factors, and tumor microenvironment modulators. The lysed tumor releases neoantigens (natural vaccine), which can be recognized in the presence of immunomodulators by antigen-presenting cells or dendritic cells and promote the activity of memory T and B cells. Thus, this approach can be developed and optimized for future clinical applications.

5. Conclusions

In conclusion, EpCAM-CD3 human Fc bispecific antibodies generated with mRNA-LNP technology demonstrate high efficacy in vitro and in vivo. This study, for the first time, shows that intratumoral delivery of EpCAM-CD3 hFc mRNA-LNPs with intravenous delivery of T cells blocked xenograft tumor growth. This approach can be used against solid tumors in future clinical studies.

6. Patents

The antibody sequences are included in the patent application.

Author Contributions: Conceptualization, L.W., W.B. and V.G.; methodology, Y.H., J.S. (John Sienkiewicz), J.S. (Jinying Sun), H.Z., H.H., S.X., R.B. and L.H.; software, Y.H., J.S. (John Sienkiewicz) and J.S. (Jinying Sun); validation, H.Z. and J.S. (John Sienkiewicz); formal analysis, V.G.; investigation, V.G. and L.W.; resources, L.W.; data curation, Y.H., J.S. (John Sienkiewicz) and J.S. (Jinying Sun); writing—original draft preparation, V.G.; writing—review and editing, V.G. and J.S. (John Sienkiewicz); visualization, V.G.; supervision, V.G. and L.W.; project administration, V.G. and L.W.; funding acquisition, L.W. All authors have read and agreed to the published version of the manuscript.

Funding: This research was funded by Promab Biotechnologies.

Institutional Review Board Statement: Not applicable.

Informed Consent Statement: Not applicable.

Data Availability Statement: Data are contained within the article.

Acknowledgments: We would like to thank Ed Lim and Jana Nilson for their excellent help with mouse xenograft experiments.

Conflicts of Interest: Vita Golubovskaya, John Sienkiewicz, Jinying Sun, Yanwei Huang, Hua Zhou, Lian Hu, Robert Berahovich, Hizkia Harto, and Shirley Xu are employees of Promab Biotechnologies. Lijun Wu is an employee and shareholder of Promab Biotechnologies. Dr. Walter Bodmer is a Scientific Advisor for Promab Biotechnologies.

References

1. Bodmer, W.F. Cancer genetics: Colorectal cancer as a model. *J. Hum. Genet.* **2006**, *51*, 391–396. [CrossRef] [PubMed]
2. Bray, F.; Ferlay, J.; Soerjomataram, I.; Siegel, R.L.; Torre, L.A.; Jemal, A. Global cancer statistics 2018: GLOBOCAN estimates of incidence and mortality worldwide for 36 cancers in 185 countries. *CA Cancer J. Clin.* **2018**, *68*, 394–424. [CrossRef] [PubMed]
3. Ruff, S.M.; Pawlik, T.M. A Review of Translational Research for Targeted Therapy for Metastatic Colorectal Cancer. *Cancers* **2023**, *15*, 1395. [CrossRef]
4. Ciardiello, D.; Vitiello, P.P.; Cardone, C.; Martini, G.; Troiani, T.; Martinelli, E. Immunotherapy of colorectal cancer: Challenges for therapeutic efficacy. *Cancer Treat. Rev.* **2019**, *76*, 22–32. [CrossRef] [PubMed]
5. Armstrong, A.; Eck, S.L. EpCAM: A new therapeutic target for an old cancer antigen. *Cancer Biol. Ther.* **2003**, *2*, 320–326. [CrossRef]
6. Schnell, U.; Cirulli, V.; Giepmans, B.N. EpCAM: Structure and function in health and disease. *Biochim. Biophys. Acta* **2013**, *1828*, 1989–2001. [CrossRef]
7. Imrich, S.; Hachmeister, M.; Gires, O. EpCAM and its potential role in tumor-initiating cells. *Cell Adhes. Migr.* **2012**, *6*, 30–38. [CrossRef]
8. van der Gun, B.T.; Melchers, L.J.; Ruiters, M.H.; de Leij, L.F.; McLaughlin, P.M.; Rots, M.G. EpCAM in carcinogenesis: The good, the bad or the ugly. *Carcinogenesis* **2010**, *31*, 1913–1921. [CrossRef]
9. Munz, M.; Baeuerle, P.A.; Gires, O. The emerging role of EpCAM in cancer and stem cell signaling. *Cancer Res.* **2009**, *69*, 5627–5629. [CrossRef]
10. Ntouroupi, T.G.; Ashraf, S.Q.; McGregor, S.B.; Turney, B.W.; Seppo, A.; Kim, Y.; Wang, X.; Kilpatrick, M.W.; Tsipouras, P.; Tafas, T.; et al. Detection of circulating tumour cells in peripheral blood with an automated scanning fluorescence microscope. *Br. J. Cancer* **2008**, *99*, 789–795. [CrossRef]
11. Cetin, D.; Okan, M.; Bat, E.; Kulah, H. A comparative study on EpCAM antibody immobilization on gold surfaces and microfluidic channels for the detection of circulating tumor cells. *Colloids Surf. B Biointerfaces* **2020**, *188*, 110808. [CrossRef] [PubMed]
12. Macdonald, J.; Henri, J.; Roy, K.; Hays, E.; Bauer, M.; Veedu, R.N. EpCAM Immunotherapy versus Specific Targeted Delivery of Drugs. *Cancers* **2018**, *10*, 19. [CrossRef] [PubMed]
13. Alhabbab, R.Y. Targeting Cancer Stem Cells by Genetically Engineered Chimeric Antigen Receptor T Cells. *Front. Genet.* **2020**, *11*, 312. [CrossRef] [PubMed]
14. Baeuerle, P.A.; Gires, O. EpCAM (CD326) finding its role in cancer. *Br. J. Cancer* **2007**, *96*, 417–423. [CrossRef]
15. Bremer, E.; Helfrich, W. EpCAM-targeted induction of apoptosis. *Front. Biosci.-Landmark* **2008**, *13*, 5042–5049. [CrossRef]
16. Carpenter, G.; Red Brewer, M. EpCAM: Another surface-to-nucleus missile. *Cancer Cell* **2009**, *15*, 165–166. [CrossRef]
17. Morais, P.; Adachi, H.; Yu, Y.T. The Critical Contribution of Pseudouridine to mRNA COVID-19 Vaccines. *Front. Cell Dev. Biol.* **2021**, *9*, 789427. [CrossRef]
18. Wang, C.; Zhang, Y.; Dong, Y. Lipid Nanoparticle-mRNA Formulations for Therapeutic Applications. *Acc. Chem. Res.* **2021**, *54*, 4283–4293. [CrossRef]
19. Jung, H.N.; Lee, S.Y.; Lee, S.; Youn, H.; Im, H.J. Lipid nanoparticles for delivery of RNA therapeutics: Current status and the role of in vivo imaging. *Theranostics* **2022**, *12*, 7509–7531. [CrossRef]
20. Zhou, L.; Zou, M.; Xu, Y.; Lin, P.; Lei, C.; Xia, X. Nano Drug Delivery System for Tumor Immunotherapy: Next-Generation Therapeutics. *Front. Oncol.* **2022**, *12*, 864301. [CrossRef]

21. Bacac, M.; Fauti, T.; Sam, J.; Colombetti, S.; Weinzierl, T.; Ouaret, D.; Bodmer, W.; Lehmann, S.; Hofer, T.; Hosse, R.J.; et al. A Novel Carcinoembryonic Antigen T-Cell Bispecific Antibody (CEA TCB) for the Treatment of Solid Tumors. *Clin. Cancer Res.* **2016**, *22*, 3286–3297. [CrossRef] [PubMed]
22. Wu, L.; Huang, Y.; Sienkiewicz, J.; Sun, J.; Guiang, L.; Li, F.; Yang, L.; Golubovskaya, V. Bispecific BCMA-CD3 Antibodies Block Multiple Myeloma Tumor Growth. *Cancers* **2022**, *14*, 2518. [CrossRef] [PubMed]
23. Berahovich, R.; Zhou, H.; Xu, S.; Wei, Y.; Guan, J.; Guan, J.; Harto, H.; Fu, S.; Yang, K.; Zhu, S.; et al. Golubovskaya. CAR-T Cells Based on Novel BCMA Monoclonal Antibody Block Multiple Myeloma Cell Growth. *Cancers* **2018**, *10*, 323. [CrossRef] [PubMed]
24. Berahovich, R.; Xu, S.; Zhou, H.; Harto, H.; Xu, Q.; Garcia, A.; Liu, F.; Golubovskaya, V.M.; Wu, L. FLAG-tagged CD19-specific CAR-T cells eliminate CD19-bearing solid tumor cells in vitro and in vivo. *Front. Biosci.-Landmark* **2017**, *22*, 1644–1654.
25. Berahovich, R.; Liu, X.; Zhou, H.; Tsadik, E.; Xu, S.; Golubovskaya, V. Hypoxia Selectively Impairs CAR-T Cells In Vitro. *Cancers* **2019**, *11*, 602. [CrossRef] [PubMed]
26. Spurr, N.K.; Durbin, H.; Sheer, D.; Parkar, M.; Bobrow, L.; Bodmer, W.F. Characterization and chromosomal assignment of a human cell surface antigen defined by the monoclonal antibody AUA1. *Int. J. Cancer* **1986**, *38*, 631–636. [CrossRef]
27. Wong, N.A.; Warren, B.F.; Piris, J.; Maynard, N.; Marshall, R.; Bodmer, W.F. EpCAM and gpA33 are markers of Barrett's metaplasia. *J. Clin. Pathol.* **2006**, *59*, 260–263. [CrossRef] [PubMed]
28. Almagro, J.C.; Fransson, J. Humanization of antibodies. *Front. Biosci.* **2008**, *13*, 1619–1633.
29. Golubovskaya, V.; Berahovich, R.; Zhou, H.; Xu, S.; Harto, H.; Li, L.; Chao, C.C.; Mao, M.M.; Wu, L. CD47-CAR-T Cells Effectively Kill Target Cancer Cells and Block Pancreatic Tumor Growth. *Cancers* **2017**, *9*, 139. [CrossRef]
30. Golubovskaya, V.; Zhou, H.; Li, F.; Valentine, M.; Sun, J.; Berahovich, R.; Xu, S.; Quintanilla, M.; Ma, M.C.; Sienkiewicz, J.; et al. Novel CD37, Humanized CD37 and Bi-Specific Humanized CD37-CD19 CAR-T Cells Specifically Target Lymphoma. *Cancers* **2021**, *13*, 981. [CrossRef]
31. Reinhard, K.; Rengstl, B.; Oehm, P.; Michel, K.; Billmeier, A.; Hayduk, N.; Klein, O.; Kuna, K.; Ouchan, Y.; Woll, S.; et al. An RNA vaccine drives expansion and efficacy of claudin-CAR-T cells against solid tumors. *Science* **2020**, *367*, 446–453. [CrossRef] [PubMed]
32. Zhou, P.; Wang, X.; Xing, M.; Yang, X.; Wu, M.; Shi, H. Intratumoral delivery of a novel oncolytic adenovirus encoding human antibody against PD-1 elicits enhanced antitumor efficacy. *Mol. Ther.-Oncolytics* **2022**, *25*, 236–248. [CrossRef] [PubMed]

Disclaimer/Publisher's Note: The statements, opinions and data contained in all publications are solely those of the individual author(s) and contributor(s) and not of MDPI and/or the editor(s). MDPI and/or the editor(s) disclaim responsibility for any injury to people or property resulting from any ideas, methods, instructions or products referred to in the content.

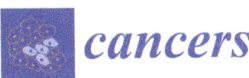

Article

Development of the Novel Bifunctional Fusion Protein BR102 That Simultaneously Targets PD-L1 and TGF-β for Anticancer Immunotherapy

Zhen-Hua Wu [1,†], Na Li [1,†], Zhang-Zhao Gao [1], Gang Chen [2], Lei Nie [1], Ya-Qiong Zhou [1], Mei-Zhu Jiang [1], Yao Chen [1], Juan Chen [1], Xiao-Fen Mei [1], Feng Hu [1] and Hai-Bin Wang [1,*]

[1] BioRay Pharmaceutical Co., Ltd., Taizhou 318000, China
[2] BioRay Pharmaceutical Corp, San Diego, CA 92121, USA
* Correspondence: haibin.wang@bioraypharm.com
† These authors contributed equally to this work.

Simple Summary: Immune checkpoint inhibitors (ICIs), such as anti-PD-1/PD-L1 antibodies, have revolutionized the therapy landscape of cancer immunotherapy. However, poor clinical response to ICIs and drug resistance are the main challenges for ICIs immunotherapy. TGF-β produced in the TME was found to confer resistance to PD-1/PD-L1-targeted immunotherapy. The independent and complementary immunosuppressive role of PD-L1 and TGF-β in cancer progression provides a rationale for simultaneously targeting TGF-β and PD-L1 to improve anti-PD-L1 therapy. Consequently, we develop and characterize a novel anti-PD-L1/TGF-β bifunctional fusion protein termed BR102. The data suggest that BR102 could simultaneously disrupt TGF-β- and PD-L1-mediated signals and display high antitumor efficacy and safety. The data support further clinical advancement of BR102 as a promising approach to cancer immunotherapy.

Abstract: Immune checkpoint inhibitors (ICIs) are remarkable breakthroughs in treating various types of cancer, but many patients still do not derive long-term clinical benefits. Increasing evidence shows that TGF-β can promote cancer progression and confer resistance to ICI therapies. Consequently, dual blocking of TGF-β and immune checkpoint may provide an effective approach to enhance the effectiveness of ICI therapies. Here, we reported the development and preclinical characterization of a novel bifunctional anti-PD-L1/TGF-β fusion protein, BR102. BR102 comprises an anti-PD-L1 antibody fused to the extracellular domain (ECD) of human TGF-βRII. BR102 is capable of simultaneously binding to TGF-β and PD-L1. Incorporating TGF-βRII into BR102 does not alter the PD-L1 blocking activity of BR102. In vitro characterization further demonstrated that BR102 could disrupt TGF-β-induced signaling. Moreover, BR102 significantly inhibits tumor growth in vivo and exerts a superior antitumor effect compared to anti-PD-L1. Administration of BR102 to cynomolgus monkeys is well-tolerated, with only minimal to moderate and reversing red cell changes noted. The data demonstrated the efficacy and safety of the novel anti-PD-L1/TGF-β fusion protein and supported the further clinical development of BR102 for anticancer therapy.

Keywords: cancer immunotherapy; PD-L1; TGF-β; bifunctional fusion protein; BR102

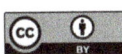

1. Introduction

Immune checkpoint molecules, including PD-1/PD-L1, CTLA-4, and LAG-3, play significant roles in mediating T-cell dysfunction during cancer progression and suppressing antitumor immunity. Cancer immunotherapy targeting immune checkpoint molecules can restore antitumor immune response to kill tumor cells. ICIs, such as monoclonal antibodies against PD-1, PD-L1 and CTLA-4, have greatly improved the clinical outcome of cancer patients [1,2], revolutionizing the treatment landscape for multiple tumor types. However, many cancer patients achieve only a short-lived clinical benefit from checkpoint blockade therapies, and some may eventually develop resistance which leads to disease progression [3–5]. This highlights the urgent need for alternative approaches to improve response rates.

TGF-β is a multifunctional cytokine involved in many developmental and metabolic processes, including proliferation, differentiation, apoptosis, angiogenesis, and cellular immune response [6]. It has three highly-conserved isoforms: TGF-β1, TGF-β2, and TGF-β3, that interact with a tetrameric receptor complex to transmit intracellular signaling. TGF-β signaling activation may lead to different effects in a context-dependent manner. In healthy and pre-malignant cells, TGF-β functions as a tumor suppressor by promoting apoptosis and cell-cycle arrest. However, cancer cells can bypass the suppressor effects of TGF-β and subvert TGF-β activity to obtain a growth advantage. TGF-β produced in the TME induces epithelial-to-mesenchymal transition (EMT), which drives migration and invasion of tumor cells [7,8]. Moreover, TGF-β also contributes to tumor progression by increasing extracellular matrix (ECM) production, activating cancer-associated fibroblasts (CAFs), promoting angiogenesis, and stimulating immune evasion [9]. High TGF-β expression correlates with poor prognosis in several tumor types [10,11]. Based on the preclinical findings that targeting TGF-β could exert antitumor activity, many pharmacological TGF-β inhibitors have been discovered and evaluated in clinical trials, including receptor kinases inhibitors, neutralizing antibodies, antisense oligonucleotides, and ligand traps. However, the tumor suppressive activity of TGF-β and its pleiotropic nature prevented rapid clinical translation of anti-TGF-β therapies [12]. In light of insights into the immunosuppressive function of TGF-β, the combined blockade of immune checkpoint and TGF-β is under intensive investigation.

TGF-β and PD-L1 act as parallel immunosuppressors through distinct mechanisms. Moreover, it has been revealed that TGF-β could upregulate PD-L1 and PD-1 expression in tumor and T cells, respectively, which serve as additional mechanisms of TGF-β-induced immune suppression [13,14]. In addition, the activation of the TGF-β pathway was linked to a lack of response to PD-1/PD-L1-targeting cancer therapy [15,16], suggesting that inhibition of TGF-β may overcome resistance to anti-PD-1/PD-L1. Furthermore, combining PD-1/PD-L1 inhibition with TGF-β blockade displays synergistic antitumor activity in vivo [15,17,18]. M7824, a recombinant anti-PD-L1/TGF-β bifunctional molecular, demonstrated stronger antitumor efficacy compared to either TGF-β or PD-L1 inhibition [19]. Considering that TGF-β and PD-L1 pathways contribute to suppressing immune response via independent and complementary pathways, simultaneous targeting TGF-β and PD-L1 represents an alternative approach to enhance antitumor immune response and improve PD-1/PD-L1-targeting therapy.

We previously reported the optimization strategies for expressing the bifunctional fusion protein, designated BR102, which simultaneously inhibited TGF-β and PD-L1 signaling [20]. BR102 consists of an anti-PD-L1 antibody fused to the ECD of human TGF-βRII. Three amino acid mutations were introduced into the N-terminus of the TGF-βRII moiety in BR102 to avoid proteolytic degradation and improve druggability [20]. Here, we characterized the preclinical efficacy and safety of BR102 in vitro and in vivo. BR102 can simultaneously disrupt TGF-β and PD-L1 signal and exert greater antitumor efficacy compared with anti-PD-L1 alone. We further demonstrate that BR102 has a good safety profile in an NHP toxicity study. These data suggest that BR102 may provide a promising approach to cancer immunotherapy and improve the efficacy of anti-PD-1/PD-L1.

2. Materials and Methods

2.1. Antibody Generation and Purification

Anti-PD-L1 antibodies were selected by binding to recombinant human PD-L1 ectodomain in a human library expressed in a phage presentation system. One positive clone, HS636, was obtained and generated on a human IgG1 backbone with N297A mutation to inactivate the Fc-mediated effect function. BR102 was designed by fusing the C-terminus of the HC of HS636 to the N-terminus of the TGF-βRII ectodomain sequence via the (GGGGS)$_4$G linker. Amino acid mutations were introduced into the N-terminus of the ectodomain of TGF-βRII to avoid proteolytic degradation. CHO-K1 cells were transfected with vectors encoding HS636 and BR102, respectively. After cell cultures, HS636 and BR102 were purified from cell supernatants by affinity chromatography. Atezolizumab was from Genentech Inc (San Francisco, CA, USA). Human IgG1 isotype control was expressed by Biointron Biological (Taizhou, China).

2.2. Cell Lines and Cell Culture

Dendritic cells (DCs) and peripheral blood mononuclear cells (PBMCs) were purchased from AllCells (Shanghai, China). TF-1 cells were from the American Type Culture Collection (Manassas, VA, USA). TGF-β reporter gene HEK-293 cells were purchased from Genomeditech (Shanghai, China). PD-L1 aAPC/CHO-K1 cells and PD-1 Effector cells were purchased from Promega (Madison, WI, USA). Cells were propagated in culture conditions as recommended by the manufacturer.

2.3. Antibody Affinity Measurement

The binding affinity of HS636 to PD-L1 was performed on a Biacore X100 instrument (GE Healthcare, Chicago, IL, USA). The anti-human antibody (human antibody capture kit; GE Healthcare) was immobilized on a CM5 sensor chip using the amine coupling kit (GE Healthcare). HS636 (1.0 μg/mL) was captured on the CM5 chip at the rate of 10 μL/min. A dilution of PD-L1-His (R&D Systems, Minneapolis, MN, USA) was injected for 180 s at a flow rate of 30 μL/min. The dissociation phase was monitored for 300 s. The sensor chip was regenerated with 3M $MgCl_2$ at a flow rate of 20 μL/min for 60 s. The binding kinetics was recorded and analyzed using Biacore X100 evaluation software.

2.4. Binding ELISA Assay

PD-L1 (ACROBiosystems, Beijing, China), TGF-β1 (ACROBiosystems), TGF-β2 (Novoprotein, Shanghai, China), TGF-β3 (R&D Systems), cynomolgus monkey PD-L1 (ACROBiosystems), or TGF-β1 (Sino Biological, Beijing, China) were coated onto high-binding microtiter plates (Corning Inc., Corning, NY, USA) in PBS at 4 °C overnight. The plates were blocked with 5% BSA in PBS and incubated with serially diluted test mAbs. HRP-labeled goat-anti-human IgG (Sigma, St.Louis, MO, USA, 1:5000) was added to the plates and incubated for 1 h at 37 °C. TMB (Huzhou InnoReagents, Huzhou, China) chromogenic reaction was stopped with 1M H_2SO_4, and the absorbance at 450 nm was determined using a Spectramax M5 microplate reader (Molecular Devices, San Jose, CA, USA). A dose response curve was fitted by 4-parameter logistic (4PL) regression (Prism 8; GraphPad, San Diego, CA, USA).

The ability of BR102 to simultaneously recognize PD-L1 and TGF-β1 was also tested by ELISA. BR102 was added to TGF-β1-coated plates, followed by biotinylated PD-L1 (ACROBiosystems) detected with streptavidin-HRP (Abcam, Cambridge, MA, USA, 1:1000). The remaining steps followed the ELISA procedure described above.

2.5. Competition ELISA Assay

The blocking ability of HS636 and BR102 was tested in competition ELISA assays. Fc-tagged human PD-1 (ACROBiosystems) was absorbed into high-binding microtiter plates (Corning) at 0.25 μg/mL in PBS at 4 °C overnight. The plates were blocked with 5% BSA in PBST. Biotinylated PD-L1 (ACROBiosystems) and serially diluted HS636 or BR102 were added to the plates. The samples were then incubated with Streptavidin-HRP (Abcam). TMB color development was stopped with 1M H_2SO_4, and the absorbance was detected at 450 nm using a Spectramax M5 microplate reader (Molecular Devices). For CD80/PD-L1 blocking assay, Fc-tagged human CD80 (ACROBiosystems) was coated at 0.5 μg/mL, and biotinylated PD-L1 was added at 4 μg/mL.

For the TGF-β1/TGF-βRII blocking assay, varying amounts of BR102 and biotinylated TGF-βRII (ACROBiosystems) were added to 96-well plates pre-coated with TGF-β1 (ACRO-Biosystems). Bound TGF-βRII was detected by adding streptavidin-HRP (Abcam) followed by TMB. Absorbance at 450 nm was read on a microplate reader (Molecular Devices).

2.6. PD-1/PD-L1 Reporter Gene Assay

PD-L1 aAPC/CHO-K1 cells were seeded in 96-well plates at a density of 4×10^4 cells per well. After incubation overnight at 37 °C, PD-1 effector cells and serially diluted HS636 or BR102 were added to the plate and incubated at 37 °C for 6 h. Thereafter, Bio-Lite Luciferase Reagent (Vazyme, Nanjing, China) was added, and the luminescence was measured after 10 min. Data were analyzed using GraphPad Prism software.

2.7. TGF-β Reporter Gene Assay

TGF-β reporter gene HEK-293 cells were designed for monitoring the activity of the SMAD signal induced by TGF-β. Cells were seeded at a density of 1.25×10^4 cells per well in 96-well plates and incubated overnight at 37 °C. 0.2 ng/mL TGF-β1 and serially diluted BR102 were added and incubated for 7 h. Bio-Lite Luciferase Reagent (Vazyme) was added, and the luminescence was measured.

2.8. TF-1 Cell Proliferation

TF-1 cells were incubated with serially diluted BR102 in the presence of 5 ng/mL IL-4 (Sino Biological) and 0.25 ng/mL TGF-β1 (ACROBiosystems) for 2 days at 37 °C. The proliferation of TF-1 cells was measured by a CellTiter-Glo kit (Promega).

2.9. Allogeneic Mixed Lymphocyte Reaction

Mixed lymphocyte reaction (MLR) was utilized to determine T cell activation induced by HS636 and BR102. For HS636, monocytes were isolated from PBMCs using CD14 microbeads (Miltenyi Biotec, Bergisch Gladbach, Germany) and grown in Mo-DC differentiation medium (Miltenyi Biotec) and Mo-DC maturation medium (Miltenyi Biotec) to generate immature dendritic cells (DCs). Human CD4 + T cells isolated from a different PBMC donor were co-cultured with the DCs in a 96-well plate, and indicated antibodies were added. Alternatively, DCs were stimulated with Mitomycin C (50 µg/mL, Selleck, Houston, TX, USA) at 37 °C for 30 min. Subsequently, DCs (5×10^3 cells) were co-cultured with allogeneic PBMCs (1×10^5) in the presence of BR102 or HS636. After 3 days of culture, IFN-γ or IL-2 secretion in cell supernatants were analyzed by ELISA.

2.10. Mouse Tumor Xenograft Models

For the human PD-L1 humanized MC38 (MC38/hPD-L1) colorectal syngeneic model, 5×10^5 MC38/hPD-L1 cells (Biocytogen, Beijing, China) were implanted subcutaneously into the right flank of PD-1-humanized C57BL/6 mice (Biocytogen). The mice were randomized into five groups (vehicle control; 1, 3 and 10 mg/kg HS636; 10 mg/kg Atezolizumab; n = 10 for each group) when mean tumor volume reached approximately 160 mm^3. Mice were intraperitoneally injected with vehicle control, Atezolizumab or HS636, every other day for a total of 8 times.

For the HCC827 non–small cell lung cancer model, NCG mice (Gempharmatech, Nanjing, China) were injected subcutaneously in the right flank at day 0 with 5×10^6 HCC827 cells. At day 5, mice were intravenously injected with 1×10^7 PBMCs. HS636 (1.5 mg/kg) or hIgG1 were intraperitoneally injected at days 5, 8, 12, 15, 19, 22 (n = 6 for each group).

MC38/hPD-L1 model was used to evaluate the antitumor efficacy of BR102 and HS636. 1×10^6 MC38/hPD-L1 cells were injected subcutaneously into C57BL/6JNifdc mice (Vital River, Beijing, China). The mice were injected intraperitoneally with PBS, HS636 (1 mg/kg), or BR102 (1.22 mg/kg, 3.66 mg/kg) twice a week, beginning when tumors had achieved an average size of 50 mm^3 (n = 8 for each group). For all the models, tumor volume was measured twice per week. The tumor volume (TV) was measured and calculated using the formula: TV (mm^3) = $1/2 \times$ length $\times$ width^2.

2.11. Toxicity Study in Non-Human Primates

The toxicology study in cynomolgus monkeys was conducted at Joinn Laboratories (Taicang, China). Animals (5 animals/gender per group) were administered intravenous (i.v.) infusion of BR102 (15, 50 or 100 mg/kg) or vehicle control (20 mM citrate pH 6.0) once weekly for 4 weeks (D1, D8, D15, D22, and D29). 3 animals/gender/group were euthanized at the end of the dosing period (D30). Following the dosing period, the last 2 animals/gender/group were maintained for a 6-week recovery period and euthanized at the end of the recovery period (D71). In-life evaluations included clinical observations, body weight, food consumption, cardiovascular safety pharmacology evaluations, and clinical pathology. Cytokines, including TNF-a, IFN-γ, IL-2, IL-4, IL-5, and IL-6, were analyzed on a FACSCalibur flow cytometer (BD Biosciences, San Jose, CA, USA) using a cytometric bead array (CBA) Kit (BD Biosciences). Following euthanasia, animals were examined for gross pathology, relative organ weight, and histopathology.

2.12. Statistics

Data were presented as mean ± standard error of the mean (SEM) unless otherwise indicated. Statistical significance was analyzed by the Student's *t*-test. *p* values were considered statistically significant below 0.05 (* $p < 0.05$; ** $p < 0.01$; *** $p < 0.001$; **** $p < 0.0001$).

3. Results

3.1. Screen and Biological Activity Evaluation of An Anti-PD-L1 Antibody

Anti-PD-L1 antibodies were screened to recognize a recombinant human PD-L1 ectodomain fusion protein in a human library expressed in a phage presentation system. One of the positive clones, designated HS636, was obtained and generated on a human IgG1 backbone with N297A mutation to inactivate Fc-mediated effect function, such as ADCC or CDC. HS636 exhibited high affinity to human PD-L1 with a equilibrium dissociation constant (KD) of 4.4 nM, as determined by SPR (Figure 1A). HS636 was also confirmed to bind to PD-L1 by ELISA (Figure 1B). Moreover, HS636 could inhibit PD-L1 binding to both of its receptors, CD80 and PD-1, in a dose-dependent manner (Figure 1C,D). We further evaluated the in vitro potency of HS636. HS636 restored PD-1/PD-L1-dependent NFAT pathway activation in an NFAT-driven luciferase reporter assay (Figure 1E) and induced the release of IL-2 and IFNγ in an MLR assay (Figure 1F). PD-1 humanized C57BL/6 mice xenografted with PD-L1 humanized MC38 colorectal cancer cell line were used to evaluate the in vivo antitumor activity induced by HS636 treatment. Treatment with HS636 significantly inhibited tumor growth compared to the control group (Figure 1G). Similar results were obtained in an NCG mice model using an NSCLC cancer cell line (HCC827 cells) with PBMC cell engraftment plus HS636, which delayed tumor growth ($p < 0.05$) (Figure 1H). We compared HS636 with the FDA-approved anti-PD-L1 antibody, Atezolizumab, concerning efficacy in vitro and in vivo. HS636 displayed similar activities with Atezolizumab (Figure 1B,C,G).

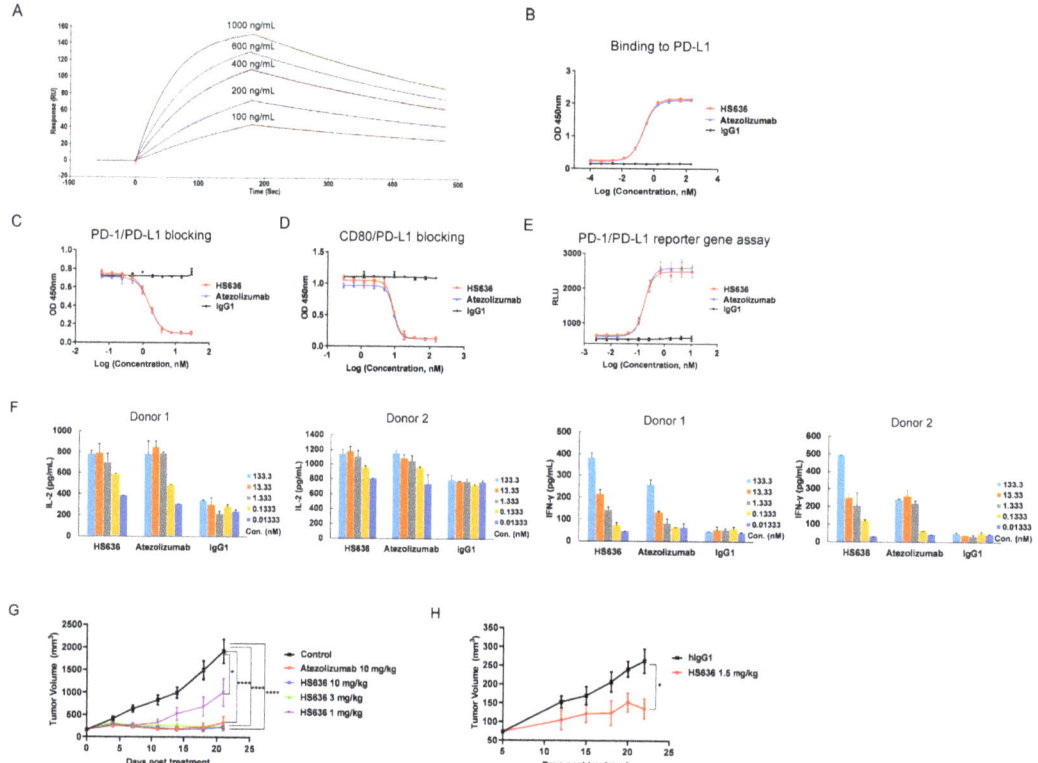

Figure 1. In vitro functional activity and in vivo antitumor efficacy of HS636. (**A**) The affinity of HS636 to PD-L1 was detected by Surface plasmon resonance (SPR). (**B**) The binding activity of HS636 to human PD-L1 was determined by ELISA. The blocking activity of HS636 towards PD-1/PD-L1 interaction (**C**) and CD80/PD-L1 interaction (**D**) was determined by competition ELISA. (**E**) The bioactivity of HS636 on PD-1/PD-L1 signaling was performed by the PD-1/PD-L1 NFAT reporter gene assay. (**F**) The T cell activation effect of HS636 was determined in MLR assay. CD4 + T cells from 2 donors and allogeneic DCs were co-cultured in the presence of indicated concentrations of HS636 for 3 days, then IL-2 and IFN-γ secretion were quantified by ELISA. (**G**) PD-1 humanized C57BL/6 mice bearing MC38/hPD-L1 tumors were treated with HS636, Atezolizumab, or vehicle control (n = 10 for each group). The tumor volume was measured twice per week. (**H**) NCG mice bearing HCC827 tumors were injected with human PBMCs (1×10^7/mouse) and HS636 or isotype control hIgG1 (n = 6 for each group). The tumor volume was measured twice per week.

3.2. BR102 Could Simultaneously Recognize TGF-β and PD-L1

BR102 is a bifunctional fusion protein composed of the anti-PD-L1 antibody HS636, fused at the C-terminus of HC to the ectodomain of TGF-βRII. BR102 bound to PD-L1 with comparable affinity compared to HS636 (Figure 2A). In addition, BR102 could recognize TGF-β1, TGF-β2, and TGF-β3 (Figure 2B), which were the three highly structurally related mammalian TGF-β isoforms. We next evaluate whether the bifunctional molecule BR102 could simultaneously bind to TGF-β1 and PD-L1, and BR102 was confirmed to simultaneously target both the two proteins in an indirect ELISA (Figure 2C).

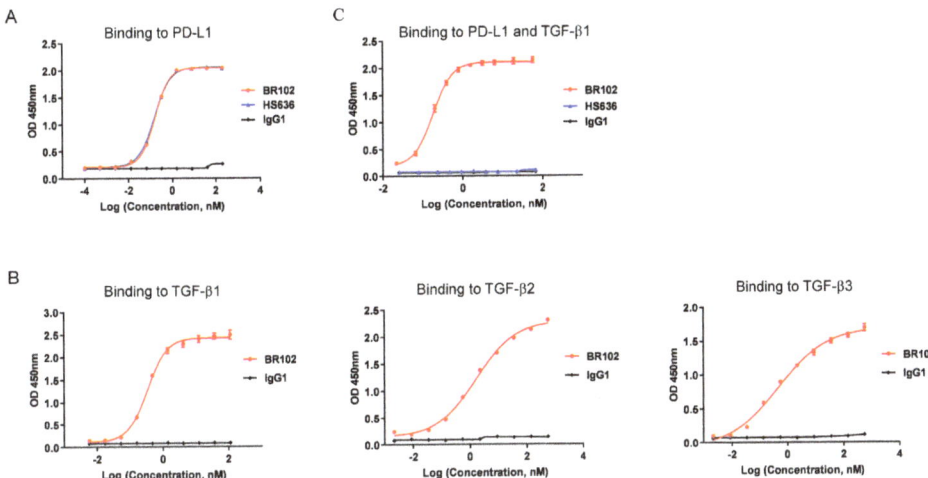

Figure 2. BR102 specifically binds to PD-L1 and TGF-β. The binding of BR102 to PD-L1 (**A**) and various human TGF-β isoforms (β1, β2, and β3) (**B**) was determined by ELISA. (**C**) The simultaneous binding of BR102 to PD-L1 and TGF-β1.

3.3. BR102 Disrupts PD-L1-Mediated Signal and Induces Activation of T Cell

The effects of BR102 on PD-L1-mediated downstream signal and T cell activation were further characterized. BR102 could block PD-L1 binding to CD80 and PD-1 (Figure 3A,B). Moreover, BR102 relieved the PD-1/PD-L1-induced blockade of NFAT signaling in a luciferase reporter assay (Figure 3C). Then, we evaluated BR102-induced activation of T cells in an MLR assay. BR102 treatment led to the enhancement of IL-2 release (Figure 3D). The in vitro potency of BR102 was similar to that of HS636 (Figure 3A–D), indicating that fusion of TGFβRII ectodomain did not affect the potency of HS636 moiety in BR102. These results suggest that BR102 could block PD-L1-induced immunosuppressive signaling and promote T cell activation.

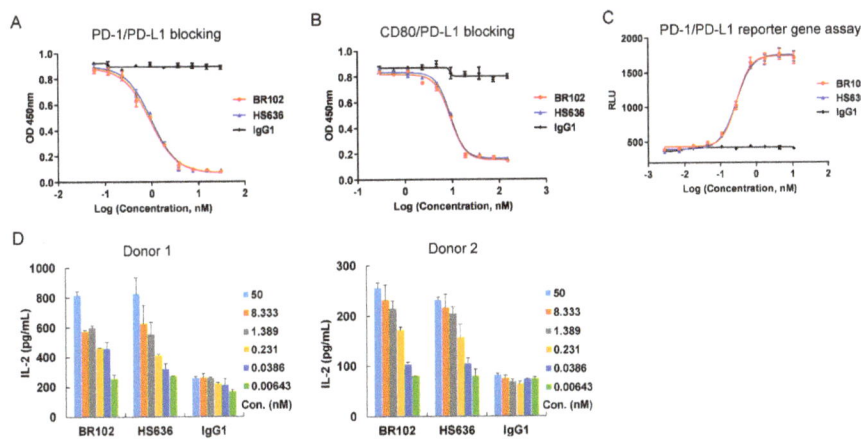

Figure 3. BR102 reversed PD-L1/PD-1 mediated immunosuppression and enhanced T cell activation. BR102 blocked PD-1/PD-L1 interaction (**A**) and CD80/ PD-L1 interaction (**B**) in competition ELISA assays. (**C**) The blockade ability of HS636 on PD-1/PD-L1 signaling was determined by the NFAT reporter gene assay. (**D**) DCs and allogeneic PBMC from 2 donors were co-cultured in the presence of indicated concentrations of BR102 or HS636 for 3 days. IL-2 secretion was analyzed by ELISA.

3.4. BR102 Inhibits TGF-β Signal In Vitro

The effects of BR102 on TGF-β-induced signal transduction and cellular function were evaluated. BR102 showed potent antagonism of TGF-β, as determined by inhibiting the interaction between TGF-β and its receptor TGF-βRII (Figure 4A). TGF-β could elicit canonical SMAD pathway upon TGF-β ligand binding with TGF-βRII. The blocking activity of BR102 on TGF-β-mediated SMAD signal was then evaluated using a TGF-β/SMAD luciferase reporter assay, and our data showed that BR102 inhibited SMAD signaling mediated by TGF-β in a dose-dependent manner (Figure 4B). In addition, BR102 also relieved TGF-β-induced growth inhibition in a human erythroleukemic cell line, TF-1 (Figure 4C). The above results suggest that BR102 could act as a potent TGF-β inhibitor.

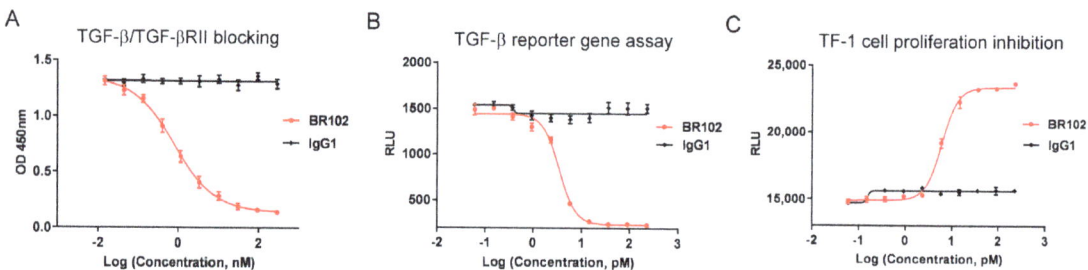

Figure 4. The inhibition effect of BR102 on TGF-β signaling pathway. (**A**) BR102 blocked the interaction of TGF-β1 with TGF-βRII. (**B**) BR102 inhibited TGF-β1-induced SMAD signaling in a TGF-β/SMAD luciferase reporter gene assay. (**C**) BR102 reversed TGF-β1 induced proliferation inhibition of TF-1 cells.

3.5. BR102 Treatment Inhibits Tumor Growth In Vivo

We next evaluated the in vivo efficacy of BR102 in a syngeneic mice model. C57BL/6JNifdc mice implanted subcutaneously with the colon adenocarcinoma MC38/hPD-L1 cell line were assigned to treatment with either PBS (vehicle) or BR102, and the anti-PD-L1 mAb HS636 was included for comparison. Compared with the control group, mice receiving intraperitoneal administration of BR102 showed significant tumor growth inhibition (Figure 5, Figure S2). Moreover, BR102 led to a more potent inhibition of tumor growth compared to the equimolar dose of HS636 (Figure 5). No significant weight loss was observed in mice treated with BR102 (Figure S2).

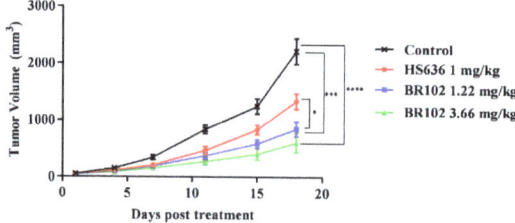

Figure 5. BR102 inhibited tumor growth in a murine tumor model. C57BL/6JNifdc mice were subcutaneously injected with MC38/hPD-L1 cells. When tumor volumes reached 50 mm^3, mice were treated with PBS, HS636, or BR102 (n = 8 for each group). The tumor volume was measured twice per week.

3.6. BR102 Shows A Favorable Safety Profile In Vivo

The safety concerns regarding anti-TGF-β therapies limit their therapy window and challenge the clinical development of TGF-β inhibitors. It was reported that administration of a neutralizing pan-TGF-β antibody in cynomolgus monkeys resulted in adverse effects, including generalized bleeding, cardiovascular toxicity, pathologic changes in the bone, and even mortality [21]. We next investigated whether BR102 would display an improved safety profile. BR102 could bind to cynomolgus TGF-β and PD-L1 (Figure S1), confirming that cynomolgus monkey is a relevant species for in vivo safety study of BR102. A repeat-dose toxicity study of BR102 in cynomolgus monkeys was performed. BR102 was well tolerated at all dose levels tested (15, 50, or 100 mg/kg). The administration of BR102 led to a minimal to moderate decrease in red blood cells (RBCs), hemoglobin (HGB), and hematocrit (HCT), and a corresponding increase in reticulocytes (Figure 6). Importantly, the levels of RBCs, HGB, HCT, and reticulocytes returned to baseline values by the end of the recovery period (Figure 6). No other BR102-related effects were detected on hematology parameters. BR102 treatment did not elicit cardiovascular toxicity, observed with pan-TGF-β antibody or TGF-βR small molecule inhibitors in animal studies [21,22]. There were no BR102-related changes in clinical observations, body weight, food consumption, clinical chemistry parameters, coagulation parameters, gross pathology, relative organ weights, or histopathology. No changes in cytokine release were noted. These data suggest that BR102 has a favorable safety profile in vivo.

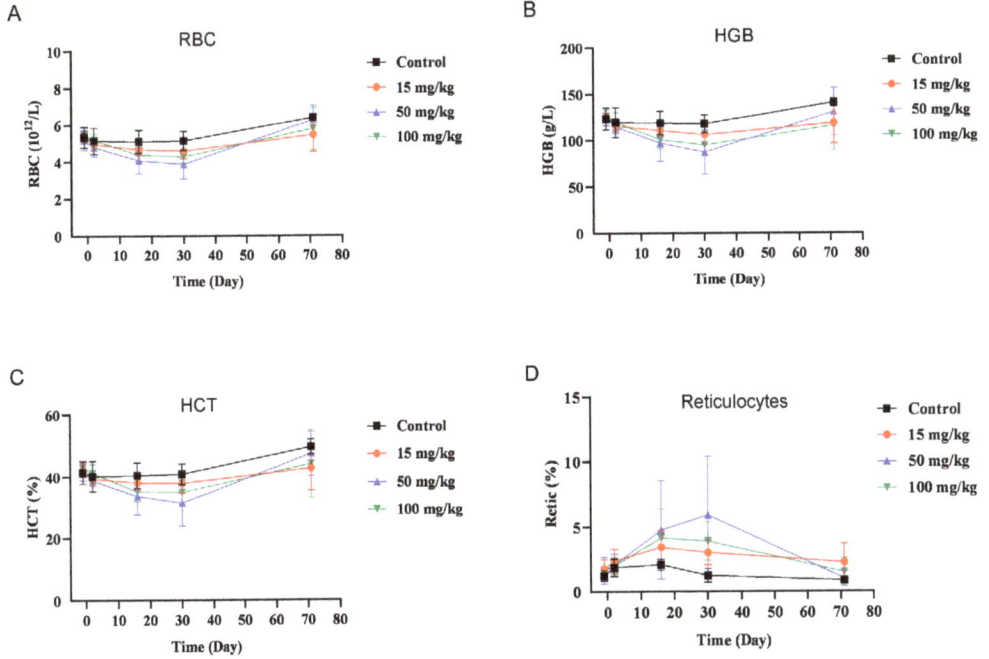

Figure 6. Treatment with BR102 is well tolerated in non-human primates. BR102 was administered to cynomolgus monkeys at 15, 50, and 100 mg/kg (five males and five females for each group) once weekly for a total of 4 weeks. Peripheral blood was collected for hematology during the pre-dose phase; on Days 2 and 16 of the dosing phases; and on Days 30 and 71 of the recovery periods. Hematology parameters, including RBC (**A**), HGB (**B**), HCT (**C**), and reticulocytes (**D**) were measured. Values are presented as mean ± SD.

4. Discussion

Poor response and resistance are the main challenges for PD-1/PD-L1-targeted immunotherapy. Other immunosuppressive regulators within TME may promote immune escape and suppress anticancer immune response [23]. TGF-β is secreted by multiple cell types in TME, which includes tumor cells, T cells, macrophages, and MDSCs. TGF-β exerts immune suppression and promotes tumor progression through its effects on both the innate and adaptive immune systems. It was shown that TGF-β could promote the expansion of

Treg cells and inhibit the function of cytotoxic T cells and DCs [24,25]. In addition, TGF-β could also impair NK function and drive myeloid cell-mediated tumor metastasis [26–28]. Moreover, TME-derived TGF-β could augment the expression of PD-1 in tumor-infiltrating lymphocytes, which causes CD8+ T cell suppression and immune resistance [14]. These indicated that TGF-β functions as a critical immune-suppressive cytokine in TME and may engage in crosstalk with PD-1/PD-L1 signal to promote immune escape. These provide a biological rationale for simultaneously targeting PD-L1 and TGF-β immunosuppressive signaling pathway, which could enhance antitumor immunity and overcome resistance to anti-PD-1/PD-L1 therapies.

We developed and characterized the novel bifunctional protein BR102, composed of an anti-PD-L1 antibody (HS636) fused to the ECD of human TGF-βRII. Amino acid mutations were introduced into the N-terminus of the ectodomain of TGF-βRII to avoid proteolytic degradation [20]. BR102 inhibits the binding of PD-L1 to both of its receptors, CD80 and PD-1. Furthermore, BR102 disrupts PD-L1-mediated downstream signaling and induces activation of T cells. The biological activity of BR102 is comparable to that of HS636, indicating that the fusion of TGF-βRII ECD does not affect the efficacy of the anti-PD-L1 antibody moiety. We found that the TGF-βRII moiety of BR102 could bind to the three TGF-β isoforms, TGF-β1, TGF-β2, and TGF-β3, and inhibit TGF-β-mediated signaling. Moreover, BR102 displays more potent antitumor activity compared to HS636 alone. Disruption of both TGF-β and PD-L1 signaling may contribute to the antitumor efficacy of BR102. These results indicate that BR102 could deliver the therapeutic benefit of simultaneously targeting TGF-β and PD-L1 signaling and support further exploiting BR102 as a novel therapy for advanced malignancies. In addition, it was shown that TGF-β-induced immunosuppression contributed to resistance to multiple antitumor treatments, such as radiotherapy, chemotherapy, immunotherapy, and targeted therapy [29]. Consequently, BR102 has the potential to be combined with these therapies to overcome therapy resistance and enhance treatment efficacy in cancer patients.

Besides BR102, other anti-PD-L1/TGF-β bifunctional proteins have been developed, including M7824 and YM101 [19,30]. Both BR102 and M7824 consist of an anti-PD-L1 antibody fused to the ECD of human TGF-βRII, while YM101 is a bispecific antibody developed with the Check-BODY™ platform [19,30]. Compared with M7824, BR102 has three amino acid mutations in the N-terminus of the ECD of TGF-βRII. We previously reported that the introduced amino acid mutations in BR102 could effectively decrease proteolytic degradation and improve druggability [20]. The anti-PD-L1 moieties of BR102 and M7824 are based on HS636 and avelumab, respectively. Although a head-to-head comparison of HS636 and avelumab was not conducted, HS636 displays similar in vitro and in vivo efficacy with another approved-anti-PD-L1, Atezolizumab. This supports that HS636 is a potent PD-L1 antagonist and HS636 is suitable for use as the anti-PD-L1 moiety of BR102. The anti-TGF-β moieties of BR102 and M7824 are based on the ECD of human TGF-βRII, designed as a trap for TGF-β, and the anti-TGF-β moiety of YM101 is based on a TGF-β antibody GC1008 [19,30]. However, the three anti-PD-L1/TGF-β bifunctional proteins could bind all three TGF-β isoforms (TGF-β1, TGF-β2, and TGF-β3). Moreover, BR102, M7824, and YM101 exhibit potent antitumor activity in syngeneic mouse models. Studies revealed that M7824 and YM101 promoted the immune-supportive TME by increased T cell infiltration into tumors, induction of an enhanced DCs density, and polarization of macrophages [19,30]. Further studies are needed to evaluate the effect of BR102 on TME regulation. Regarding safety, M7824 shows a manageable safety profile in clinical trials [31,32], and our data in the preclinical toxicity study also support the favorable safety profile of BR102. No YM101-related safety data have been disclosed or published. The molecular structure, specificity, and affinity of the anti-PD-L1 and anti-TGF-β moieties, may play key roles in determining the efficacy and safety of the anti-PD-L1/TGF-β bifunctional proteins.

Due to the accumulated evidence about the implication of TGF-β in tumor progression, various strategies, including antibodies against TGF-β or TGF-βR, ligand traps, TGF-βRI inhibitors, and antisense oligonucleotides have been explored to target TGF-β signaling and are being evaluated in clinical trials. However, only a minor clinical benefit and limited success using these TGF-β-targeting therapies were observed in the clinical setting. Moreover, adverse effects are another issue that challenges the clinical development of TGF-β-targeting therapies. It has been shown that blocking the TGF-β signaling with antibodies or TGF-βR kinase inhibitors resulted in cardiovascular toxicity in animals [21,22]. The cardiac side effects may be mitigated by employing an intermittent dosing schedule in human clinical trials using galunisertib, a TGF-βRI kinase inhibitor [33–35]. This indicated that optimal dosing regimens are needed to decrease toxicity for exploring TGF-β-targeted therapies. In addition, reversible cutaneous keratoacanthomas and squamous-cell carcinomas were observed in patients administrated with fresolimumab (GC1008), a TGF-β antibody [36]. In a phase I study evaluating the safety of an anti-TGF-βRII antibody (LY3022859) to treat patients with solid tumors, the maximum tolerated dose was not defined because of negative symptoms, such as uncontrolled cytokine release, despite prophylaxis [37]. The challenges for clinical development of TGF-β pathway antagonists may be largely due to the pleiotropic effect and dual function of TGF-β. TGF-β plays a significant role in embryonic development and maintenance of adult tissue homeostasis by transmitting its canonical and non-canonical signals. TGF-β functions as a tumor suppressor in the early stages and as a tumor promoter in the late stages. Mutations of various components of TGF-β signals may prompt the conversion of the TGF-β role in different tumor stages [38,39]. The pleiotropic nature of TGF-β restricts the clinical development of pharmacological TGF-β-targeted agents, which can affect normal tissue and lead to unwanted side effects. Considering the high PD-L1 expression within TME, the bifunctional anti-PD-L1/TGF-βRII fusion protein BR102 could be anticipated to lead to a more tumor-targeted inhibition of TGF-β within the TME and reduce safety concerns associated with some TGF-β targeted therapies. In the preclinical NHP toxicity study, BR102 displays a favorable safety profile. BR102 treatment does not cause cardiovascular toxicity and does not induce enhanced cytokine release. The red cell changes induced by BR102 are reversible. BR102 is being evaluated in clinical trials to test the safety and preliminary efficacy in advanced-stage cancer patients.

BR102 consists of the TGF-βRII moiety, which recognizes TGF-β1, TGF-β2, and TGF-β3. BR102 would likely block signals downstream of TGF-βR mediated by all three TGF-β isoforms. These isoforms are highly similar in sequence and structure, but show differential expression patterns in vivo. Studies reveal that TGF-β1 is the most prevalent member responsible for TGF-β pathway activity in many human tumor types. Selective TGF-β1 blocking could overcome resistance to ICIs in a mouse tumor model [40]. Although TGF-β2 and TGF-β3 are less frequently expressed in tumors, they may also be implicated in the progression of certain cancers. For example, TGF-β2 is overexpressed in glioblastoma and has been associated with poor clinical outcomes [41], and expression of TGF-β3 is shown to promote head and neck cancer growth and metastasis [42]. However, the role of TGF-β2 and TGF-β3 in tumor development must be better determined. Some Pan-TGF-β inhibitors that target all three TGF-β isoforms have been developed and are evaluated in clinical trials. In addition, isoform-selective inhibitors are also identified and selected for clinical evaluation, with the rational that that selectively targeting the cancer-relevant TGF-β pathway may avoid the side effects of broad TGF-β inhibition and benefit most from the TGF-β targeting. A specifically anti-TGF-β1 neutralizing antibody did not show clinical efficacy in the clinical evaluation as a monotherapy [43]. AVID200, an engineered TGF-β ligand trap that selectively binds and neutralizes TGF-β1 and TGF-β3, is currently in phase 1 trial for patients with advanced solid tumors (NCT03834662). NIS793 is an anti-TGF-β1/2 antibody combined with chemotherapy in a phase 2 trial patients with solid metastatic tumors (NCT04390763). More clinical outcomes are needed to evaluate whether these isoform-selective inhibitors could lead to a more favorable clinical benefit. In addition, considering that the PD-L1 and TGF-β are nonredundant pathways mediating immunosuppressive activity within TME, it is suggestive that BR102, the bifunctional molecular that simultaneously targets PD-L1 and TGF-β, may provide an alternative strategy to improve anti-TGF-β therapies. Furthermore, it is crucial to uncover biomarkers for defining patients who will benefit from TGF-β-targeted treatment. Several reports indicate that high expression of TGF-β target genes and mesenchymal subtypes correlate with poor prognosis in patients with many different cancer types, including CRC, hepatocellular carcinoma, and lung cancer [44–46]. A better understanding of the underlying mechanisms by which TGF-β signaling regulates normal and malignant processes will facilitate appropriate patient selection in clinical trials and advance the development of TGF-β antagonists.

5. Conclusions

BR102 is a novel bifunctional molecule that could simultaneously target the two immunosuppressors TGF-β and PD-L1. BR102 shows a higher antitumor efficacy than the anti-PD-L1 antibody, as well as a more favorable safety profile compared with some TGF-β-target therapies. The data support further development of BR102 for treating various tumor types.

6. Patents

Patent applications related to this work have been filed by BioRay (WO/2022/063114).

Supplementary Materials: The following supporting information can be downloaded at: https://www.mdpi.com/article/10.3390/cancers14194964/s1, Figure S1: Binding of BR102 to cynomolgus monkey PD-L1 and TGF-β1 were assessed by ELISA. Figure S2: Tumor weights (A), tumor images (B), and body weights (C) of MC38/hPD-L1-bearing mice treated with HS636 or BR102.

Author Contributions: Conceptualization, H.-B.W. and Z.-H.W.; methodology, Z.-H.W. and N.L.; validation, Z.-H.W., Z.-Z.G., G.C. and Y.-Q.Z.; formal analysis, Z.-H.W. and N.L.; investigation, N.L., M.-Z.J., Y.C., J.C., X.-F.M. and F.H.; data curation, Z.-H.W. and N.L.; visualization, N.L.; writing—original draft preparation, Z.-H.W.; writing—review and editing, G.C.; supervision, H.-B.W. and Z.-H.W.; project administration, Z.-H.W., N.L. and L.N.; funding acquisition, L.N. All authors have read and agreed to the published version of the manuscript.

Funding: This work was supported by the Key Research and Development Program of Zhejiang Province funded by the Science and Technology Department of Zhejiang Province, China (grant number 2021C03089).

Institutional Review Board Statement: The animal study protocol was approved by the Institutional Animal Care and Use Committee of Biocytogen (Approval number: 0078-17025-AN-01; 20170428), Crown Bioscience (Approval number: AN-1507-009-657; 20160620), and Joinn (Approval number: ACU20-2060; 20200721).

Informed Consent Statement: Not applicable.

Data Availability Statement: All data in the current study are available from the corresponding author upon reasonable request.

Conflicts of Interest: Z.-H.W., N.L., Z.-Z.G., L.N., Y.-Q.Z., M.-Z.J., Y.C., J.C., X.-F.M., F.H. and H.-B.W. are employees of BioRay Co., Ltd. G.C. is an employee of BioRay Corp.

References

1. Hodi, F.S.; O'Day, S.J.; McDermott, D.F.; Weber, R.W.; Sosman, J.A.; Haanen, J.B.; Gonzalez, R.; Robert, C.; Schadendorf, D.; Hassel, J.C.; et al. Improved survival with ipilimumab in patients with metastatic melanoma. N. Engl. J. Med. 2010, 363, 711–723. [CrossRef] [PubMed]
2. Robert, C.; Ribas, A.; Hamid, O.; Daud, A.; Wolchok, J.D.; Joshua, A.M.; Hwu, W.J.; Weber, J.S.; Gangadhar, T.C.; Joseph, R.W.; et al. Durable Complete Response After Discontinuation of Pembrolizumab in Patients With Metastatic Melanoma. J. Clin. Oncol. 2018, 36, 1668–1674. [CrossRef] [PubMed]
3. Reck, M.; Rodriguez-Abreu, D.; Robinson, A.G.; Hui, R.; Csoszi, T.; Fulop, A.; Gottfried, M.; Peled, N.; Tafreshi, A.; Cuffe, S.; et al. Pembrolizumab versus Chemotherapy for PD-L1-Positive Non-Small-Cell Lung Cancer. N. Engl. J. Med. 2016, 375, 1823–1833. [CrossRef] [PubMed]

4. Restifo, N.P.; Smyth, M.J.; Snyder, A. Acquired resistance to immunotherapy and future challenges. *Nat. Rev. Cancer* **2016**, *16*, 121–126. [CrossRef]
5. Sharma, P.; Hu-Lieskovan, S.; Wargo, J.A.; Ribas, A. Primary, Adaptive, and Acquired Resistance to Cancer Immunotherapy. *Cell* **2017**, *168*, 707–723. [CrossRef]
6. Derynck, R.; Akhurst, R.J.; Balmain, A. TGF-beta signaling in tumor suppression and cancer progression. *Nat. Genet.* **2001**, *29*, 117–129. [CrossRef]
7. Derynck, R.; Muthusamy, B.P.; Saeteurn, K.Y. Signaling pathway cooperation in TGF-beta-induced epithelial-mesenchymal transition. *Curr. Opin. Cell Biol.* **2014**, *31*, 56–66. [CrossRef]
8. Hao, Y.; Baker, D.; Ten Dijke, P. TGF-beta-Mediated Epithelial-Mesenchymal Transition and Cancer Metastasis. *Int. J. Mol. Sci.* **2019**, *20*, 2767. [CrossRef]
9. Batlle, E.; Massague, J. Transforming Growth Factor-beta Signaling in Immunity and Cancer. *Immunity* **2019**, *50*, 924–940. [CrossRef]
10. Lin, R.L.; Zhao, L.J. Mechanistic basis and clinical relevance of the role of transforming growth factor-beta in cancer. *Cancer Biol. Med.* **2015**, *12*, 385–393. [CrossRef]
11. Calon, A.; Lonardo, E.; Berenguer-Llergo, A.; Espinet, E.; Hernando-Momblona, X.; Iglesias, M.; Sevillano, M.; Palomo-Ponce, S.; Tauriello, D.V.; Byrom, D.; et al. Stromal gene expression defines poor-prognosis subtypes in colorectal cancer. *Nat. Genet.* **2015**, *47*, 320–329. [CrossRef] [PubMed]
12. Ciardiello, D.; Elez, E.; Tabernero, J.; Seoane, J. Clinical development of therapies targeting TGFbeta: Current knowledge and future perspectives. *Ann. Oncol.* **2020**, *31*, 1336–1349. [CrossRef] [PubMed]
13. David, J.M.; Dominguez, C.; McCampbell, K.K.; Gulley, J.L.; Schlom, J.; Palena, C. A novel bifunctional anti-PD-L1/TGF-beta Trap fusion protein (M7824) efficiently reverts mesenchymalization of human lung cancer cells. *Oncoimmunology* **2017**, *6*, e1349589. [CrossRef]
14. Park, B.V.; Freeman, Z.T.; Ghasemzadeh, A.; Chattergoon, M.A.; Rutebemberwa, A.; Steigner, J.; Winter, M.E.; Huynh, T.V.; Sebald, S.M.; Lee, S.J.; et al. TGFbeta1-Mediated SMAD3 Enhances PD-1 Expression on Antigen-Specific T Cells in Cancer. *Cancer Discov.* **2016**, *6*, 1366–1381. [CrossRef]
15. Mariathasan, S.; Turley, S.J.; Nickles, D.; Castiglioni, A.; Yuen, K.; Wang, Y.; Kadel, E.E., III; Koeppen, H.; Astarita, J.L.; Cubas, R.; et al. TGFbeta attenuates tumour response to PD-L1 blockade by contributing to exclusion of T cells. *Nature* **2018**, *554*, 544–548. [CrossRef] [PubMed]
16. Hugo, W.; Zaretsky, J.M.; Sun, L.; Song, C.; Moreno, B.H.; Hu-Lieskovan, S.; Berent-Maoz, B.; Pang, J.; Chmielowski, B.; Cherry, G.; et al. Genomic and Transcriptomic Features of Response to Anti-PD-1 Therapy in Metastatic Melanoma. *Cell* **2016**, *165*, 35–44. [CrossRef]
17. Tauriello, D.V.F.; Palomo-Ponce, S.; Stork, D.; Berenguer-Llergo, A.; Badia-Ramentol, J.; Iglesias, M.; Sevillano, M.; Ibiza, S.; Canellas, A.; Hernando-Momblona, X.; et al. TGFbeta drives immune evasion in genetically reconstituted colon cancer metastasis. *Nature* **2018**, *554*, 538–543. [CrossRef]
18. de Streel, G.; Bertrand, C.; Chalon, N.; Lienart, S.; Bricard, O.; Lecomte, S.; Devreux, J.; Gaignage, M.; De Boeck, G.; Marien, L.; et al. Selective inhibition of TGF-beta1 produced by GARP-expressing Tregs overcomes resistance to PD-1/PD-L1 blockade in cancer. *Nat. Commun.* **2020**, *11*, 4545. [CrossRef]
19. Lan, Y.; Zhang, D.; Xu, C.; Hance, K.W.; Marelli, B.; Qi, J.; Yu, H.; Qin, G.; Sircar, A.; Hernandez, V.M.; et al. Enhanced preclinical antitumor activity of M7824, a bifunctional fusion protein simultaneously targeting PD-L1 and TGF-beta. *Sci. Transl. Med.* **2018**, *10*, eaan5488. [CrossRef]
20. Gao, Z.Z.; Li, C.; Chen, G.; Yuan, J.J.; Zhou, Y.Q.; Jiao, J.Y.; Nie, L.; Qi, J.; Yang, Y.; Chen, S.Q.; et al. Optimization strategies for expression of a novel bifunctional anti-PD-L1/TGFBR2-ECD fusion protein. *Protein. Expr. Purif.* **2022**, *189*, 105973. [CrossRef]
21. Mitra, M.S.; Lancaster, K.; Adedeji, A.O.; Palanisamy, G.S.; Dave, R.A.; Zhong, F.; Holdren, M.S.; Turley, S.J.; Liang, W.C.; Wu, Y.; et al. A Potent Pan-TGFbeta Neutralizing Monoclonal Antibody Elicits Cardiovascular Toxicity in Mice and Cynomolgus Monkeys. *Toxicol. Sci.* **2020**, *175*, 24–34. [CrossRef] [PubMed]
22. Anderton, M.J.; Mellor, H.R.; Bell, A.; Sadler, C.; Pass, M.; Powell, S.; Steele, S.J.; Roberts, R.R.; Heier, A. Induction of heart valve lesions by small-molecule ALK5 inhibitors. *Toxicol. Pathol.* **2011**, *39*, 916–924. [CrossRef] [PubMed]
23. Kim, J.M.; Chen, D.S. Immune escape to PD-L1/PD-1 blockade: Seven steps to success (or failure). *Ann. Oncol.* **2016**, *27*, 1492–1504. [CrossRef] [PubMed]
24. Thomas, D.A.; Massague, J. TGF-beta directly targets cytotoxic T cell functions during tumor evasion of immune surveillance. *Cancer Cell* **2005**, *8*, 369–380. [CrossRef]
25. Chen, W.; Jin, W.; Hardegen, N.; Lei, K.J.; Li, L.; Marinos, N.; McGrady, G.; Wahl, S.M. Conversion of peripheral CD4+CD25- naive T cells to CD4+CD25+ regulatory T cells by TGF-beta induction of transcription factor Foxp3. *J Exp Med* **2003**, *198*, 1875–1886. [CrossRef]
26. Viel, S.; Marcais, A.; Guimaraes, F.S.; Loftus, R.; Rabilloud, J.; Grau, M.; Degouve, S.; Djebali, S.; Sanlaville, A.; Charrier, E.; et al. TGF-beta inhibits the activation and functions of NK cells by repressing the mTOR pathway. *Sci. Signal.* **2016**, *9*, ra19. [CrossRef]
27. Motz, G.T.; Coukos, G. Deciphering and reversing tumor immune suppression. *Immunity* **2013**, *39*, 61–73. [CrossRef]
28. Pang, Y.; Gara, S.K.; Achyut, B.R.; Li, Z.; Yan, H.H.; Day, C.P.; Weiss, J.M.; Trinchieri, G.; Morris, J.C.; Yang, L. TGF-beta signaling in myeloid cells is required for tumor metastasis. *Cancer Discov.* **2013**, *3*, 936–951. [CrossRef]

29. Derynck, R.; Turley, S.J.; Akhurst, R.J. TGFbeta biology in cancer progression and immunotherapy. *Nat. Rev. Clin. Oncol.* **2021**, *18*, 9–34. [CrossRef]
30. Yi, M.; Zhang, J.; Li, A.; Niu, M.; Yan, Y.; Jiao, Y.; Luo, S.; Zhou, P.; Wu, K. The construction, expression, and enhanced anti-tumor activity of YM101: A bispecific antibody simultaneously targeting TGF-beta and PD-L1. *J. Hematol. Oncol.* **2021**, *14*, 27. [CrossRef]
31. Strauss, J.; Heery, C.R.; Schlom, J.; Madan, R.A.; Cao, L.; Kang, Z.; Lamping, E.; Marte, J.L.; Donahue, R.N.; Grenga, I.; et al. Phase I Trial of M7824 (MSB0011359C), a Bifunctional Fusion Protein Targeting PD-L1 and TGFbeta, in Advanced Solid Tumors. *Clin. Cancer Res.* **2018**, *24*, 1287–1295. [CrossRef] [PubMed]
32. Khasraw, M.; Weller, M.; Lorente, D.; Kolibaba, K.; Lee, C.K.; Gedye, C.; La Fuente, M.I.; Vicente, D.; Reardon, D.A.; Gan, H.K.; et al. Bintrafusp alfa (M7824), a bifunctional fusion protein targeting TGF-beta and PD-L1: Results from a phase I expansion cohort in patients with recurrent glioblastoma. *Neurooncol. Adv.* **2021**, *3*, vdab058. [CrossRef] [PubMed]
33. Gueorguieva, I.; Cleverly, A.L.; Stauber, A.; Sada Pillay, N.; Rodon, J.A.; Miles, C.P.; Yingling, J.M.; Lahn, M.M. Defining a therapeutic window for the novel TGF-beta inhibitor LY2157299 monohydrate based on a pharmacokinetic/pharmacodynamic model. *Br. J. Clin. Pharm.* **2014**, *77*, 796–807. [CrossRef] [PubMed]
34. Kovacs, R.J.; Maldonado, G.; Azaro, A.; Fernandez, M.S.; Romero, F.L.; Sepulveda-Sanchez, J.M.; Corretti, M.; Carducci, M.; Dolan, M.; Gueorguieva, I.; et al. Cardiac Safety of TGF-beta Receptor I Kinase Inhibitor LY2157299 Monohydrate in Cancer Patients in a First-in-Human Dose Study. *Cardiovasc. Toxicol.* **2015**, *15*, 309–323. [CrossRef] [PubMed]
35. Rodon, J.; Carducci, M.A.; Sepulveda-Sanchez, J.M.; Azaro, A.; Calvo, E.; Seoane, J.; Brana, I.; Sicart, E.; Gueorguieva, I.; Cleverly, A.L.; et al. First-in-human dose study of the novel transforming growth factor-beta receptor I kinase inhibitor LY2157299 monohydrate in patients with advanced cancer and glioma. *Clin. Cancer Res.* **2015**, *21*, 553–560. [CrossRef] [PubMed]
36. Lacouture, M.E.; Morris, J.C.; Lawrence, D.P.; Tan, A.R.; Olencki, T.E.; Shapiro, G.I.; Dezube, B.J.; Berzofsky, J.A.; Hsu, F.J.; Guitart, J. Cutaneous keratoacanthomas/squamous cell carcinomas associated with neutralization of transforming growth factor beta by the monoclonal antibody fresolimumab (GC1008). *Cancer Immunol. Immunother.* **2015**, *64*, 437–446. [CrossRef]
37. Tolcher, A.W.; Berlin, J.D.; Cosaert, J.; Kauh, J.; Chan, E.; Piha-Paul, S.A.; Amaya, A.; Tang, S.; Driscoll, K.; Kimbung, R.; et al. A phase I study of anti-TGFbeta receptor type-II monoclonal antibody LY3022859 in patients with advanced solid tumors. *Cancer Chemother. Pharmacol.* **2017**, *79*, 673–680. [CrossRef]
38. de Miranda, N.F.; van Dinther, M.; van den Akker, B.E.; van Wezel, T.; ten Dijke, P.; Morreau, H. Transforming Growth Factor beta Signaling in Colorectal Cancer Cells with Microsatellite Instability Despite Biallelic Mutations in TGFBR2. *Gastroenterology* **2015**, *148*, 1427–1437.e8. [CrossRef]
39. Yakicier, M.C.; Irmak, M.B.; Romano, A.; Kew, M.; Ozturk, M. Smad2 and Smad4 gene mutations in hepatocellular carcinoma. *Oncogene* **1999**, *18*, 4879–4883. [CrossRef]
40. Martin, C.J.; Datta, A.; Littlefield, C.; Kalra, A.; Chapron, C.; Wawersik, S.; Dagbay, K.B.; Brueckner, C.T.; Nikiforov, A.; Danehy, F.T., Jr.; et al. Selective inhibition of TGFbeta1 activation overcomes primary resistance to checkpoint blockade therapy by altering tumor immune landscape. *Sci. Transl. Med.* **2020**, *12*, eaay8456. [CrossRef]
41. Rodon, L.; Gonzalez-Junca, A.; Inda Mdel, M.; Sala-Hojman, A.; Martinez-Saez, E.; Seoane, J. Active CREB1 promotes a malignant TGFbeta2 autocrine loop in glioblastoma. *Cancer Discov.* **2014**, *4*, 1230–1241. [CrossRef]
42. Qin, X.; Yan, M.; Zhang, J.; Wang, X.; Shen, Z.; Lv, Z.; Li, Z.; Wei, W.; Chen, W. TGFbeta3-mediated induction of Periostin facilitates head and neck cancer growth and is associated with metastasis. *Sci. Rep.* **2016**, *6*, 20587. [CrossRef] [PubMed]
43. Cohn, A.; Lahn, M.M.; Williams, K.E.; Cleverly, A.L.; Pitou, C.; Kadam, S.K.; Farmen, M.W.; Desaiah, D.; Raju, R.; Conkling, P.; et al. A phase I dose-escalation study to a predefined dose of a transforming growth factor-beta1 monoclonal antibody (TbetaM1) in patients with metastatic cancer. *Int. J. Oncol.* **2014**, *45*, 2221–2231. [CrossRef]
44. De Sousa, E.M.F.; Wang, X.; Jansen, M.; Fessler, E.; Trinh, A.; de Rooij, L.P.; de Jong, J.H.; de Boer, O.J.; van Leersum, R.; Bijlsma, M.F.; et al. Poor-prognosis colon cancer is defined by a molecularly distinct subtype and develops from serrated precursor lesions. *Nat. Med.* **2013**, *19*, 614–618. [CrossRef]
45. Fessler, E.; Drost, J.; van Hooff, S.R.; Linnekamp, J.F.; Wang, X.; Jansen, M.; De Sousa, E.M.F.; Prasetyanti, P.R.; JE, I.J.; Franitza, M.; et al. TGFbeta signaling directs serrated adenomas to the mesenchymal colorectal cancer subtype. *EMBO Mol. Med.* **2016**, *8*, 745–760. [CrossRef] [PubMed]
46. Coulouarn, C.; Factor, V.M.; Thorgeirsson, S.S. Transforming growth factor-beta gene expression signature in mouse hepatocytes predicts clinical outcome in human cancer. *Hepatology* **2008**, *47*, 2059–2067. [CrossRef] [PubMed]

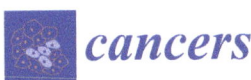

Article

Bispecific BCMA-CD3 Antibodies Block Multiple Myeloma Tumor Growth

Lijun Wu [1,2], Yanwei Huang [1], John Sienkiewicz [1], Jinying Sun [1], Liselle Guiang [1], Feng Li [1], Liming Yang [1] and Vita Golubovskaya [1,*]

[1] Promab Biotechnologies, 2600 Hilltop Drive, Richmond, CA 94806, USA; john@promab.com (L.W.); yanwei.huang@promab.com (Y.H.); john.sienkiewicz@promab.com (J.S.); sunnie.sun@promab.com (J.S.); liselle.guiang@promab.com (L.G.); feng.li@promab.com (F.L.); liming.yang@promab.com (L.Y.)
[2] Forevertek Biotechnology, Janshan Road, Changsha Hi-Tech Industrial Development Zone, Changsha 410205, China
* Correspondence: vita.gol@promab.com; Tel.: +1-510-974-0697

Citation: Wu, L.; Huang, Y.; Sienkiewicz, J.; Sun, J.; Guiang, L.; Li, F.; Yang, L.; Golubovskaya, V. Bispecific BCMA-CD3 Antibodies Block Multiple Myeloma Tumor Growth. *Cancers* 2022, 14, 2518. https://doi.org/10.3390/cancers14102518

Academic Editors: Sylvie Hermouet and Taketo Yamada

Received: 1 April 2022
Accepted: 18 May 2022
Published: 20 May 2022

Publisher's Note: MDPI stays neutral with regard to jurisdictional claims in published maps and institutional affiliations.

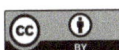

Copyright: © 2022 by the authors. Licensee MDPI, Basel, Switzerland. This article is an open access article distributed under the terms and conditions of the Creative Commons Attribution (CC BY) license (https://creativecommons.org/licenses/by/4.0/).

Simple Summary: Multiple myeloma accounts for approximately 10% of hematological cancers in the United States. It is a malignancy of plasma cells which accumulate in the bone marrow and produce a monoclonal protein. Novel treatments are needed to cure multiple myeloma patients. The goal of this report was to develop novel bispecific BCMA-CD3 antibodies targeting a B cell maturation antigen, BCMA, which is overexpressed in multiple myeloma. The data demonstrated high efficacy of BCMA-CD3 antibodies in multiple myeloma cell lines in vitro and in vivo. The data provide a basis for future clinical studies.

Abstract: BCMA antigen is overexpressed in multiple myeloma cells and has been shown to be a promising target for novel cellular and antibody therapeutics. The humanized BCMA (clone 4C8A) antibody that effectively targeted multiple myeloma in a CAR (chimeric antigen receptor) format was used for designing several formats of bispecific BCMA-CD3 antibodies. Several different designs of univalent and bivalent humanized BCMA-CD3 CrossMAB and BCMA-FAB-CD3 ScFv-Fc antibodies were tested for binding with BCMA-positive cells and T cells and for killing by real time cytotoxic activity and IFN-gamma secretion with CHO-BCMA target cells and with multiple myeloma MM1S and H929 cell lines. All BCMA-CD3 antibodies demonstrated specific binding by FACS to CHO-BCMA, multiple myeloma cells, and to T cells with affinity Kd in the nM range. All antibodies with T cells specifically killed CHO-BCMA and multiple myeloma cells in a dose-dependent manner. The BCMA-CD3 antibodies with T cells secreted IFN-gamma with EC_{50} in the nM range. In addition, three BCMA bispecific antibodies had high in vivo efficacy using an MM1S xenograft NSG mouse model. The data demonstrate the high efficacy of novel hBCMA-CD3 antibodies with multiple myeloma cells and provide a basis for future pre-clinical and clinical development.

Keywords: multiple myeloma; BCMA; bispecific antibody

1. Introduction

Multiple myeloma accounts for 1.3% of all cancers and more than 10% of hematological diseases in the USA [1,2]. Multiple myeloma (MM) is characterized by clonal expansion of plasma cells in the bone marrow resulting in the expression of myeloma M protein (also called monoclonal protein) and causing different organ damage [1]. Although current therapies for multiple myeloma cause remission, most of the patients will eventually die due to relapse [3]. Novel immunotherapy treatments are needed for multiple myeloma with novel monoclonal antibodies, antibody drug conjugates, ADC, CAR (chimeric antigen receptor)-T cell therapy, or bispecific antibodies targeting specific multiple myeloma antigens [3–13].

BCMA (CD269 or tumor necrosis factor receptor superfamily member 17 (TNFRSF17)) is a B cell maturation antigen that is overexpressed in malignant plasma B cells [14]. BCMA is one of the multiple myeloma antigens which has emerged as a promising therapeutic target [6,15–17]. BCMA binds several ligands including APRIL (a proliferation-inducing ligand) and BAFF (B cell-activating factor) [18,19] and plays an important role in survival signaling mediated by NF-kappa B, STAT3, ERK1/2, and AKT/PI3K signaling pathways [13,14,19,20].

In this report, we generated novel BCMA-CD3 antibodies using several different designs and tested their efficacy in vitro and in vivo. The data demonstrate the functional activity of novel BCMA-CD3 bispecific antibodies which can be used in future pre-clinical and clinical studies.

2. Materials and Methods

2.1. Cell Lines

Multiple myeloma H929, RPMI8226, and MM1S cell lines and lymphoblast K562 cell lines were purchased from the ATCC (Manassas, VA, USA) and cultured in RPMI-1640 medium (Thermo Fisher, Waltham, MA, USA) with 10% FBA (AmCell, Mountain View, CA, USA). CHO cells were cultured in DMEM (GE Healthcare, Chicago, IL, USA) containing 10% FBS (AmCell, Mountain View, CA, USA). CHO-BCMA cells were purchased from BPS Bioscience (San Diego, CA, USA) and cultured in Ham's F12K medium containing 10% FBS with 1 mg/mL Geneticin (Thermo Fisher). Human peripheral blood mononuclear cells (PBMC) were isolated from whole blood at the Stanford Hospital Blood Center according to IRB-approved protocol (#13942). PBMC were isolated by density sedimentation over Ficoll-Paque (GE Healthcare). B cells were isolated from PBMC using a human B cell isolation kit according to the manufacturer's protocol (Myltenyi Biotech, Bergisch Gladbach, Germany). B cells were expanded for 7 days using IMDM (Iscove's Modified Dulbecco's Medium) with 10% human AB serum, IL-21 (50 ng/mL), CD40 ligand (100 ng/mL), and anti-HA antibody (200 ng/mL). B cell marker was detected on B cells by FACS with an anti-CD20 antibody.

2.2. Cloning of Bispecific Antibodies

Different designs of BCMA CrossMab KIH IgG1 bivalent and univalent were constructed according to [21]. The Fc region contained P329G mutation and L234AL235A (LALA) mutations to silence Fc by preventing binding to Fc gamma receptors and activating innate immune cells [21]. Humanized BCMA VH and VL from antibody 4C8A clones were used for bispecific antibody generation [22,23]. CD3 Scfv and VH and VL humanized sequences were from CD3e antibodies [21]. Another design was triple chain with BCMA univalent part and CD3 ScFv with KIH and LALA mutations. For one of triple chain designs antibody differently humanized CD3 e was used. All three or four subunits of bispecific antibody were subcloned into pYD11 vector and DNA constructs used for co-transfection of 293 cells at equal ratio. The four subunits of PF3135 (PF-06863135) bispecific BCMA-CD3 antibody sequences were obtained from https://drugs.ncats.io/drug/L0HR9A577V (accessed on 18 May 2022) and each subunit was subcloned into PYD11 vector and engineered antibody (PBM0057) was used as a positive control. The sequences of all antibodies are shown in Supplemental Table S1.

2.3. Transfection of 293 Cells, Isolation and Purification of Bispecific Antibodies

293S cells were transfected using DNA constructs of bispecific antibodies and Nano-Fect transfection agent and incubated in Freestyle F17 medium with 8 mM Glutamine and 0.1% Pluronic F68 surfactant in suspension bottles using shaker at 37 °C and 5% CO_2. The supernatant was collected at days 3–7 for antibody purification by centrifugation for 12 min at $3000 \times g$. The filtered supernatant was used for the isolation of antibody using column with protein A beads (Millipore, Burlington, MA, USA). After washing column with 1× PBS, the antibody was eluted with Pierce IgG elution buffer (ThermoFisher). The concentration of bispecific antibody was estimated with Nanodrop instrument and BCA protein assay kit (Thermo Fisher). The purified antibodies were run on SDS gel and used for functional analyses.

2.4. Flow Cytometry

To measure binding of bispecific antibodies 0.25 million cells were suspended in 100 µL of buffer (PBS containing 2 mM EDTA pH 8 and 0.5% BSA) and incubated on ice with 1 µL of human serum (Jackson Immunoresearch, West Grove, PA, USA) for 10 min. Then different dilutions of antibody were added, and the cells were incubated on ice for 30 min. The cells were rinsed with FACS buffer and suspended in 100 µL of buffer. Then 1 µL of phycoerythrin (PE) or APC-conjugated secondary antibody (BD Biosciences, San Jose, CA, USA) was added, and the cells were incubated on ice for 30 min. The cells were rinsed and suspended in buffer for analysis on a FACSCalibur (BD Biosciences). Affinity (Kd) was measured with GraphPad software. CAR-positive cells were detected by FACS with anti-mouse F(ab)'2 antibody and biotin-conjugated recombinant BCMA protein added with CD3-APC-conjugated mouse anti-CD3 antibody and PE-conjugated streptavidin at 1:100 dilution. After 30 min incubation at 4 °C, the cells were rinsed, stained with 7-AAD, suspended in the FACS buffer, and analyzed on a FACSCalibur (BD Biosciences).

2.5. Real-Time Cytotoxicity Assay (RTCA)

Adherent target cells (CHO or CHO-BCMA) were seeded into 96-well E-plates (Acea Biosciences, San Diego, CA, USA) at 1×10^4 cells per well and monitored in culture overnight with the impedance-based real-time cell analysis (RTCA) × CELLigence system (Acea Biosciences). The next day, the medium was removed and replaced with AIM V-AlbuMAX medium containing 10% FBS $\pm$ 1×10^5 effector cells (CAR-T cells, non-transduced T cells, or T cells with BCMA-CD3 bispecific antibodies), in triplicate. The cells in the E-plates were monitored for another one to two days with the RTCA system, and impedance was plotted over time.

2.6. ELISA (Enzyme-Linked Immunoassay)

Target cells (H929, RPMI8226, and MM1S) were cultured with different dilutions of BCMA-CD3 antibodies in U-bottom 96-well plates with 200 µL of AIM V-AlbuMAX medium containing 10% FBS, in triplicate and then analyzed by ELISA for human IFN-γ levels using a kit from R&D Systems (Minneapolis, MN, USA) according to the manufacturer's protocol. For adherent CHO and CHO-BCMA supernatant after cytotoxicity assay was collected and analyzed as above by ELISA.

2.7. Lentiviral CAR and CAR-T Cell Generation

Lentiviral CAR construct containing humanized BCMA ScFv with same VH and VL as used in BCMA-CD3 bispecific antibodies, 41BB costimulatory and CD3 activating domains was ordered from Vector Builder (Chicago, IL, USA). Lentiviral CAR was used for lentivirus generation as described in [22]. In brief, CAR-T cells were generated by transducing lentiviral CAR into PBMC pre-activated with CD3/CD28 Dynabeads from Thermo Fisher as described in [22]. CAR-T cells were expanded over 10–12 days using AIM-AlbuMAX medium (Thermo Fisher, USA) with 10% FBS and 10 ng/mL IL-2 (Thermo Fisher).

2.8. Mouse RPMI8226 Xenograft Tumors

Six-week-old NSG mice (Jackson Laboratories, Bar Harbor, ME, USA) were housed and manipulated in strict accordance with the Institutional Animal Care and Use Committee (IACUC) (#LUM-001). Each mouse was injected intravenously on day 0 with 100 µL of 2×10^6 MM1S-luciferase positive cells and 5×10^6 PBMC. Bispecific antibodies were injected intravenously (50 ug/mice) on days 4 and 11, and (100 ug/mice) on day 18 as described in [21]. A total of 2×10^6 RPMI8226-luciferase$^+$ cells were injected intravenously to NSG mice, and next day 1×10^7 CAR-T cells were injected intravenously to perform imaging and survival study. Imaging was performed using IVIS Imaging System (Perkin Elmer, Watham, MA, USA), and quantification of BLI (bioluminescence) in photons/sec was used for the analysis of xenograft tumor growth. Kaplan Myer curve was used for analysis of mice survival.

2.9. Statistical Analysis

Data were analyzed and plotted with Prism software (GraphPad, San Diego, CA, USA). Comparisons between three or more groups were performed by one-way ANOVA or two-way ANOVA with Tukey's or Sidak's post hoc test. Comparisons between two groups were performed by unpaired Student's t-test. The survival curves were compared with Log-rank Mantel-Cox test. The difference with $p < 0.05$ was considered significant, and with $p < 0.001$ was considered highly significant.

3. Results

3.1. Structures of Bispecific BCMA-CD3 Antibodies

We designed BCMA-CD3 antibodies with different structures such as univalent, bivalent BCMA-CD3 CrossMab knob-in-hole KIH and BCMA-CD3 ScFv triple chain antibodies (Figure 1). Bivalent CrossMAB and knob-in-hole KIH (IgG1) BCMA-CD3 antibodies are shown on the left upper panel, called PBM0012. The Fc part of BCMA-CD3 antibody contains modification Pro329Gly, called P329G, and Leu234Ala/Leu235Ala, called LALA mutations, as described in [21] (Figure 1). These mutations decrease the binding of BCMA-CD3 antibody to Fc gamma receptors and to complement components preventing Fc gamma receptor-mediated activation of innate immune effector cells including natural killer (NK) cells, monocytes/macrophages, and neutrophils [21]. The same structure but univalent BCMA-CD3 antibody is shown on the lower-left panel and called, PBM0056. The BCMA-CD3 antibody with univalent BCMA arm and CD3 ScFv and with KIH Fc with LALA mutations is shown in Figure 1, middle-upper panel, called PBM0060. The same structure but with a differently humanized CD3 ScFv sequence with KIH Fc with LALA mutations is shown in Figure 1, middle-lower panel, called PBM0055. The control benchmark antibody was Pfizer's PF3135 antibody with IgG2 Fc with D265A mutation, called PBM0057 (Figure 1, upper right panel).

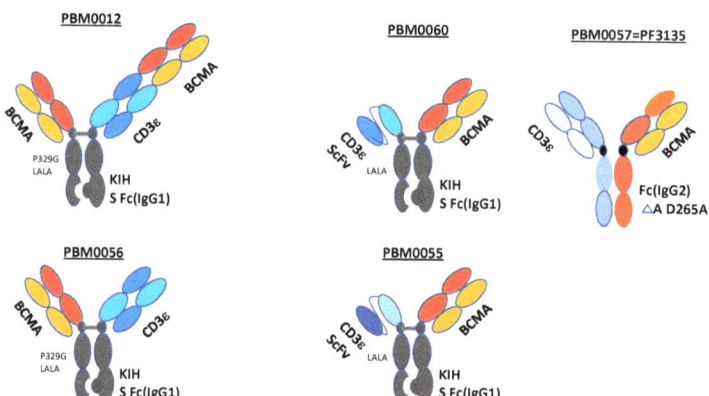

Figure 1. Different structures of BCMA-CD3 antibodies. Left panels: Bivalent PBM0012 antibody Crossmab KIH (**upper panel**) and univalent PBM0056 BCMA-CD3 CrossMAB KIH (IgG1) (**lower panel**) antibodies. Middle upper panel: BCMA-FAB-CD3 Scfv KIH, called PBM0060 (CD3 ScFv contains same heavy and light chains as for PBM0012 and PBM0056); middle lower panel: PBM0055 structure is the same as for PBM0060 antibody but with differently humanized CD3 ScFv. Right upper panel: Pfizer PF3135 control benchmark antibody, called PBM0057.

3.2. Binding of BCMA-CD3 Antibodies to BCMA-Positive Cells and T Cells

All formats of BCMA-CD3 antibodies shown in Figure 1 were tested with CHO-BCMA-positive cells by FACS for binding (Figure 2A–E). All antibodies bound CHO-BCMA cells at Kd in nM range from 0.22–4.9 nM. There was no binding of BCMA-CD3 antibodies to CHO cells (Figure S1A). These antibodies also bound to CD3-positive T cells with KD that varied from 6.2 nM to 690 nM (Figure 2F–J). Thus, BCMA-CD3 antibodies bound both BCMA-positive and CD3-positive cells.

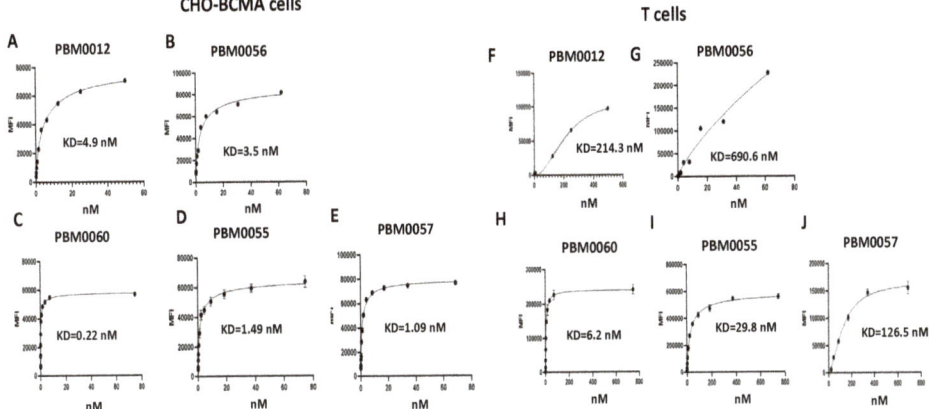

Figure 2. Binding of BCMA-CD3 antibodies to BCMA-positive CHO-BCMA cells and T cells. FACS was performed with all antibodies on BCMA-positive CHO-BCMA cells (**A–E**), and T cells (**F–J**). Representative assay is shown.

3.3. T Cells with BCMA-CD3 Antibody Kill CHO-BCMA-Positive Cells and Secrete IFN-Gamma

T cells with different dilutions of BCMA-CD3 antibodies were used in a real-time cytotoxicity assay (RTCA) with CHO-BCMA target cells (Figure 3A). All designs of BCMA-CD3 antibodies with T cells killed CHO-BCMA in a dose-dependent manner (Figure 3A). BCMA-CD3 antibody alone without T cells did not have cytotoxic activity.

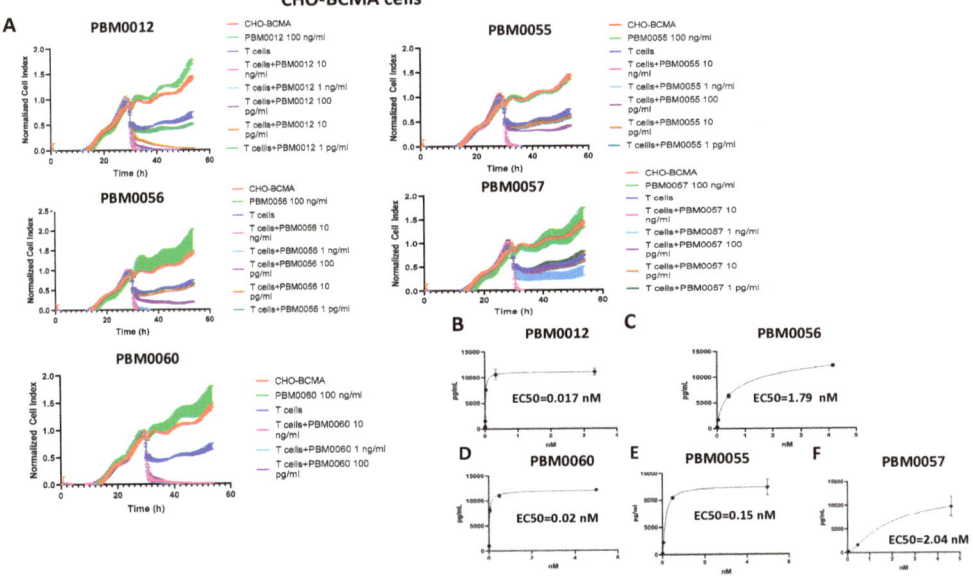

Figure 3. T cells with BCMA-CD3 antibodies effectively killed CHO-BCMA cells and secreted IFN-gamma. (**A**) RTCA killing assay with T cells and BCMA-CD3 antibodies against CHO-BCMA target cells. (**B–F**) IFN-gamma secretion by T cells with BCMA-CD3 antibodies and CHO-BCMA target cells. EC50 for each antibody is shown in nM. Representative RTCA and IFN-gamma assays are shown.

BCMA-CD3 bispecific antibodies with T cells secreted IFN-gamma with EC50 ranged from 0.017–2.04 nM (Figure 3B–F). There was no IFN-gamma secretion by BCMA-CD3 antibodies with T cells and BCMA-negative CHO cells (Figure S1B). Thus, all BCMA-CD3 antibodies had high efficacy with CHO-BCMA target cells.

3.4. BCMA-CD3 Antibodies Bind to BCMA-Positive Multiple Myeloma Cells and Cause Secretion of IFN-Gamma

BCMA-CD3 antibodies were tested for binding with MM1S and H929 multiple myeloma cell lines. FACS analysis with BCMA-CD3 antibodies demonstrated that all antibodies bound BCMA-positive multiple myeloma cell lines with KD in the nM range (Figure 4A). There was no binding of BCMA-CD3 antibodies to BCMA-negative lymphablstoid K562 cell line, while there was positive binding to RPMI8226 multiple myeloma cell line (Figure S2A).

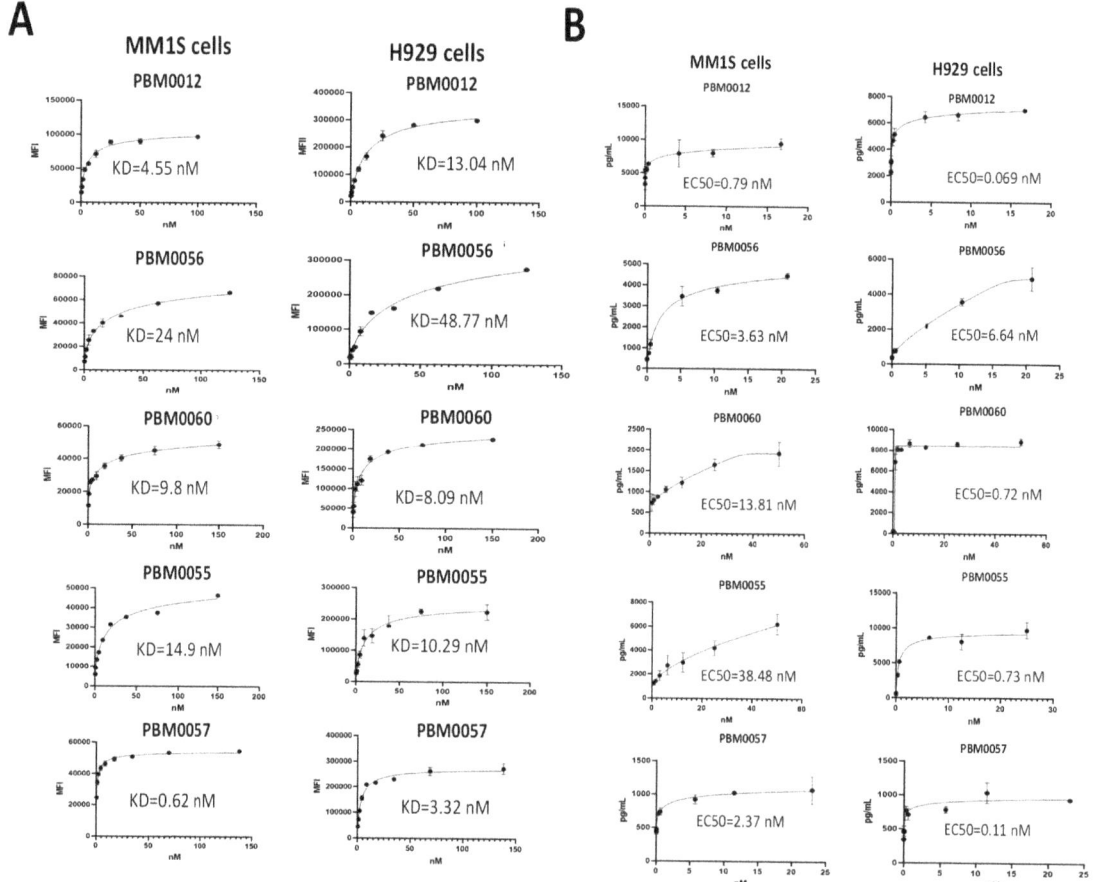

Figure 4. (**A**) BCMA-CD3 antibodies bind multiple myeloma cell lines and all bispecific antibodies with T cells secrete IFN-gamma. (**A**) Representative FACS assay with MM1S and H929 cells is shown. (**B**) BCMA-CD3 antibodies and T cells secrete IFN-gamma with multiple myeloma cells. Representative assay is shown. Bars show standard deviations from three independent measurements.

We tested these antibodies for secretion of INF-gamma with multiple myeloma cell lines (Figure 4B). All antibodies secreted high levels of IFN-gamma and EC50 was from 0.7–38 nM. There was no high secretion of IFN-gamma by T cells and BCMA-CD3 antibodies in the BCMA-negative K562 cell line (Figure S2B) and in BCMA-negative primary B cells

(Figure S3). Thus, BCMA-CD3 antibodies effectively and specifically bound BCMA-positive multiple myeloma cell lines and all antibodies with T cells secreted IFN-gamma.

3.5. BCMA-CD3 Antibodies with T Cells Effectively Block Multiple Myeloma Tumor Growth In Vivo

We tested the efficacy of BCMA-CD3 antibodies using the MM1S xenograft mouse NSG model (Figure 5). MM1S-luciferase-positive cells were injected intravenously into mice and antibodies with T cells were injected intravenously three times. All antibodies except PBM0055 significantly decreased tumor growth with $p < 0.001$ ((Figure 5A). In addition, PBM0012, PBM0056, PBM0060, and PBM0057 antibodies with T cells significantly prolonged mouse survival ($p < 0.04$) (Figure 5B). Thus, three bispecific BCMA-CD3 antibodies significantly decreased MM1S tumor growth similarly to the control PBM0057 antibody.

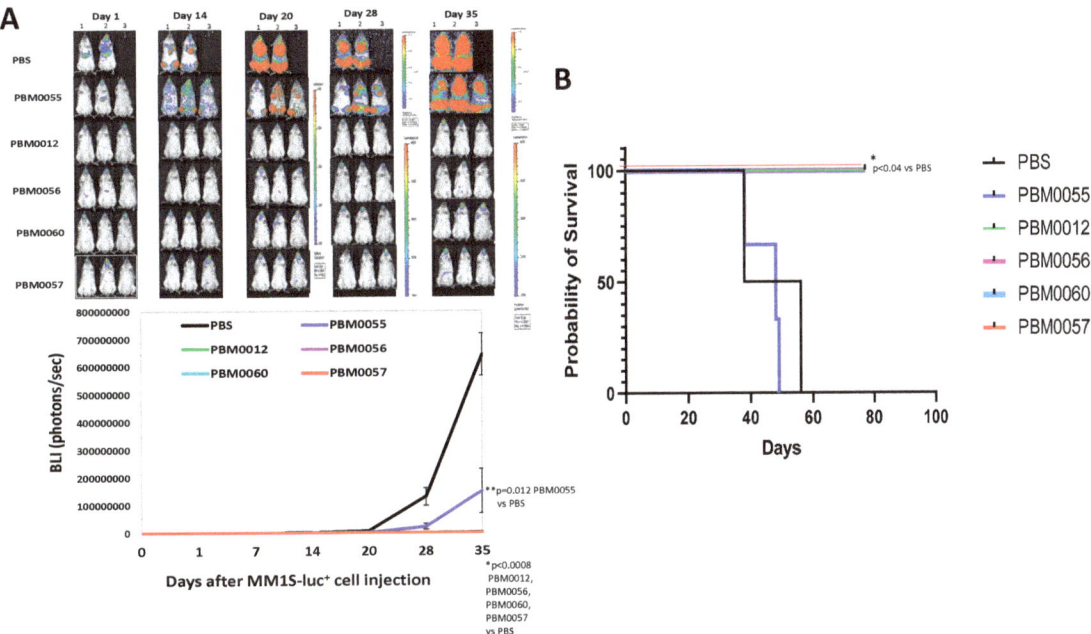

Figure 5. BCMA-CD3 antibodies with T cells significantly decrease MM1S-luciferase+ tumor growth. (**A**) Imaging of MM1S-luc xenografts with BCMA-CD3 antibodies and T cells. The PBS-treated group had two mice; all BCMA-CD3-treated groups had three mice per group ($n = 3$). Upper panel: Images of mice. Lower panel Quantification of BLI (photons/sec). $p < 0.0008$, BLI for PBM0012, PBM0056, PBM0060 and PBM0057 versus PBS group. $p = 0.012$, BLI for PBM0055 versus PBS-group, Student's t-test. (**B**) Kaplan Myer survival curve. $p < 0.04$ all antibodies vs. PBS control by Log-rank Mantel-Cox test.

In addition, we performed an additional mouse in vivo efficacy study using CAR-T cells with humanized BCMA Scfv with the same VH and VL as in BCMA-CD3 antibodies (Figure S4). We designed humanized BCMA ScFv-41BB-CD3 CAR shown in Figure S4A. The generated hBCMA-CAR-T cells expressed more than 70% BCMA-CAR-positive cells (Figure S4B). The CAR-T cells killed CHO-BCMA cells and did not kill CHO cells (Figure S4C) and secreted a high level of IFN-gamma with CHO-BCMA target cells (Figure S4D). Moreover, hBCMA-CAR-T cells significantly ($p < 0.05$) decreased RPMI8226-luciferase$^+$ multiple myeloma xenograft tumor growth by imaging (Figure S4E) and significantly prolonged mouse survival $p < 0.02$ (Figure S4E). The high in vivo efficacy of the humanized BCMA-CAR-T cells in the multiple myeloma xenograft model confirms the high in vivo efficacy of BCMA-CD3 bispecific antibodies.

4. Discussion

This report demonstrated the generation of several antibody designs bivalent, univalent BCMA-CD3 Crossmab KIH; and BCMA-CD3 ScFv KIH with two different CD3 ScFv humanized sequences. We tested these antibodies for binding with BCMA-positive cell lines and detected that all antibodies specifically bound with high KD to BCMA-positive CHO-BCMA cells. In addition, they all bound CD3-positive T cells. All antibodies also bound multiple myeloma cell lines with KD in the nM range. BCMA-CD3 antibodies did not bind CHO, K562, and primary B cells. The BCMA-CD3 antibodies with T cells killed BCMA-positive CHO-BCMA cell lines and secreted IFN-gamma with EC50 in the nM range. BCMA-CD3 with T cells did not secrete IFN-gamma with BCMA-negative cells. Moreover, three BCMA-CD3 antibodies significantly decreased MM1S-luc$^+$ xenograft tumor growth and prolonged mouse survival in vivo except for one BCMA-CD3 antibody PBM0055 which has different CD3 ScFv. Thus, this report demonstrates the high in vitro and in vivo efficacy of novel BCMA-CD3 bispecific antibodies with different designs.

In addition, we confirmed the high in vitro and in vivo efficacy of BCMA-CD3 antibodies with humanized BCMA-CAR-T cells containing the same humanized BCMA ScFv (Figure S4). Future pre-clinical studies will be performed to compare both types of therapies.

The BCMA-CD3 antibodies bound CHO-BCMA cells and did not bind CHO and K562 cells. The bivalent CrossMab and univalent CrossMab KIH bound BCMA-positive cells with similar KD with both CHO-BCMA and with multiple myeloma cell lines. These antibodies had lower binding to T cells than other designs suggesting that designs with CD3 ScFv have higher binding to T cells. PBM0055 did not have in vivo activity that can be explained by different humanized CD3 ScFv compared to other designs. The future study will detect the differences between humanized CD3 sequences and the effect of several amino-acid changes on antibody functions in vivo.

The future pre-clinical efficacy, toxicology, and pharmacokinetics studies will be performed with different doses of antibodies, larger mouse groups, and humanized mouse models to reveal differences between different designs of antibodies. This is the first study to demonstrate in vitro and in vivo functional efficacy of these novel BCMA-CD3 antibodies.

Several BCMA-CD3 antibodies were tested in clinical studies in different formats: AMG420, BITE BCMA-CD3, and AMG701, half-life extended HLE-BITE by Amgen; CC-93269, EM901 CrossMab KIH bivalent BCMA-CD3 antibody by Celgene; PF-06863135 BCMA-CD3 antibody by Pfizer; JNJ-64007957, Duobody by Janssen and REGN5458, hetero H, CL IgG4 with Fc silenced by Regeneron [24]. The AMG420 BITE BCMA-CD3 antibody had a short half-life and needed to be administered for 4 weeks, while HLE-BITE AMG701 required to be administered only once a week and now it is tested in phase I clinical trial [24]. EM-801 CrossMAB bivalent KIH BCMA-CD3 bispecific antibody has an advantage of prolonged stability and can be administered intravenously weekly [25]. The first clinical result of the related EM901 antibody showed that more than 90 percent of patients responded to the treatment [24]. Pfizer's PF-06863135 antibody showed high in vitro and in vivo efficacy [26] and is now tested in a clinical phase I trial (NCT03269136) [24]. Each of the mentioned antibodies has its own mechanism and its own advantages and disadvantages [24]. We presented novel BCMA-CD3 antibodies with high in vitro and in vivo activities. More mechanistic, efficacy and toxicology pre-clinical studies will be performed in a future report to compare present antibodies to other BCMA-CD3 antibodies. There are several challenges like cytokine release syndrome, inhibitory checkpoint signaling, inhibitory tumor microenvironment, and other factors that need to be addressed in future preclinical and clinical studies [24]. Novel bispecific BCMA-CD3 antibodies are important to develop for better therapeutic targeting of multiple myeloma.

In summary, the presented novel BCMA-CD3 antibodies with different designs containing CD3 sequences of PBM0012, PBM0056, and PBM0060 have high in vitro and in vivo activity.

5. Conclusions

This study demonstrates the high efficacy of novel BCMA-CD3 antibodies in vitro and in vivo. The data provide a basis for future pre-clinical and clinical studies.

6. Patents

Humanized BCMA VH, VL, and Scfv and bispecific antibody sequences are included in the Promab Biotechnology patent application.

Supplementary Materials: The following supporting information can be downloaded at: https://www.mdpi.com/article/10.3390/cancers14102518/s1. Table S1, Amino-acid sequence of BCMA-CD3 antibodies used in the study; Figure S1, A. FACS with BCMA-CD3 antibodies shows no binding with BCMA-negative CHO cells. B. IFN-gamma ELISA assay shows no secretion of IFN-gamma by T cells with BCMA-CD3 antibodies with CHO target cells; Figure S2, A. FACS with BCMMA-CD3 antibodies shows no binding of BCMA-CD3 antibodies to K562 lymphoblast cells. B. T cells with BCMA-CD3 antibodies don't secrete high level IFN-gamma with K562 cells; Figure S3, T cells with BCMA-CD3 antibodies secrete significantly less IFN-gamma with B cells than with MM1S multiple myeloma cells; Figure S4, Humanized BCMA-CAR-T cells significantly block RPMI8226-luciferase+ multiple myeloma xenograft tumor growth.

Author Contributions: Conceptualization, L.W. and V.G.; methodology, Y.H., J.S. (John Sienkiewicz), J.S. (Jinying Sun), L.G., F.L., L.Y.; software, Y.H., J.S. (John Sienkiewicz) and J.S. (Jinying Sun); validation, Y.H., J.S. (John Sienkiewicz), L.G. and J.S. (Jinying Sun); formal analysis, L.Y. and V.G.; investigation, V.G., and L.W.; resources, L.W.; data curation, Y.H., J.S. (John Sienkiewicz), J.S. (Jinying Sun) and L.G.; writing—original draft preparation, V.G.; writing—review and editing, V.G.; visualization, V.G.; supervision, L.Y., V.G. and L.W.; project administration, V.G., L.Y. and L.W.; funding acquisition, L.W. All authors have read and agreed to the published version of the manuscript.

Funding: This research was funded by Promab Biotechnologies.

Institutional Review Board Statement: Human peripheral blood mononuclear cells (PBMC) were isolated from whole blood from the Stanford Hospital Blood Center according to IRB-approved protocol (#13942). The mice experiments were conducted according to approved Institutional Animal Care and Use Committee (IACUC) by Lumigenix (#LUM-001).

Informed Consent Statement: Not applicable.

Data Availability Statement: Data are contained within the article.

Acknowledgments: The authors would like to acknowledge Ed Lim for help with mice imaging and animal experiments. We would like to thank Dr. Robert Berahovich for providing expanded B cells. We would like to thank Dr. Walter Bodmer (Weatherall Institute of Molecular Medicine John Radcliffe Hospital, Oxford, UK) for discussions and suggestions with bispecific antibodies. We would like to thank Hua Zhou for functional analysis of hBCMA-CAR-T cells.

Conflicts of Interest: Lijun Wu is CEO of Promab Biotechnologies, and the co-authors are employees of Promab Biotechnologies.

References

1. Das, S.; Juliana, N.; Yazit, N.A.A.; Azmani, S.; Abu, I.F. Multiple Myeloma: Challenges Encountered and Future Options for Better Treatment. *Int. J. Mol. Sci.* **2022**, *23*, 1649. [CrossRef] [PubMed]
2. Dhodapkar, M.V.; Borrello, I.; Cohen, A.D.; Stadtmauer, E.A. Hematologic Malignancies: Plasma Cell Disorders. *Am. Soc. Clin. Oncol. Educ. Book* **2017**, *37*, 561–568. [CrossRef]
3. Carpenter, R.O.; Evbuomwan, M.O.; Pittaluga, S.; Rose, J.J.; Raffeld, M.; Yang, S.; Gress, R.E.; Hakim, F.T.; Kochenderfer, J.N. B-cell maturation antigen is a promising target for adoptive T-cell therapy of multiple myeloma. *Clin. Cancer Res.* **2013**, *19*, 2048–2060. [CrossRef] [PubMed]

4. Chen, K.H.; Wada, M.; Pinz, K.; Liu, H.; Shuai, X.; Chen, X.; Yan, L.E.; Petrov, J.C.; Salman, H.; Senzel, L.; et al. A compound chimeric antigen receptor strategy for targeting multiple myeloma. *Leukemia* **2018**, *32*, 402–412. [CrossRef] [PubMed]
5. Chu, J.; He, S.; Deng, Y.; Zhang, J.; Peng, Y.; Hughes, T.; Yi, L.; Kwon, C.H.; Wang, Q.E.; Devine, S.M.; et al. Genetic modification of T cells redirected toward CS1 enhances eradication of myeloma cells. *Clin. Cancer Res.* **2014**, *20*, 3989–4000. [CrossRef] [PubMed]
6. Cronk, R.J.; Zurko, J.; Shah, N.N. Bispecific Chimeric Antigen Receptor T Cell Therapy for B Cell Malignancies and Multiple Myeloma. *Cancers* **2020**, *12*, 2523. [CrossRef]
7. Timmers, M.; Roex, G.; Wang, Y.; Campillo-Davo, D.; Van Tendeloo, V.F.I.; Chu, Y.; Berneman, Z.N.; Luo, F.; Van Acker, H.H.; Anguille, S. Chimeric Antigen Receptor-Modified T Cell Therapy in Multiple Myeloma: Beyond B Cell Maturation Antigen. *Front. Immunol.* **2019**, *10*, 1613. [CrossRef]
8. Zah, E.; Nam, E.; Bhuvan, V.; Tran, U.; Ji, B.Y.; Gosliner, S.B.; Wang, X.; Brown, C.E.; Chen, Y.Y. Systematically optimized BCMA/CS1 bispecific CAR-T cells robustly control heterogeneous multiple myeloma. *Nat. Commun.* **2020**, *11*, 2283. [CrossRef]
9. Zhou, Z.H.; Zhang, L.; Pan, Q.Y.; Huang, B.H.; Zheng, D.; Liu, J.R.; Li, J.; Luo, S.K. BAFF level in bone marrow and expression of BAFF receptor on B cells in multiple myeloma patients. *Zhongguo Shi Yan Xue Ye Xue Za Zhi* **2012**, *20*, 1131–1134.
10. Garcia-Guerrero, E.; Sierro-Martinez, B.; Perez-Simon, J.A. Overcoming Chimeric Antigen Receptor (CAR) Modified T-Cell Therapy Limitations in Multiple Myeloma. *Front. Immunol.* **2020**, *11*, 1128. [CrossRef]
11. Garfall, A.L.; Fraietta, J.A.; Maus, M.V. Immunotherapy with chimeric antigen receptors for multiple myeloma. *Discov. Med.* **2014**, *17*, 37–46.
12. Hipp, S.; Tai, Y.T.; Blanset, D.; Deegen, P.; Wahl, J.; Thomas, O.; Rattel, B.; Adam, P.J.; Anderson, K.C.; Friedrich, M. A novel BCMA/CD3 bispecific T-cell engager for the treatment of multiple myeloma induce, s selective lysis in vitro and in vivo. *Leukemia* **2017**, *31*, 1743–1751. [CrossRef] [PubMed]
13. Yu, G.; Boone, T.; Delaney, J.; Hawkins, N.; Kelley, M.; Ramakrishnan, M.; McCabe, S.; Qiu, W.; Kornuc, M.; Xia, X.Z.; et al. APRIL and TALL-I and receptors BCMA and TACI: System for regulating humoral immunity. *Nat. Immunol.* **2000**, *1*, 252–256. [CrossRef] [PubMed]
14. Novak, A.J.; Darce, J.R.; Arendt, B.K.; Harder, B.; Henderson, K.; Kindsvogel, W.; Gross, J.A.; Greipp, P.R.; Jelinek, D.F. Expression of BCMA, TACI, and BAFF-R in multiple myeloma: A mechanism for growth and survival. *Blood* **2004**, *103*, 689–694. [CrossRef] [PubMed]
15. Tai, Y.T.; Anderson, K.C. Targeting B-cell maturation antigen in multiple myeloma. *Immunotherapy* **2015**, *7*, 1187–1199. [CrossRef]
16. Cohen, A.D.; Garfall, A.L.; Stadtmauer, E.A.; Melenhorst, J.J.; Lacey, S.F.; Lancaster, E.; Vogl, D.T.; Weiss, B.M.; Dengel, K.; Nelson, A.; et al. B cell maturation antigen-specific CAR T cells are clinically active in multiple myeloma. *J. Clin. Investig.* **2019**, *130*, 2210–2221. [CrossRef]
17. D'Agostino, M.; Boccadoro, M.; Smith, E.L. Novel Immunotherapies for Multiple Myeloma. *Curr. Hematol. Malig. Rep.* **2017**, *12*, 344–357. [CrossRef]
18. Moreaux, J.; Legouffe, E.; Jourdan, E.; Quittet, P.; Reme, T.; Lugagne, C.; Moine, P.; Rossi, J.F.; Klein, B.; Tarte, K. BAFF and APRIL protect myeloma cells from apoptosis induced by interleukin 6 deprivation and dexamethasone. *Blood* **2004**, *103*, 3148–3157. [CrossRef]
19. Notas, G.; Alexaki, V.-I.; Kampa, M.; Pelekanou, V.; Charalampopoulos, I.; Sabour-Alaoui, S.; Pediaditakis, I.; Dessirier, V.; Gravanis, A.; Stathopoulos, E.; et al. APRIL binding to BCMA activates a JNK2-FOXO3-GADD45 pathway and induces a G2/M cell growth arrest in liver cells. *J. Immunol.* **2012**, *189*, 4748–4758. [CrossRef]
20. Nobari, S.T.; Nojadeh, J.N.; Talebi, M. B-cell maturation antigen targeting strategies in multiple myeloma treatment, advantages and disadvantages. *J. Transl. Med.* **2022**, *20*, 82. [CrossRef]
21. Bacac, M.; Fauti, T.; Sam, J.; Colombetti, S.; Weinzierl, T.; Ouaret, D.; Bodmer, W.; Lehmann, S.; Hofer, T.; Hosse, R.J.; et al. A Novel Carcinoembryonic Antigen T-Cell Bispecific Antibody (CEA TCB) for the Treatment of Solid Tumors. *Clin. Cancer Res.* **2016**, *22*, 3286–3297. [CrossRef] [PubMed]
22. Berahovich, R.; Zhou, H.; Xu, S.; Wei, Y.; Guan, J.; Guan, J.; Harto, H.; Fu, S.; Yang, K.; Zhu, S.; et al. CAR-T Cells Based on Novel BCMA Monoclonal Antibody Block Multiple Myeloma Cell Growth. *Cancers* **2018**, *10*, 323. [CrossRef] [PubMed]
23. Berahovich, R.; Liu, X.; Zhou, H.; Tsadik, E.; Xu, S.; Golubovskaya, V.; Wu, L. Hypoxia Selectively Impairs CAR-T Cells In Vitro. *Cancers* **2019**, *11*, 602. [CrossRef] [PubMed]
24. Lejeune, M.; Kose, M.C.; Duray, E.; Einsele, H.; Beguin, Y.; Caers, J. Bispecific, T-Cell-Recruiting Antibodies in B Cell Malignancies. *Front. Immunol.* **2020**, *11*, 762. [CrossRef]
25. Seckinger, A.; Delgado, J.A.; Moser, S.; Moreno, L.; Neuber, B.; Grab, A.; Lipp, S.; Merino, J.; Prosper, F.; Emde, M.; et al. Target Expression, Generation, Preclinical Activity, and Pharmacokinetics of the BCMA-T Cell Bispecific Antibody EM801 for Multiple Myeloma Treatment. *Cancer Cell* **2017**, *31*, 396–410. [CrossRef]
26. Panowski, S.H.; Kuo, T.C.; Zhang, Y.; Chen, A.; Geng, T.; Aschenbrenner, L.; Kamperschroer, C.; Pascua, E.; Chen, W.; Delaria, K.; et al. Preclinical Efficacy and Safety Comparison of CD3 Bispecific and ADC Modalities Targeting BCMA for the Treatment of Multiple Myeloma. *Mol. Cancer Ther.* **2019**, *18*, 2008–2020. [CrossRef]

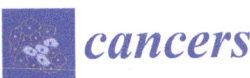

Article

Glofitamab Treatment in Relapsed or Refractory DLBCL after CAR T-Cell Therapy

Vera Rentsch [1], Katja Seipel [2], Yara Banz [3], Gertrud Wiedemann [4], Naomi Porret [4], Ulrike Bacher [5] and Thomas Pabst [1,*]

1. Department of Medical Oncology, Inselspital, Bern University Hospital, 3010 Bern, Switzerland; vera.rentsch@students.unibe.ch
2. Department of Biomedical Research, University of Bern, 3008 Bern, Switzerland; katja.seipel@dbmr.unibe.ch
3. Institute of Pathology, Inselspital, University of Bern, 3008 Bern, Switzerland; yara.banz@pathology.unibe.ch
4. Center of Laboratory Medicine (ZLM), Inselspital, Bern University Hospital, 3010 Bern, Switzerland; gertrud.wiedemann@insel.ch (G.W.); naomiazur.porret@insel.ch (N.P.)
5. Department of Hematology, Inselspital, Bern University Hospital, 3010 Bern, Switzerland; veraulrike.bacher@insel.ch
* Correspondence: thomas.pabst@insel.ch; Tel.: +41-31-632-8430; Fax: +41-31-632-3410

Simple Summary: CAR T-cell therapies represent a major advance in the treatment of relapsed B-cell non-Hodgkin lymphomas. Nevertheless, a significant proportion of these patients will experience disease progression following CAR T treatment. For these patients, no standard therapeutic procedure is established so far. The novel bispecific antibody glofitamab has shown promising activity in the treatment of refractory or relapsed B-cell non-Hodgkin lymphomas. In this study, we provide evidence for good tolerance and promising efficacy of glofitamab administration in patients relapsing after CAR T-cell therapy.

Abstract: Chimeric antigen receptor T-cells (CAR T) treatment has become a standard option for patients with diffuse large B-cell lymphomas (DLBCL), which are refractory or relapse after two prior lines of therapy. However, little evidence exists for treatment recommendations in patients who relapse after CAR T-cell treatment and the outcome for such patients is poor. In this study, we evaluated the safety and efficacy of a monotherapy with the bispecific CD20xCD3 antibody glofitamab in patients who progressed after CAR T treatment. We report nine consecutive patients with progressive DLBCL after preceding CAR T-cell therapy. The patients received a maximum of 12 cycles of glofitamab after a single obinutuzumab pre-treatment at an academic institution. CRS was observed in two patients (grade 2 in both patients). We observed an overall response rate of 67%, with four patients achieving a complete response and a partial remission in two patients. Interestingly, we identified increased persistence of circulating CAR T-cells in peripheral blood in three of the five patients with measurable CAR T-cells. Our data suggest that glofitamab treatment is well tolerated and effective in patients with DLBCL relapsing after CAR T-cell therapy and can enhance residual CAR T-cell activity.

Keywords: CAR T-cell therapy; glofitamab; diffuse large B-cell lymphoma (DLBCL); relapse

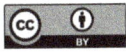

1. Introduction

The most common type of aggressive non-Hodgkin Lymphomas is diffuse large B-cell lymphoma (DLBCL) [1]. Whereas most patients achieve a complete remission following first-line therapy with chemotherapy and rituximab, approximately 40% will, ultimately, relapse [2,3]. Such patients usually undergo salvage therapy, with a proportion of 30–40% of them responding [4,5], and these patients are candidates for consolidation with autologous stem cell transplantation (ASCT). Among them, up to 50% may relapse after ASCT [6–8]. For DLBCL patients who relapse or are refractory after at least two lines of prior therapy, treatment with chimeric antigen receptor T-cells (CAR T) has become the standard option [9,10]. Registration studies reported an overall response rate (ORR) of 52–82% after CAR T treatment, with complete response (CR) rates of 40–52% [11–13]. Remarkably, real-world studies reported comparable outcomes [14–16]. Clinical response rates were reported to correlate with expansion levels and the duration of persistence of CAR T-cells [17,18]. In addition, varying outcomes after CAR T therapy seem to be associated to different DLBCL subtypes [19].

However, along with the increased use of this innovative therapy, the number of patients relapsing after CAR T-cell treatment is emerging as a novel challenge. Various approaches are being explored for patients with relapses following established CD19 targeted CAR T-cell therapy, e.g., CD19-specific CAR T-cells that express a PD-1/CD28 chimeric switch receptor [20]. So far, the survival of patients relapsing after CAR T therapy is poor [21,22], and treatment recommendations for these patients are largely lacking [23,24]. Treatment with bispecific antibodies is a prominent option, and recent studies reported ORR ranging from 60% to 90%, with CR rates between 40% and 60% [25]. Importantly, bispecific antibody treatment also appears to be effective in patients relapsing after CAR T-cell therapy [26–28]. Among these compounds, glofitamab is a bispecific T-cell engager (BiTEs) consisting of two variable fragments joined by a flexible glycine-serine linker. They express two binding domains, with one of them recognizing CD3 on T-cells and the other binding to the target tumor antigen CD20 on (malignant and normal) B-cells. Thereby, immune response is enhanced and effector T-cells are directed to exert cytotoxicity against cells bearing the target antigen [29]. Glofitamab differs from other bispecific antibodies by its 2:1 configuration, which mediates enhanced anti-lymphoma efficacy and a prolonged half-life [30].

In the first in-human phase I dose-escalation study NP30179 (NCT03075696), the recommended phase II dose (RP2D) of increasingly applied 2.5 mg/10 mg/30 mg dose steps was established. The study reported an ORR of 65.7% and a CR rate of 57.1%, while toxicities were manageable. The most common adverse event was cytokine release syndrome (CRS), occurring in 50.3% of the patients [31]. CRS is the result of a hyperactivated immune response and is associated with enhanced production of inflammatory cytokines, including interleukin (IL)-6 [32]. The IL-6-receptor antagonist tocilizumab and steroids are used as standard treatment against CRS [33].

Apart from the promising results in phase I studies with glofitamab, its availability off the shelf makes it an attractive option as a rescue treatment after CAR T failure. In addition, due to its targeted mode of action, it has the potential to avoid toxic effects on residual circulating CAR T-cells' possible enabling synergistic effects. In this retrospective study, we analyzed the safety and efficacy of administering monotherapy with glofitamab in DLBCL patients relapsing after CAR T treatment, and we specifically investigated the effects of glofitamab treatment on the remaining CAR T-cells in the peripheral blood.

2. Materials and Methods

In this single-center study, we retrospectively analyzed real-world experiences of consecutive DLBCL patients receiving glofitamab monotherapy after CAR T treatment at the Inselspital, University Hospital in Bern, Switzerland. Glofitamab was provided free as part of the standardized pre-approval access program (PAA) of the manufacturing company (Roche Pharma), as the compound is not yet approved in Switzerland. We included the data of all consecutive patients with relapsed or refractory DLBCL after CAR T treatment, who received at least one dose of glofitamab monotherapy as the next line after CAR T treatment at our institution between September 2020 and March 2022. All patients gave written informed consent, and the study was approved by a decision of the local ethics committee of Bern, Switzerland.

The treatment comprised pretreatment with a single dose of obinutuzumab (Gazyvaro®) 1000 mg in cycle 1 on day 1 (C1D1), thereby depleting B-cells in the peripheral blood and lymphoid organs resulting in reduced T-cell activation and cytokine release [30]. In order to mitigate eventual side effects, glofitamab was applied using a standard step-up dosing mode. The first dose of 2.5 mg was applied on day 8 of cycle 1 (C1D8) and the second dose (10 mg) was given on day 15 of cycle 1 (C1D15). The first cycle lasted 21 days. From day 1 of cycle 2 (C2D1) until day 1 of cycle 12 (C12D1) 30 mg of glofitamab was applied every 21 days. The initial doses of glofitamab on C1D8 and C1D15 were administered to adequately pre-hydrated patients as 4 h infusions. In the absence of infusion-related symptoms, subsequent doses of glofitamab were given as 2 h infusions.

The Ann Arbor classification was used to define initial tumor stages while risk assessments were determined by the International Prognostic Index (IPI). Tissue biopsies served to assess tumor antigens such as CD20 positivity using routine immunohistochemistry (IHC) and to verify lymphoma histology. Bone marrow infiltration was assessed by standard aspiration and biopsy. Lymphomas that occupied at least one-third of the chest width or that had a diameter larger than 7 cm were assessed as bulky diseases.

We measured the occurrence of CAR T-cell-specific DNA in the peripheral blood by digital-droplet PCR (ddPCR) technology [31,33]. Peak IL-6 and C-reactive protein (CRP) serum levels were recorded during the treatment, in order to evaluate the occurrence of CRS and infections [32]. Toxicities were graded using CTCAE 4.0 criteria (Common Terminology Criteria for Adverse Events). Remission status was based on CT or PET assessments and classified by the RECIST 1.1 criteria.

All statistical analyses were performed using GraphPad Prism® Version 8. Progression-free survival (PFS) was defined as the time between C1D1 and death, progression, or last follow-up, whichever occurred first. Overall survival (OS) was defined as the time between C1D1 and death from any cause or last follow-up. Survival curves were estimated using the Kaplan–Meier method and differences were evaluated by the log-rank test. Patients being alive and progression free were censored at the time of the last follow-up.

3. Results

3.1. Clinical Characteristics of the Patients

Between September 2020 and March 2022, nine patients with CAR T failure were treated with a monotherapy of glofitamab at our institution. All of them had DLBCL, relapsing after previous CAR T treatment. DLBCL was transformed in five cases (here, the limited patient number has to be seen) from follicular lymphoma (FL) and in one patient from marginal zone lymphoma (MZL). At first diagnosis, four patients had stage IV disease, three patients had stage III, and two patients had stage II disease. All lymphomas were high-intermediate risk or high risk. Detailed patient characteristics at diagnosis are summarized in Table 1.

Table 1. Patient characteristics at diagnosis.

Patient Characteristics		
Age, years, median (range)	60	(41–73)
Gender, male, n (%)	5	56%
Histology Diffuse large B cell lymphoma (DLBCL), n (%)	9	100%
De Novo, n (%)	3	33%
Transformed DLBCL, n (%)	6	64%
-from follicular lymphoma (FL), n (%)	5	56%
-from marginal zone lymphoma (MZL), n (%)	1	11%
Elevated LDH, n (%)	9	100%
Disease Stage, n (%)		
II	2	22%
III	3	33%
IV	4	44%
IPI, n (%)		
3 (high-intermediate risk)	5	56%
4–5 (high risk)	4	44%

Table 1. Cont.

Patient Characteristics		
Bone marrow infiltration, no of pts (%)	5	56%
Infiltration, % of cells, median (range)	50	(10–90)
Bulky disease, n (%)	2	22%
CNS infiltration, n (%)	0	0%
B symptoms, n (%)	1	11%
Immunohistochemistry CD20+, n (%)		100%

Elevated LDH: Lactate dehydrogenase > 480 U/L; IPI: International prognostic index; CNS: Central nervous system.

Table 2 reports patient characteristics at the start of glofitamab treatment. The median age at glofitamab therapy was 66 years, and the median time from diagnosis to the beginning of the treatment was 3.8 years. Patients had a median of three previous lines of therapy, which included a median of three prior anti-CD20 therapies. All patients underwent previous CAR T-cell therapy as the last preceding line of treatment. The median time between CAR T-cell infusion and glofitamab treatment was six months. The median peak expansion of CAR T-cells was 3260 copies/µg DNA after CAR T treatment. In contrast, the median level of circulating CAR T-cells before the first glofitamab administration was reduced to 34 copies/µg DNA. In three (33%) patients, no circulating CAR T-cells were detectable at all. After CAR T-cell therapy, complete response (CR) was achieved in two patients, six patients were in partial response (PR) and one patient had stable disease (SD). Before glofitamab therapy, all patients had PET-CT-documented relapsed DLBCL, and relapsing disease was verified in six (67%) of them.

Table 2. Patient characteristics at start of Glofitamab therapy.

Patient Characteristics		
Age at glofitamab therapy, median (range)	66	(41–75)
Time from diagnosis to glofitamab, months, median (range)	45	(9–284)
Previous therapy lines before glofitamab, median (range)	3	(2–7)
Anti CD-20 therapies before glofitamab, median (range)	3	(1–6)
Previous autologous stem cell transplantation, n (%)	5	(56%)
Previous CAR T cell therapy, n (%)	9	100%
tisagenlecleucel, n (%)	6	67%
axicabtagene ciloleucel, n (%)	3	33%
CAR T toxicities, n (%)		
CRS	6	67%
Neurotoxicity	2	22%
Best response to CAR T cell therapy, n (%)		
SD	1	11%
PR	6	67%
CR	2	22%
Interval CAR T-cell infusion to glofitamab, days, median (range)	187	(86–655)
Peak expansion of CAR T cells, copies/µg DNA, median (range)	3260	(54–12,578)
CAR T cell expansion before glofitamab, copies/µg DNA, median (range)	34	(0–1470)
Patients without detectable CAR T cells before glofitamab, n (%)	3	33%
Bulky disease, n (%)	2	22%
CNS infiltration, n (%)	1	11%
B symptoms, n (%)	3	33%

CAR T: Chimeric antigen receptor T-cells; CRS: Cytokine release syndrome; SD: Stable disease; PR: Partial response; CR: Complete response; CNS: Central nervous system.

3.2. Therapeutic Course and Safety

All nine patients completed at least one cycle of glofitamab treatment. Two patients had ongoing progression and ultimately died after the first cycle due to lymphoma progression. Lymphoma progression led to cessation of glofitamab treatment in one patient each after cycles 3, 9, and 10. Four (44%) patients completed the planned 12 cycles. Treatment characteristics are listed in Table 3.

Table 3. Glofitamab treatment characteristics and adverse events.

Treatment Characteristics		
Glofitamab given, n (%)	9	100%
Number of cycles completed, n (%)		
1 cycle	2	22%
3 cycles	1	11%
9 cycles	1	11%
10 cycles	1	11%
12 cycles	4	44%
Premature termination of treatment, n (%)	5	56%
-due to lymphoma progression, n (%)	5	
Peak IL-6 after glofitamab, pg/mL, median (range)	43	(7–1975)
Peak expansion of CAR T cells after glofitamab, copies/µg DNA, median (range)	66	(0–340)
Adverse events, n (%)		
CRS	2	22%
-Grade II	2	
Neurotoxicity	0	0%
Tumor lysis syndrome	1	11%
Anemia	1	11%
Neutropenia	3	33%
Thrombocytopenia	1	11%
Fatigue	7	78%
Nausea	4	44%
Emesis	1	11%
Diarrhea	3	33%
Obstipation	4	44%
Dyspnea	2	22%
Cough	2	22%
At least one febrile episode of ≥38 °C	6	67%
Days with fever, n, median (range)	1	(1–3)
Infections, n (%)		
Patients with at least one identified pathogen	4	44%
Bacteria, gram-positive	1	
Viral infection	3	

CRP: C-reactive protein; IL-6: Interleukin 6; CRS: Cytokine release syndrome. Bacteria: staphylococcus; Viral: Enterovirus (two patients), Varicella Zoster Virus (one patient).

Glofitamab was generally well tolerated, and there were no discontinuations or dose reductions due to treatment-related adverse events (AEs). All AEs that occurred during the treatment period are summarized in Table 3. The majority of the patients (7 of 9) experienced fatigue, three of them regularly during the first few days after the infusion of the medication.

CRS was observed in two patients during cycle 1, both being grade II. One patient was treated with tocilizumab and dexamethasone. Biomarkers for CRS, such as IL-6 and CRP, were elevated in cycle 1, with median peak levels of 43 pg/mL and 131 mg/L. Peak IL-6 values during all cycles are shown in Figure 1.

One patient experienced symptoms of tumor lysis syndrome after the first administration of obinutuzumab, with emesis, diarrhea, and abdominal pain for 2 days. Transient neutropenia occurred in three patients (grade 1 in one patient and grade 3 in two patients). One patient each experienced anemia (grade 1) and thrombocytopenia (grade 1), conditions that were not previously known. Other AEs included obstipation (grade 1) in four patients, diarrhea in three patients (grade 1 in two patients and grade 2 in one patient), nausea (grade 2) in four patients, emesis (grade 1) in one patient, dyspnea in two patients (grade 1 in one patient and grade 2 in one patient), and cough (grade 1) in two patients.

Infections with at least one febrile episode of ≥38 °C were detected in six patients, while the median number of days with fever was only one day. Infections, with at least one identified germ, were seen in four patients, three of which were viral (Enterovirus (two patients), Varicella Zoster Virus (one patient)). One infection was bacterial (Staphylococcus), detected by blood culture.

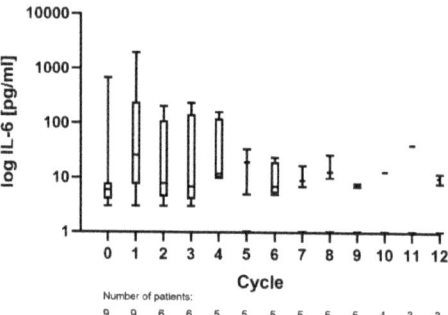

Figure 1. Peak IL-6 measurements of all treated patients during each cycle.

3.3. Efficacy of Glofitamab Therapy

All patients were evaluable for response, and response rates are summarized in Table 4. The overall response rate after glofitamab treatment was 67%. CR assessed by PET-CT was achieved in four patients and partial response (PR) was seen in two patients. We had stable disease (SD) in one patient and progressive disease (PD) in two patients. The median time between the first treatment infusion and CR was 8.3 months. One patient achieved CR after only cycle 1 of the treatment. In three patients with ultimate CR, PR occurred first. Achievement of PR was documented after cycles 2 or 3, after a median of 56 days. Two patients with PR relapsed after a median of 142 days after the first Glofitamab infusion and, therefore, terminated the treatment prematurely.

Table 4. Outcomes of Glofitamab treatment.

Outcome Parameter			
Follow-up, median days (range)		246	(15–482)
Patients without relapse at last follow-up, no (%)		4/9 (44%)	
-PFS, days, median		161	
Relapse, n (%)		2	22%
-Time since glofitamab, days, median (range)		142	(123–161)
Patients alive at last follow-up, no (%)		5/9 (56%)	
Median OS		n.r.	
Deaths, n (% of all pts)		4	44%
-Time since glofitamab, days, median (range)		70	(15–246)
-Due to progression, n (%)		4	44%
Best overall response rate (ORR), %		67%	
Best CR rate, %		44%	
Remission status	First response	Best response	Last follow-up
CR	1	4	4
PR	5	2	0
SD	1	1	0
PD	2	2	5

OS: Overall survival; PFS: Progression-free survival; CR: Complete response; PR: Partial response; SD: Stable disease; PD: Progressive disease; First response: After cycle 1, 2 or 3. n.r.: not reached.

During the study period, four deaths occurred. All patients died due to lymphoma progression, and two of them received only one cycle of treatment. The median time from treatment beginning until death was 70 days. A summary of treatment outcomes is depicted in Figure 2.

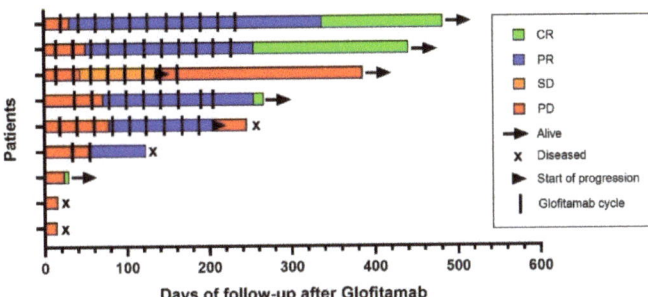

Figure 2. Swimmer plot illustrating outcomes after glofitamab therapy.

The median time until the last follow-up was 246 days. Response at the last follow-up was CR in four patients and PD in five patients. Progression-free survival (PFS) was 44%, and 5/9 (56%) of the patients were alive at the last follow-up. The median PFS was 161 days, and median OS was not reached. PFS and OS are presented in Figure 3.

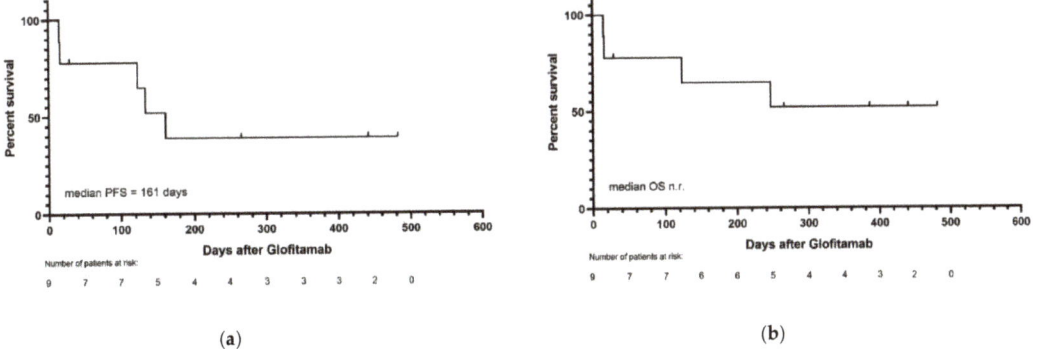

Figure 3. (a) Progression-free and (b) overall survival of all patients.

3.4. Effects of Glofitamab on CAR T-Cells

All nine patients had previously received CAR T-cell therapy. The kinetics of CAR T-cell-specific DNA in peripheral blood was assessed before, during, and after glofitamab treatment. One patient died before the measurement of CAR T-cells in the peripheral blood during cycle 1. In the three patients without detectable CAR T-cells before the therapy, CAR T-cells in the peripheral blood remained undetectable during glofitamab therapy. The decrease in CAR T-cells after CAR T-cell therapy continued following glofitamab in two patients. However, three patients experienced a re-expansion of CAR T-cells in the peripheral blood after glofitamab infusions. Peak CAR T-cell expansion by digital-droplet PCR (ddPCR) occurred after a median of 35 days from the start of glofitamab treatment. Later, during glofitamab treatment, the initially enhanced cell expansion decreased again; however, it did not fall below the levels seen before the start of glofitamab therapy.

The median peak CAR T-cell expansion of all evaluable patients during glofitamab treatment was 66 copies/µg DNA. No association between CAR T-cell expansion and response to glofitamab could be observed, as three patients with CR did not have any detectable CAR T-cells before and after treatment. Only one patient with CR experienced a CAR T-cell expansion during glofitamab therapy. CAR T-cell expansion after glofitamab is illustrated in Figure 4. Given the small numbers, any correlation between CAR T-cell levels and response during glofitamab treatment remains speculative at this moment.

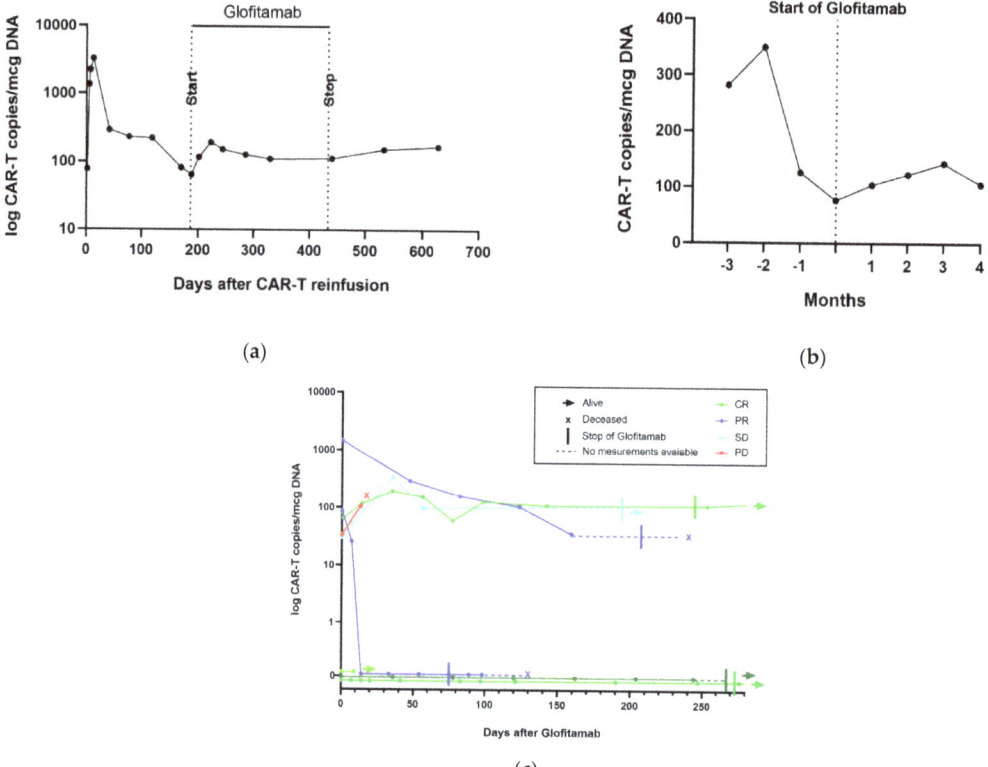

Figure 4. CAR T-cell expansion during glofitamab therapy. (**a**) CAR T-cell copies/mcg DNA in one patient who had CR and experienced a re-expansion of CAR T-cells after glofitamab; (**b**) median CAR T-cell copies/mcg DNA before and after glofitamab in all patients who had measurable CAR T-cells; (**c**) CAR T-cell copies/mcg DNA for each patient after the administration of glofitamab.

4. Discussion

In this study, we investigated patients with refractory or relapsed DLBCL, who received glofitamab as the next line of treatment, after relapse following CAR T treatment, at a single academic institution. All patients were heavily pre-treated and had exhausted the available options. Our study intended to provide information on the safety of glofitamab after CAR T-cell infusion, preliminary evidence of efficacy, and the ability of glofitamab to eventually enhance the declining activity of residual CAR T-cells.

In our study cohort, glofitamab application turned out to be safe and was generally well tolerated. We did not record unexpected new adverse events during glofitamab therapy. In particular, the incidence of infections and the observed germs, as well as the rate of glofitamab-related neutropenia and thrombocytopenia, were comparable to the phase I dose-escalation study. In contrast, the occurrence of CRS was significantly lower in our cohort with 22%, as compared to 71% in the phase 1 study [31]. CRS after glofitamab treatment does not seem to be associated with persisting CAR T-cells, as one patient out of two patients with CRS in our cohort did not have persisting CAR T-cells in the peripheral blood at all. Furthermore, no CRS was observed in patients with enhanced circulating CAR T-cell levels.

Our data suggest that glofitamab therapy resulted in significant clinical response in a subset of patients with DLBCL relapsing after CAR T treatment. This supports earlier reports of the efficacy of BsAbs [25]. Furthermore, our results propose that BsAbs can be effective in patients who experienced CAR T failure, supporting previous reports on mosunetuzumab and odronextamab, which are other CD3/CD20 BiTE antibodies [27,28,34]. Schuster et al. reported a CR rate of 22.2% in 18 patients treated with mosunetuzumab who relapsed after CAR T-cell therapy and had at least 3 months of follow-up [27], while Bannerji et al. reported a CR rate of 27% in 30 patients treated with odronextamab after CAR-T failure [28].

To our knowledge, no information on the efficacy of glofitamab administration in DLBCL patients relapsing after CAR T-cell therapy is yet available. The ORR and CR rates in our cohort after glofitamab treatment were similar to those observed in the phase I dose-escalation trial of glofitamab, in which patients achieved an ORR of 65.7% with a CR rate of 57.1% when treated with the RP2D [31]; however, most of these patients had no CAR-T therapy.

The median OS in DLBCL patients progressing after CAR-T treatment is poor. Two studies reported overall survival of 161 and 180 days only [20,21]. Our data suggest that glofitamab therapy can prolong survival in patients failing CAR T therapy, since we observed a median OS not reached after a median follow-up of 246 days. However, our data need longer follow-up and confirmation in larger series of patients, preferably in a prospective comparative study. Even though the results of our retrospective analysis seem promising, it will be necessary to investigate the administration of Glofitamab after failed CAR T-cell therapy in a larger number of patients in prospective studies. A French phase II study (NCT04703686) is investigating glofitamab in patients with relapsed or refractory non-Hodgkin lymphoma after CAR T therapy [35]. This study and other investigations are needed to establish recommendations for patients with progressive DLBCL after CAR T-cell therapy.

Finally, we found evidence that Glofitamab administration may enhance circulating CAR T-cells in the peripheral blood assessed by ddPCR. This effect was similarly observed following mosunetuzumab treatment [27], but has not been described so far for glofitamab. Among the patients with re-expansion of CAR T-cells in our study, only one achieved CR, making it impossible to draw conclusions between CAR T-cell re-expansion and response. However, given the relevance of the level of CAR T-cell expansion and persistence for the effectiveness of CAR T-cell therapy [17,18], it is tempting to speculate that the effectiveness of glofitamab treatment after CAR T failure may, in part, be due to its potential to induce CAR T-cell re-expansion. One may hypothesize that this could be due to lymphoma burden reduction and thereby, antigen reduction, leading to the proliferation of "less exhausted" CAR T-cells. However, we favor the concept that the main therapeutic effect of glofitamab in this patient series is due to CD3 cytotoxicity, rather than residual CAR T cells, as the efficacy of glofitamab was not limited to patients with CAR-T cell expansion in the peripheral blood following glofitamab application.

5. Conclusions

In conclusion, treatment with glofitamab in patients with refractory or relapsed DLBCL after CAR T-cell therapy seems to be safe and effective. Additionally, our data suggest that the administration of glofitamab can lead to an expansion of residual CAR T-cells. However, larger studies are needed to assess whether this effect contributes to the responses observed and in order to propose an improved management of patients after CAR T-cell failure.

Author Contributions: Design of study: T.P.; data analysis: V.R., K.S., T.P. and U.B.; statistics: V.R. and T.P.; writing of the manuscript: V.R., U.B. and T.P.; providing material: T.P., K.S., G.W. and N.P.; histopathology: Y.B.; review of manuscript and approval of final version: all authors. All authors have read and agreed to the published version of the manuscript.

Funding: This research received no external funding.

Institutional Review Board Statement: The study was conducted according to the guidelines of the Declaration of Helsinki and approved by the Ethics Committee in Bern, Switzerland (decision number 2021-01294 and date of approval 9 December 2021).

Informed Consent Statement: Informed consent was obtained from all subjects involved in the study.

Data Availability Statement: Data can be acquired from the corresponding author by email.

Conflicts of Interest: The authors declare no conflict of interest. No financial support was received from Roche Pharma; data were analyzed and the manuscript was written completely independently from the company.

References

1. Swerdlow, S.H.; Campo, E.; Pileri, S.A.; Harris, N.L.; Stein, H.; Siebert, R.; Advani, R.; Ghielmini, M.; Salles, G.A.; Zelenetz, A.D.; et al. The 2016 Revision of the World Health Organization Classification of Lymphoid Neoplasms. *Blood* **2016**, *127*, 2375–2390. [CrossRef] [PubMed]
2. International Non-Hodgkin's Lymphoma Prognostic Factors Project A Predictive Model for Aggressive Non-Hodgkin's Lymphoma. *N. Engl. J. Med.* **1993**, *329*, 987–994. [CrossRef] [PubMed]
3. Sehn, L.H.; Berry, B.; Chhanabhai, M.; Fitzgerald, C.; Gill, K.; Hoskins, P.; Klasa, R.; Savage, K.J.; Shenkier, T.; Sutherland, J.; et al. The Revised International Prognostic Index (R-IPI) Is a Better Predictor of Outcome than the Standard IPI for Patients with Diffuse Large B-Cell Lymphoma Treated with R-CHOP. *Blood* **2007**, *109*, 1857–1861. [CrossRef] [PubMed]
4. Gisselbrecht, C.; Glass, B.; Mounier, N.; Singh Gill, D.; Linch, D.C.; Trneny, M.; Bosly, A.; Ketterer, N.; Shpilberg, O.; Hagberg, H.; et al. Salvage Regimens with Autologous Transplantation for Relapsed Large B-Cell Lymphoma in the Rituximab Era. *J. Clin. Oncol.* **2010**, *28*, 4184–4190. [CrossRef]
5. Van Den Neste, E.; Schmitz, N.; Mounier, N.; Gill, D.; Linch, D.; Trneny, M.; Milpied, N.; Radford, J.; Ketterer, N.; Shpilberg, O.; et al. Outcome of Patients with Relapsed Diffuse Large B-Cell Lymphoma Who Fail Second-Line Salvage Regimens in the International CORAL Study. *Bone Marrow Transpl.* **2016**, *51*, 51–57. [CrossRef]
6. Gisselbrecht, C.; Schmitz, N.; Mounier, N.; Singh Gill, D.; Linch, D.C.; Trneny, M.; Bosly, A.; Milpied, N.J.; Radford, J.; Ketterer, N.; et al. Rituximab Maintenance Therapy after Autologous Stem-Cell Transplantation in Patients with Relapsed CD20+ Diffuse Large B-Cell Lymphoma: Final Analysis of the Collaborative Trial in Relapsed Aggressive Lymphoma. *J. Clin. Oncol.* **2012**, *30*, 4462–4469. [CrossRef]
7. Hamadani, M.; Hari, P.N.; Zhang, Y.; Carreras, J.; Akpek, G.; Aljurf, M.D.; Ayala, E.; Bachanova, V.; Chen, A.I.; Chen, Y.-B.; et al. Early Failure of Frontline Rituximab-Containing Chemo-Immunotherapy in Diffuse Large B Cell Lymphoma Does Not Predict Futility of Autologous Hematopoietic Cell Transplantation. *Biol. Blood Marrow Transpl.* **2014**, *20*, 1729–1736. [CrossRef]
8. Mathys, A.; Bacher, U.; Banz, Y.; Legros, M.; Mansouri Taleghani, B.; Novak, U.; Pabst, T. Outcome of Patients with Mantle Cell Lymphoma after Autologous Stem Cell Transplantation in the Pre-CAR T-Cell Era. *Hematol. Oncol.* **2021**, *40*, 292–296. [CrossRef]
9. Novartis Receives First Ever FDA Approval for a CAR-T Cell Therapy, Kymriah(TM) (CTL019), for Children and Young Adults with B-Cell ALL That Is Refractory or Has Relapsed at Least Twice. Available online: https://www.novartis.com/news/media-releases/novartis-receives-first-ever-fda-approval-car-t-cell-therapy-kymriahtm-ctl019-children-and-young-adults-b-cell-all-refractory-or-has-relapsed-least-twice (accessed on 22 March 2022).
10. Kite's YescartaTM (Axicabtagene Ciloleucel) Becomes First CAR T Therapy Approved by the FDA for the Treatment of Adult Patients with Relapsed or Refractory Large B-Cell Lymphoma after Two or More Lines of Systemic Therapy. Available online: https://www.gilead.com/news-and-press/press-room/press-releases/2017/10/kites-yescarta-axicabtagene-ciloleucel-becomes-first-car-t-therapy-approved-by-the-fda-for-the-treatment-of-adult-patients-with-relapsed-or-refrac (accessed on 22 March 2022).
11. Neelapu, S.S.; Locke, F.L.; Bartlett, N.L.; Lekakis, L.J.; Miklos, D.B.; Jacobson, C.A.; Braunschweig, I.; Oluwole, O.O.; Siddiqi, T.; Lin, Y.; et al. Axicabtagene Ciloleucel CAR T-Cell Therapy in Refractory Large B-Cell Lymphoma. *N. Engl. J. Med.* **2017**, *377*, 2531–2544. [CrossRef]
12. Schuster, S.J.; Bishop, M.R.; Tam, C.S.; Waller, E.K.; Borchmann, P.; McGuirk, J.P.; Jäger, U.; Jaglowski, S.; Andreadis, C.; Westin, J.R.; et al. Tisagenlecleucel in Adult Relapsed or Refractory Diffuse Large B-Cell Lymphoma. *N. Engl. J. Med.* **2019**, *380*, 45–56. [CrossRef]
13. Abramson, J.S.; Palomba, M.L.; Gordon, L.I.; Lunning, M.A.; Wang, M.; Arnason, J.; Mehta, A.; Purev, E.; Maloney, D.G.; Andreadis, C.; et al. Lisocabtagene Maraleucel for Patients with Relapsed or Refractory Large B-Cell Lymphomas (TRANSCEND NHL 001): A Multicentre Seamless Design Study. *Lancet* **2020**, *396*, 839–852. [CrossRef]
14. Jacobson, C.A.; Hunter, B.D.; Redd, R.; Rodig, S.J.; Chen, P.-H.; Wright, K.; Lipschitz, M.; Ritz, J.; Kamihara, Y.; Armand, P.; et al. Axicabtagene Ciloleucel in the Non-Trial Setting: Outcomes and Correlates of Response, Resistance, and Toxicity. *J. Clin. Oncol.* **2020**, *38*, 3095–3106. [CrossRef]
15. Nastoupil, L.J.; Jain, M.D.; Feng, L.; Spiegel, J.Y.; Ghobadi, A.; Lin, Y.; Dahiya, S.; Lunning, M.; Lekakis, L.; Reagan, P.; et al. Standard-of-Care Axicabtagene Ciloleucel for Relapsed or Refractory Large B-Cell Lymphoma: Results From the US Lymphoma CAR T Consortium. *J. Clin. Oncol.* **2020**, *38*, 3119–3128. [CrossRef]
16. Iacoboni, G.; Villacampa, G.; Martinez-Cibrian, N.; Bailén, R.; Lopez Corral, L.; Sanchez, J.M.; Guerreiro, M.; Caballero, A.C.; Mussetti, A.; Sancho, J.-M.; et al. Real-World Evidence of Tisagenlecleucel for the Treatment of Relapsed or Refractory Large B-Cell Lymphoma. *Cancer Med.* **2021**, *10*, 3214–3223. [CrossRef]
17. Kochenderfer, J.N.; Somerville, R.P.T.; Lu, T.; Shi, V.; Bot, A.; Rossi, J.; Xue, A.; Goff, S.L.; Yang, J.C.; Sherry, R.M.; et al. Lymphoma Remissions Caused by Anti-CD19 Chimeric Antigen Receptor T Cells Are Associated with High Serum Interleukin-15 Levels. *JCO* **2017**, *35*, 1803–1813. [CrossRef]

18. Turtle, C.J.; Hanafi, L.-A.; Berger, C.; Hudecek, M.; Pender, B.; Robinson, E.; Hawkins, R.; Chaney, C.; Cherian, S.; Chen, X.; et al. Immunotherapy of Non-Hodgkin's Lymphoma with a Defined Ratio of CD8+ and CD4+ CD19-Specific Chimeric Antigen Receptor–Modified T Cells. *Sci. Transl. Med.* **2016**, *8*, 355ra116. [CrossRef]
19. Nydegger, A.; Novak, U.; Kronig, M.-N.; Legros, M.; Zeerleder, S.; Banz, Y.; Bacher, U.; Pabst, T. Transformed Lymphoma Is Associated with a Favorable Response to CAR-T-Cell Treatment in DLBCL Patients. *Cancers* **2021**, *13*, 6073. [CrossRef]
20. Liang, Y.; Liu, H.; Lu, Z.; Lei, W.; Zhang, C.; Li, P.; Liang, A.; Young, K.H.; Qian, W. CD19 CAR-T Expressing PD-1/CD28 Chimeric Switch Receptor as a Salvage Therapy for DLBCL Patients Treated with Different CD19-Directed CAR T-Cell Therapies. *J. Hematol. Oncol.* **2021**, *14*, 26. [CrossRef]
21. Spiegel, J.Y.; Dahiya, S.; Jain, M.D.; Tamaresis, J.; Nastoupil, L.J.; Jacobs, M.T.; Ghobadi, A.; Lin, Y.; Lunning, M.; Lekakis, L.; et al. Outcomes of Patients with Large B-Cell Lymphoma Progressing after Axicabtagene Ciloleucel Therapy. *Blood* **2021**, *137*, 1832–1835. [CrossRef]
22. Chow, V.A.; Gopal, A.K.; Maloney, D.G.; Turtle, C.J.; Smith, S.D.; Ujjani, C.S.; Shadman, M.; Cassaday, R.D.; Till, B.G.; Tseng, Y.D.; et al. Outcomes of Patients with Large B-Cell Lymphomas and Progressive Disease Following CD19-Specific CAR T-Cell Therapy. *Am. J. Hematol.* **2019**, *94*, E209–E213. [CrossRef]
23. EHA Guidance Document The Process of CAR-T Cell Therapy in Europe. *Hemasphere* **2019**, *3*, e280. [CrossRef]
24. Byrne, M.; Oluwole, O.O.; Savani, B.; Majhail, N.S.; Hill, B.T.; Locke, F.L. Understanding and Managing Large B Cell Lymphoma Relapses after Chimeric Antigen Receptor T Cell Therapy. *Biol. Blood Marrow Transplant.* **2019**, *25*, e344–e351. [CrossRef]
25. Schuster, S.J. Bispecific Antibodies for the Treatment of Lymphomas: Promises and Challenges. *Hematol. Oncol.* **2021**, *39*, 113–116. [CrossRef]
26. Hutchings, M. Subcutaneous Epcoritamab Induces Complete Responses with an Encouraging Safety Profile across Relapsed/Refractory B-Cell Non-Hodgkin Lymphoma Subtypes, Including Patients with Prior CAR-T Therapy: Updated Dose Escalation Data. ASH, December 6 2020. *Blood* **2020**, *136*, 45–46. [CrossRef]
27. Schuster, S.J.; Bartlett, N.L.; Assouline, S.; Yoon, S.-S.; Bosch, F.; Sehn, L.H.; Cheah, C.Y.; Shadman, M.; Gregory, G.P.; Ku, M.; et al. Mosunetuzumab Induces Complete Remissions in Poor Prognosis Non-Hodgkin Lymphoma Patients, Including Those Who Are Resistant to or Relapsing after Chimeric Antigen Receptor T-Cell (CAR-T) Therapies, and Is Active in Treatment through Multiple Lines. *Blood* **2019**, *134*, 6. [CrossRef]
28. Bannerji, R.; Arnason, J.E.; Advani, R.H.; Brown, J.R.; Allan, J.N.; Ansell, S.M.; Barnes, J.A.; O'Brien, S.M.; Chávez, J.C.; Duell, J.; et al. Odronextamab, a Human CD20×CD3 Bispecific Antibody in Patients with CD20-Positive B-Cell Malignancies (ELM-1): Results from the Relapsed or Refractory Non-Hodgkin Lymphoma Cohort in a Single-Arm, Multicentre, Phase 1 Trial. *Lancet Haematol.* **2022**, *9*, e327–e339. [CrossRef]
29. Huehls, A.M.; Coupet, T.A.; Sentman, C.L. Bispecific T-Cell Engagers for Cancer Immunotherapy. *Immunol. Cell Biol.* **2015**, *93*, 290–296. [CrossRef]
30. Bacac, M.; Colombetti, S.; Herter, S.; Sam, J.; Perro, M.; Chen, S.; Bianchi, R.; Richard, M.; Schoenle, A.; Nicolini, V.; et al. CD20-TCB with Obinutuzumab Pretreatment as Next-Generation Treatment of Hematologic Malignancies. *Clin. Cancer Res.* **2018**, *24*, 4785–4797. [CrossRef]
31. Hutchings, M.; Morschhauser, F.; Iacoboni, G.; Carlo-Stella, C.; Offner, F.C.; Sureda, A.; Salles, G.; Martínez-Lopez, J.; Crump, M.; Thomas, D.N.; et al. Glofitamab, a Novel, Bivalent CD20-Targeting T-Cell-Engaging Bispecific Antibody, Induces Durable Complete Remissions in Relapsed or Refractory B-Cell Lymphoma: A Phase I Trial. *J. Clin. Oncol.* **2021**, *39*, 1959–1970. [CrossRef]
32. Pabst, T.; Joncourt, R.; Shumilov, E.; Heini, A.; Wiedemann, G.; Legros, M.; Seipel, K.; Schild, C.; Jalowiec, K.; Mansouri Taleghani, B.; et al. Analysis of IL-6 Serum Levels and CAR T Cell-Specific Digital PCR in the Context of Cytokine Release Syndrome. *Exp. Hematol.* **2020**, *88*, 7.e3–14.e3. [CrossRef]
33. Messmer, A.S.; Que, Y.-A.; Schankin, C.; Banz, Y.; Bacher, U.; Novak, U.; Pabst, T. CAR T-Cell Therapy and Critical Care: A Survival Guide for Medical Emergency Teams. *Wien. Klin Wochenschr.* **2021**, *133*, 1318–1325. [CrossRef]
34. Flach, J.; Shumilov, E.; Joncourt, R.; Porret, N.; Novak, U.; Pabst, T.; Bacher, U. Current Concepts and Future Directions for Hemato-Oncologic Diagnostics. *Crit. Rev. Oncol. Hematol.* **2020**, *151*, 102977. [CrossRef]
35. The Lymphoma Academic Research Organisation. A Phase II Trial Evaluating Glofitamab, a Bispecific CD3xCD20 Antibody for Relapse/Refractory Lymphomas after CAR T-Cells Therapy. 2021. Available online: https://clinicaltrials.gov/ct2/show/NCT04703686 (accessed on 26 April 2022).

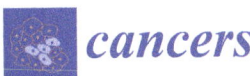

Article

IgG-Based Bispecific Anti-CD95 Antibodies for the Treatment of B Cell-Derived Malignancies and Autoimmune Diseases

Sebastian Hörner [1,2], Moustafa Moustafa-Oglou [1], Karin Teppert [1], Ilona Hagelstein [2,3], Joseph Kauer [1,2], Martin Pflügler [1,2,3], Kristina Neumann [1], Hans-Georg Rammensee [1,3], Thomas Metz [4], Andreas Herrmann [5], Helmut R. Salih [2,3], Gundram Jung [1,3] and Latifa Zekri [1,2,3,*]

1. Department of Immunology, Institute for Cell Biology, Eberhard Karls University Tuebingen, German Cancer Consortium (DKTK), Partner Site Tuebingen, 72076 Tuebingen, Germany
2. Clinical Collaboration Unit Translational Immunology, German Cancer Consortium (DKTK), Department of Internal Medicine, University Hospital Tuebingen, 72076 Tuebingen, Germany
3. DFG Cluster of Excellence 2180 "Image-guided and Functional Instructed Tumor Therapy" (iFIT), Eberhard Karls University Tuebingen, 72076 Tuebingen, Germany
4. Charles River Discovery Research Services Germany GmbH, 79108 Freiburg, Germany
5. Baliopharm AG, 4051 Basel, Switzerland
* Correspondence: latifa.zekri@ifiz.uni-tuebingen.de; Tel.: +49-(0)-7071-29-87630

Simple Summary: Therapeutic antibodies have become a crucial cornerstone of the standard therapy for lymphoma and autoimmune diseases. However, the respective target antigens are also expressed on healthy B cells resulting in unspecific effects. In this article, we present a novel approach to selectively induce apoptosis in lymphoma cells and autoreactive B cells that express the CD95 death receptor. Therefore, we developed an improved IgG-based bispecific antibody format with favorable production properties and pharmacokinetics for CD20- and CD19-directed induction of apoptosis via CD95. We could show that our bispecific anti-CD95 antibodies are very efficient in the depletion of malignant and autoreactive B cells in vitro and in vivo. Therefore, our antibodies could help to provide a more selective therapy for patients with B cell-derived malignancies and autoimmune diseases.

Abstract: Antibodies against the B cell-specific antigens CD20 and CD19 have markedly improved the treatment of B cell-derived lymphoma and autoimmune diseases by depleting malignant and autoreactive B cells. However, since CD20 and CD19 are also expressed on healthy B cells, such antibodies lack disease specificity. Here, we optimize a previously developed concept that uses bispecific antibodies to induce apoptosis selectively in malignant and autoreactive B cells that express the death receptor CD95. We describe the development and characterization of bispecific antibodies with CD95xCD20 and CD95xCD19 specificity in a new IgG-based format. We could show that especially the CD95xCD20 antibody mediated a strong induction of apoptosis in malignant B cells in vitro. In vivo, the antibody was clearly superior to the previously used Fabsc format with identical specificities. In addition, both IgGsc antibodies depleted activated B cells in vitro, leading to a significant reduction in antibody production and cytokine secretion. The killing of resting B cells and hepatocytes that lack CD95 and CD20/CD19, respectively, was marginal. Thus, our results imply that bispecific anti-CD95 antibodies in the IgGsc format are an attractive tool for a more selective and efficient depletion of malignant as well as autoreactive B cells.

Keywords: bispecific antibodies; lymphoma; autoimmune diseases; apoptosis; CD20; CD19; CD95

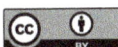

1. Introduction

B cells play a central role in the adaptive immune system. Differentiated into plasma cells, they produce antibodies. In addition, they act as antigen-presenting cells (APC) that produce a variety of cytokines and support T cell activation. Disrupting the finely balanced

B cell homeostasis can lead to cancer or autoimmune diseases. Recombinant antibodies targeting B cell-associated antigens, such as CD20 and CD19, are successfully used for the treatment of B cell-derived malignancies and autoimmune diseases.

The anti-CD20 antibody Rituximab was the first recombinant antibody to be approved by the FDA in 1997 for the treatment of non-Hodgkin lymphoma (NHL) [1,2] and later for the treatment of chronic lymphocytic leukemia (CLL). Due to its profound potential to deplete CD20-positive B cells, it is now also successfully used to treat autoimmune diseases such as rheumatoid arthritis (RA) [3], Wegener's granulomatosis [4], Sjögren syndrome [5], or multiple sclerosis (MS) [6]. Rituximab induces profound B cell depletion by mediating antibody-dependent cellular cytotoxicity (ADCC) and complement-dependent cytotoxicity (CDC). Although the antibody is relatively well tolerated, an increased risk of infections resulting from profound B cell depletion is a major concern [7]. Although CD19 appears to be more attractive than CD20 with respect to its broader expression on immature and differentiated B cells (plasma cells), clinical development of monospecific anti-CD19 antibodies is far less advanced [8]. Possibly due to its less pronounced expression, CD19 targeting was mainly used by T cell recruiting strategies, where limited numbers of target molecules per cell are less critical. Blinatumomab, a CD19xCD3 bispecific antibody (bsAb), which is used for the treatment of acute lymphoblastic leukemia (ALL), is the most prominent example [9,10]. Likewise, CD19 is successfully used as a target antigen for CAR T cells that are functionally closely related to bsAbs [11].

CD95 (Apo-1, Fas) is a member of the tumor necrosis factor superfamily (TNF) with an intracellular death domain for the induction of apoptosis [12]. In combination with its ligand FasL, it plays an important role in B and T cell homeostasis as these cell types increase CD95 expression in response to activation and become susceptible to the CD95-mediated apoptosis [13,14]. In addition, many cancer cells express CD95, although during disease progression it is frequently downregulated [15–17]. In fact, it had been the effective killing of lymphoma cells by an antibody (Apo-1) with—at that time—unknown specificity that allowed the identification of CD95 as a prototypical death receptor [18]. Thus, it appeared tempting to use CD95 agonists (either antibodies or FasL fusion proteins) to induce CD95-mediated apoptosis in cancer cells. However, it was soon recognized that the systemic administration of agonistic antibodies induces severe liver damage in mice [19–21]. This dramatically highlighted the need for more selective induction of apoptosis. In 2001, Jung et al. demonstrated that chemically hybridized bispecific F(ab)$_2$ fragments with CD95xtarget specificity induce apoptosis selectively in tumor cells expressing the selected target antigen [22]. More recently, Nalivaiko et al. showed that recombinant bsAbs with CD95xCD20 specificity in the Fabsc-format were selectively inducing apoptosis not only in CD20 expressing tumor cells but also in normal, activated B cells expressing CD95 [23].

BsAbs that lack functional Fc parts such as Fabsc molecules or BiTEs (bispecific T cell engagers) suffer from a low serum half-life that may seriously limit therapeutic efficiency. Here, we introduce an IgG-based format (IgGsc) for target cell-restricted activation of CD95 [24]. We evaluated the ability of the IgGsc molecules to induce apoptosis in different lymphoma cell lines and in activated B cells in vitro. In addition, the CD95xCD20 IgGsc molecule was found to be superior to a Fabsc-molecule with identical specificity in an established lymphoma xenograft model.

2. Materials and Methods

2.1. Cells and Reagents

Daudi, Jurkat, SKW6.4, JY, C1R, Raji, and LX-1 cells were purchased from the American Type Culture Collection (ATCC, Manassas, VA, USA). Density-gradient centrifugation (Biocoll separating solution, Biochrom, Berlin, Germany) was used to isolate PBMCs from heparinized blood of healthy donors. All cells were cultured in RPMI 1640 compl. medium (Thermo Fisher Scientific, Darmstadt, Germany) containing 1x MEM-NEAA (Thermo Fisher Scientific), 10% FCS (Sigma-Aldrich, Hamburg, Germany), 100 U/mL penicillin, and 100 µg/mL streptomycin (Sigma-Aldrich), 1x sodium-pyruvate (Sigma-Aldrich) and 50 µM β-mercaptoethanol (Merck, Darmstadt, Germany). All cell lines were regularly tested for mycoplasma contamination and were cultured at 37 °C and 5% CO_2.

The expression of CD20, CD19, and CD95 on different cell lines was determined by flow cytometry using QIFIKIT calibration beads (Agilent, Santa Clara, CA, USA) according to the manufacturer's instructions. The hybridoma-derived antibodies 2H7, 4G7, and Apo-1 were used for quantification. Binding of bsAbs to Daudi and Jurkat cells was determined using flow cytometry. PE-conjugated goat anti-human F(ab)$_2$ fragments were used to detect primary antibodies (Jackson ImmunoResearch, West Grove, PA, USA). Flow analysis was performed using the BD FACSCanto™ II and BD FACSCalibur™ systems (BD Biosciences, Heidelberg, Germany). Data were analyzed using FlowJo (FlowJo LLC, Ashland, OR, USA). EC_{50} values were calculated using GraphPad Prism9 (GraphPad Software, Inc., San Diego, CA, USA).

2.2. Generation and Purification of Recombinant Antibodies

The variable domains of the humanized Apo-1 antibody (EP2920210B1), the humanized 2H7 antibody (EP2920210B1), the 4G7 antibody (GenBank no.: AJ555479 and AJ555622), and the MOPC-21 antibody (GenBank no.: AAD15290.1 and AAA39002.1) were codon-optimized using the GeneArt GeneOptimizer tool for the transfection of CHO cells (Thermo Fisher Scientific). V_H, V_L, and scFv sequences were synthesized de novo at GeneArt (Thermo Fisher Scientific). As previously described, the variable domains were inserted into a human IgGγ1sc backbone, which is designed to abolish FcR-binding and complement fixation [24]. IgGsc molecules were produced in the ExpiCHO™ Expression System (Thermo Fisher Scientific) according to the manufacturer's instructions and then purified by HiTrap™ MabSelect™ SuRe columns (Cytiva, Freiburg, Germany), before being subjected to preparative and analytical size exclusion chromatography (SEC) using HiLoad™ 16/600 Superdex 200 pg and Superdex™ 200 Increase 10/300 GL columns (Cytiva), respectively. Sodium dodecyl sulfate-polyacrylamide gel electrophoresis (SDS-PAGE) was performed as previously described [25]. The generation and purification of Fabsc molecules were described by Nalivaiko and colleagues [23].

2.3. Induction of Apoptosis and Caspase-3 Activation in Lymphoma Cells

The induction of apoptosis was evaluated by incubating 50,000 lymphoma cells/well (SKW6.4, JY, C1R, and Raji) in 96-well plates for 24 h with varying concentrations of different bsAbs before they were pulsed with 0.5 μCi/well ^{3}H-thymidine (Hartmann Analytics, Braunschweig, Germany). After 20 h, cells were harvested on filter mats (Perkin Elmer, Waltham, MA, USA), and precipitated radioactivity was determined in a liquid scintillation counter (MicroBeta, Perkin Elmer).

SKW6.4 cells were also incubated with LX-1 hepatic stellate cells (50,000 cell/well each) for 20 h, before assessing viability with 7-AAD (BioLegend, San Diego, CA, USA) by flow cytometry. Absolute cell counts were calculated using equal numbers of latex beads (3 μm particle size, Sigma-Aldrich). LX-1 were distinguished from SKW6.4 using PE-EpCAM (clone 9C4, BioLegend).

For the determination of caspase-3 activity, 100,000 target cells were incubated for 20 h with 0.3 nM of bispecific antibody. Subsequent intracellular staining was performed using the Cytofix/Cytoperm buffer and Perm/wash solution (BD Biosciences) with an anti-active caspase-3 antibody (BD Biosciences) according to the manufacturer's instructions. Samples were then analyzed by flow cytometry.

2.4. Depletion of Activated B Cells and Inhibition of IgG and Cytokine Production

For the bsAb-induced depletion of activated B cells, PBMCs from healthy donors (400,000 cells/well in 96-well plates) were stimulated with 0.1 μM ODN2006 (Miltenyi Biotec, Bergisch Gladbach, Germany) for 7 days [26]. Cells were then washed twice with DPBS before they were treated with 0.1 nM bsAb for 2 days. Lymphocytes were detected using CD4-FITC (clone OKT4), CD8-APC/Cy7 (clone SK1), CD19-PE/Cy7 (clone HIB19) or

CD20-PE/Cy7 (clone 2H7), CD56-Brilliant Violet 421 (clone HCD56), CD69-PE (clone FN50) and CD95-APC (clone EH12.2H7). Cell viability was assessed using 7-AAD. All directly labeled antibodies were purchased from BioLegend. Equal numbers of latex beads (3 µm particle size, Sigma-Aldrich) were used to calculate absolute cell numbers.

Cytokines were measured using the Th1 LEGENDplex™ multiplex kit (BioLegend) according to the manufacturer's instructions. Only positive donors were used for analysis. The inhibition of IgG production of activated B cells after treatment with bsAbs was assessed by ELISA as previously described [23].

2.5. Animal Experiments

All experiments and protocols were approved by the animal welfare body at Charles River Discovery Research Services, Freiburg, Germany, and the local authorities, and were conducted in accordance with all applicable international, national, and local laws and guidelines (study number P500A4A). Only animals with unobjectionable health were selected to enter testing procedures.

To assess the activity of bsAbs against established tumors, 10^7 SKW6.4 cells were injected subcutaneously into the left flank of female CB17 SCID mice. Mice were randomized if they bore a tumor of 50–250 mm^3. The Fabsc molecule was administered intraperitoneal at 100 µg/mouse (twice daily for 10 days), while the IgGsc molecule was administered at 50 µg/mouse (on days 0 and 3). The animals were monitored at least once daily and were weighed three times a week. Blood was collected by retro-orbital sinus puncture and mice were sacrificed when their tumor had grown to a size limit of 2000 mm^3. Tumor volumes were calculated according to the formula: tumor volume = (a × b^2) × 0.5.

The serum concentrations of bsAb were measured by ELISA. An amount of 1 µg/mL CD95-Fc fusion protein was coated in 96-Well Half Area Microplates (Greiner Bio-One), before adding various dilutions of sera. Primary antibodies were detected using HRP-conjugated goat anti-human F(ab)2 specific antibodies (Jackson ImmunoResearch) and the TMB Peroxidase Substrate Kit (Seracare). The optical density at 450 nm was determined using a Spectra Max 340 (Molecular devices). Serum concentrations were interpolated by nonlinear regression using GraphPad Prism9.

2.6. Statistics

Data are presented as means ± SD or SEM as stated in the figure legends. Statistical significance was calculated with GraphPad Prism version 9.4 (GraphPad Software, San Diego, CA, USA) as indicated in the figure legends, with $p < 0.05$ considered statistically significant. ns $p > 0.05$, * $p < 0.05$, ** $p < 0.01$, *** $p < 0.001$, **** $p < 0.0001$.

3. Results

3.1. Construction of Improved Anti-CD95 bsAbs Targeting CD20 or CD19

Two different anti-CD95 antibodies in the IgGsc format were constructed (Figure 1a). The IgGsc format was originally published by Coloma and Morrison [27]. It contains two single-chain fragments variable (scFv) attached to the C-termini of an IgG1 antibody and was then further optimized in our group with a combination of multiple point mutations or deletions to eliminate the Fc receptor (FcR)-mediated multimerization of CD95 [24]. The F(ab)2 and the single-chain moiety of both molecules contained the CD95 agonist Apo-1 [18] and the anti-CD20 clone 2H7 [28] or the anti-CD19 clone 4G7 [29], respectively. This particular orientation was chosen because the Apo-1 antibody cannot be expressed as a single chain [23]. Analysis of both proteins by SDS-PAGE (Figure 1b) revealed the expected molecular weights of the heavy chain (75 kDa), the light chain (25 kDa), and the intact IgGsc molecule (200 kDa). Since the IgGsc format was previously designed for minimal aggregation, it lacked significant amounts of aggregates (less than 4%) as can be seen in gel filtration (Figure 1c). In addition, a CD95xMOPC control was generated to assess CD20- and CD19-independent effects (Figure S1a).

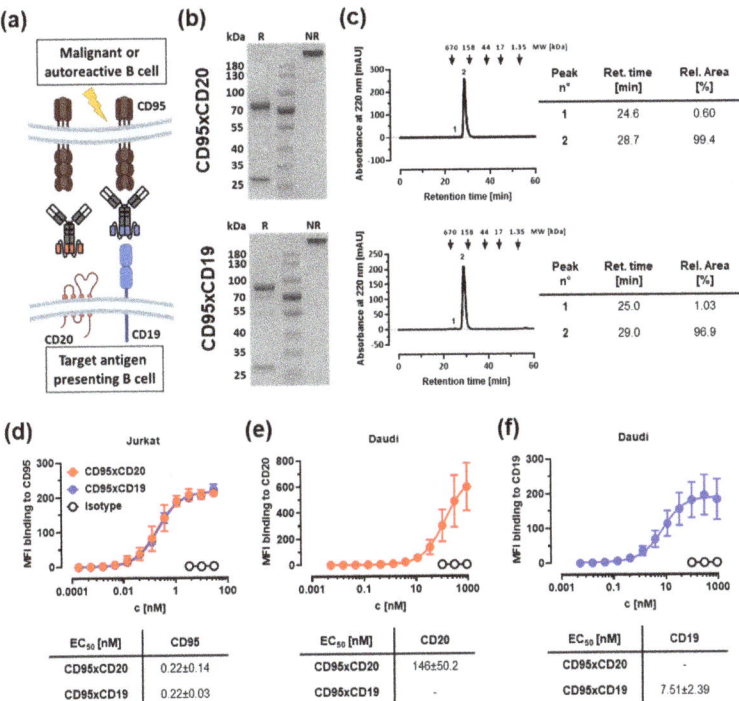

Figure 1. Characterization of improved anti-CD95 bsAbs targeting CD20 or CD19. (**a**) Schematic representation of how the bsAbs induce a target-mediated clustering of the Fas receptor and ultimately lead to apoptosis of the target cell. Created with BioRender.com (accessed on 18 May 2022). (**b**) SDS-PAGE of the bispecific CD95xCD20 (top) and CD95xCD19 (bottom) molecules. R: reduced; NR: non-reduced. (**c**) Both antibodies were subjected to analytical size exclusion chromatography (SEC). The corresponding analysis is presented in the tables on the right. (**d–f**) Binding to CD95-expressing Jurkats (**d**) and Daudi cells expressing CD20 (**e**) and CD19 (**f**) was assessed by flow cytometry. Mean ± SD, n = 3.

The binding of the molecules to CD95$^+$ Jurkat cells (CD20$^-$ and CD19$^-$, Figure S1b) was evaluated by flow cytometry (Figure 1d) and revealed a binding affinity in a low nanomolar range (EC$_{50}$ = 0.2 nM). Binding to CD20 and CD19 was assessed using double positive Daudi cells (Figure S1b). Although the expression of the CD20 antigen was higher than that of CD19, the binding affinity of the CD20 binding moiety was rather low. Saturation could not be reached for concentrations up to 900 nM (Figure 1e). Obviously, conversion of the anti-CD20 clone into an scFv resulted in a significant loss of affinity compared to the parental antibody as previously described by Nalivaiko and colleagues [23]. In contrast, the binding affinity to CD19 revealed an EC$_{50}$ value of approximately 7.5 nM (Figure 1f).

3.2. In Vitro Activity against Malignant B Cells

The ability of the CD95xCD20 and CD95xCD19 constructs to induce apoptosis was assessed using the B cell lymphoma cell lines SKW6.4, JY, C1R, and Raji. All cells tested positive for CD95, expressing at least 90,000 molecules per cell (Figure 2a and Table 1). The expression of the target molecules CD20 and CD19 revealed significant differences. CD20 expression was 3–10-fold higher on all cell lines tested. Only Raji cells expressed more than 20,000 CD19 molecules per cell, while expression of CD20 was higher than 190,000 molecules per cell on all lymphoma cell lines tested in this work.

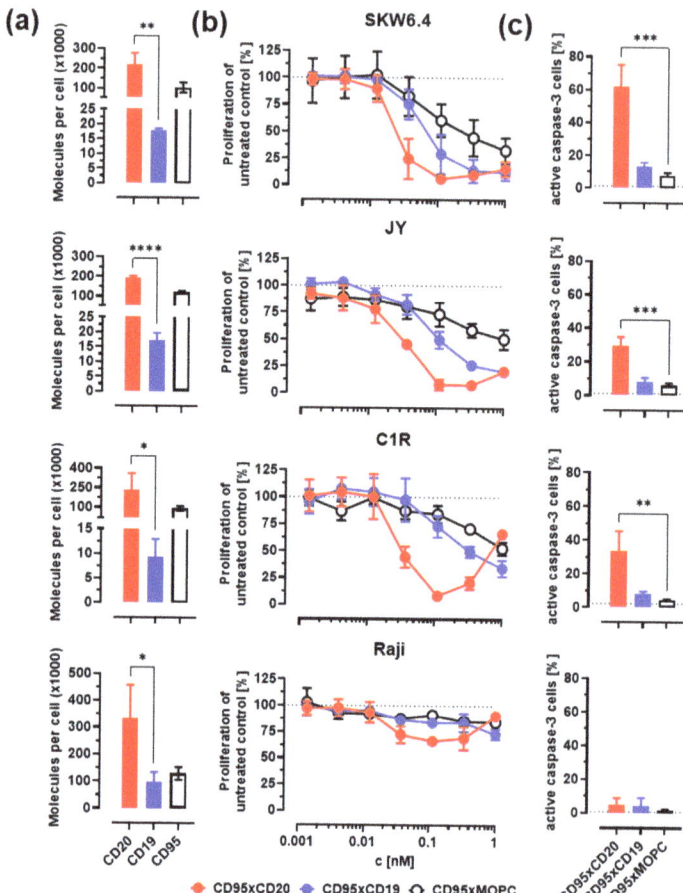

Figure 2. Bispecific CD95 antibodies induce depletion of lymphoma cells via apoptosis. The target antigen-mediated induction of apoptosis was evaluated on SKW6.4, JY, C1R, and Raji cells. (**a**) The antigen density of CD95, CD20, and CD19 on the cell surface of different cell lines was calculated using the flow cytometry-based Qifikit system. Statistics were calculated using an unpaired t-test, CD20 vs. CD19 expression. (**b**) Different lymphoma cell lines were incubated for 48 h with different concentrations of bispecific antibodies. Inhibition of cell proliferation was evaluated using a ^{3}H-thymidine uptake. (**c**) Induction of apoptosis with the indicated bsAbs (0.3 nM) was verified by intracellular active caspase-3 staining after 20 h using flow cytometry. Statistics were calculated with one-way ANOVA. Treatment versus isotype control. Mean ± SD, $n = 3$. * $p < 0.05$, ** $p < 0.01$, *** $p < 0.001$, **** $p < 0.0001$. Further analysis of (**a**,**b**) is also presented in Table 1.

We further assessed the ability of our bsAbs to inhibit cell proliferation in a ^{3}H-thymidine-based proliferation inhibition assay. SKW6.4, JY, and C1R were sensitive to antibody treatment, resulting in a concentration-dependent inhibition of proliferation, while Raji cells were CD95-resistant despite expressing sufficient levels of CD95, CD20, and CD19 (Figure 2b). The CD95xCD20 bsAb showed the most pronounced cell reduction resulting in IC$_{50}$ values between 24 and 35 pM (Table 1). In contrast, treatment with the CD95xCD19 bsAb exhibited only moderate inhibition of proliferation. This result was surprising given the higher binding affinity of the anti-CD19 clone 4G7 compared to the anti-CD20 clone 2H7 (Figure 1e,f). Our results suggest that the significantly higher expression of CD20 on lymphoma cell lines seems to be an important prerequisite for triggering efficient CD95 signaling (Figure 2a). The CD95xMOPC molecule also showed moderate inhibition of cell proliferation, but only at high concentrations, indicating that the observed effect is highly dependent on the presence of the respective target antigen.

Table 1. Antigen expression on lymphoma cell lines and IC_{50} values of bispecific antibodies. The number of CD20, CD19, and CD95 molecules expressed on different lymphoma cell lines (see also Figure 2a) as well as the absolute IC_{50} values (pM) of different bispecific antibodies (see also Figure 2b). Mean ± SD, $n = 3$.

Cell Line	Molecules/Cell (×1000)			CD95xCD20 abs. IC_{50}	CD95xCD19 abs. IC_{50}	CD95xMOPC abs. IC_{50}
	CD20	CD19	CD95			
SKW6.4	218 ± 58	18 ± 1	105 ± 26	24 ± 11	69 ± 29	481 ± 571
JY	190 ± 10	17 ± 3	122 ± 5	35 ± 1	107 ± 35	-
C1R	233 ± 124	9 ± 4	93 ± 17	32 ± 7	306 ± 154	-
Raji	332 ± 125	99 ± 36	130 ± 24	-	-	-

To further confirm that the observed inhibition of proliferation is due to apoptosis, an intracellular staining of active caspase-3 was performed using flow cytometry. The results depicted in Figure 2c demonstrated that upon treatment with CD95xCD20 bsAb a significantly higher active caspase-3 staining was observed. In contrast, no significant increase was observed with CD95xCD19 and the control bsAb.

3.3. In Vivo Activity against Malignant B Cells

Next, we decided to compare the newly generated CD95xCD20 molecule in the IgGsc format to the previously generated Fabsc molecule by Nalivaiko and colleagues in vitro and in vivo (Figure 3a) [23]. CD19 bsAbs were not included in in vivo assays as they showed no significant therapeutic effects on lymphoma cell lines. In vitro, both CD95xCD20 antibody formats induced similar killing of SKW6.4 cells (Figure 3b).

In vivo antitumor activity of CD95xCD20 was examined using established SKW6.4 tumor models in CB17 SCID mice. Antibodies in the Fabsc format were shown to have a very short serum half-life, which is greatly increased in IgGsc molecules, as the latter contains a functional CH3 that allows binding to FcRn and recycling of the molecule (Figure 3d) [23,24]. Accordingly, the IgGsc molecule was dosed twice on days 0 and 3 (50 µg per mouse, 100 µg total), while the Fabsc molecule was injected twice daily for 10 days (100 µg per mouse, 2 mg total) to compensate for the lower serum half-life. Both molecules had no side effects as the mice were monitored three times a week and no loss in weight was observed (Figure 3c). The Fabsc showed tumor regression until day ~15, but once the antibody injection was stopped the tumors started to regrow rapidly. In marked contrast, the IgGsc construct showed tumor regression until day ~40, despite a 20-fold reduced total dose compared to the Fabsc (Figure 3e). Consequentially, the IgGsc molecule resulted in improved overall survival of the mice (Figure 3f).

3.4. Depletion of Activated B Cells and Reduction of IgG and Cytokine Levels

Next, we assessed the activity of the IgGsc constructs to induce apoptosis in activated B cells. The intention was to mimic the situation in patients with autoimmune diseases, where activated B cells produce autoantibodies and cytokines or act as APCs that stimulate T cells against self-antigens. Unlike CD19, CD20 is not expressed on antibody-producing plasma cells. Therefore, the CD95xCD19 construct was again included in these experiments, even if it showed only minor activity against lymphoma cells. Peripheral blood mononuclear cells (PBMCs) from healthy individuals were stimulated for 7 days with toll-like-receptor 9 (TLR9) agonistic CpG oligodeoxynucleotides (ODN2006), before being treated with the bsAbs for 2 days [26]. ODN2006 represents a B-class ODN for the activation of B cells, leading to the upregulation of CD20, CD19, and especially CD95 (Figure S2a–c). The expression of CD20 (~124,000 molecules per cell) and CD19 (~22,000 molecules per cell) on activated B cells was comparable to lymphoma cell lines (see also Figure 2a and Table 1).

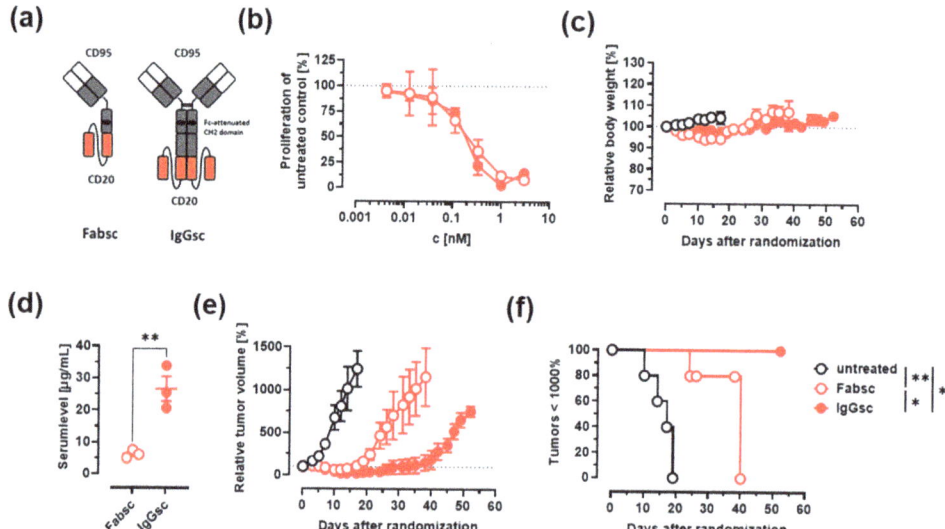

Figure 3. Antitumor activity of the bispecific Fabsc and IgGsc molecules (CD95xCD20) in immunodeficient mice. (**a**) Schematic representation of the Fabsc (left) and the IgGsc format (right). (**b**) The lymphoma cell line SKW6.4 was incubated for 48 h with different concentrations of bispecific antibodies. Inhibition of proliferation was measured using a ^{3}H-thymidine uptake. Mean ± SD, $n = 3$. (**c–f**) 10^7 SKW6.4 cells were injected s.c. in CB17 SCID mice, and antibody treatment was started when tumors reached a volume of 50–250 mm^3. The Fabsc molecule was given twice daily at 100 µg/mouse for 10 days (total dose 2 mg/mouse), while the IgGsc molecule was only dosed twice (on day 0 and day 3) at 50 µg/mouse (total dose 100 µg/mouse). Mean ± SEM, 3–5 mice per group. (**c**) The body weight of the mice was controlled 3 times per week. (**d**) Serum concentrations of the Fabsc and the IgGsc molecule 1 h after injection of the dose on day 10 or on day 3, respectively. Unpaired t-test was used for statistical analysis. (**e**) The relative tumor volume over time and (**f**) Kaplan–Meier plot of the experiment shown in (**e**). Log-rank (Mantel–Cox) test for pairwise comparisons was used for statistical analysis. * $p < 0.05$, ** $p < 0.01$.

The bispecific anti-CD95 antibodies induced a pronounced target cell-mediated depletion of activated B cells with comparable efficacy for the CD95xCD20 and CD95xCD19 construct (Figure 4a). The depletion of activated B cells also resulted in reduced IgG and cytokine (IL-6 and IL-10) levels in the supernatant (Figure 4c,d). Both cytokines are associated with different autoimmune diseases [30]. IL-2 and TNFα could not be detected. IFNγ secretion appeared to be reduced after antibody treatment but was highly donor-dependent and the effect was overall not significant (data not shown). The secretion of different cytokines most probably also led to minor activation of T and NK cells, resulting in "bystander killing" by cross-linking with CD20- and CD19-expressing B cells (Figures 4a and S2a). The killing of B cells within resting PBMC preparations was much weaker, highlighting the specificity for CD95-expressing activated lymphocytes (Figure 4b).

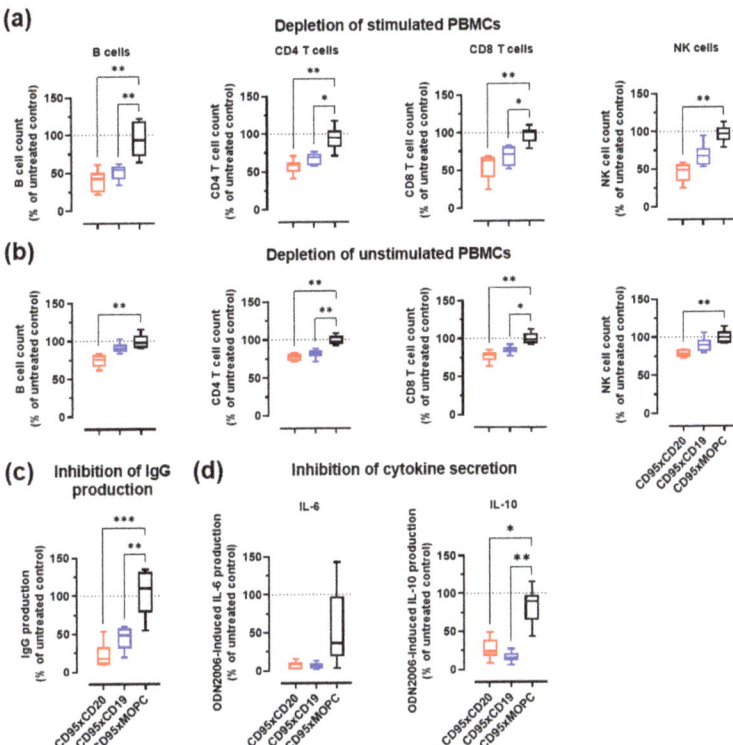

Figure 4. Bispecific CD95 antibodies induce depletion of activated B cells and reduce the production of IgG antibodies and cytokines. CD95xCD20 in red, CD95xCD19 in blue and CD95xMOPC in white. (**a**) Human PBMCs were activated with 0.1 µM ODN2006 for 7 days before they were incubated for 2 days with 0.1 nM of bispecific antibody. The viability of B cells, T cells, and NK cells was then analyzed by flow cytometry and normalized to the untreated controls. (**b**) Unstimulated human PBMCs were treated for 2 days with 0.1 nM of bispecific antibody and then analyzed as in (**a**). (**c**) The supernatant from (**a**) was analyzed for inhibition of IgG production and (**d**) for the secretion of IL-6 and IL-10 from activated B cells. Boxplot and whiskers from six different donors. Statistics were calculated with one-way ANOVA. Treatment versus isotype control. * $p < 0.05$, ** $p < 0.01$, *** $p < 0.001$.

3.5. Anti-CD95 bsAbs in the IgGsc Format Do Not Induce Apoptosis in Hepatocytes

Systemic administration of anti-CD95 antibodies can lead to fulminant hepatitis. This depends, among other reasons, on the antibody clone used and whether it stimulates type I apoptosis (mitochondria-independent) or type II apoptosis (mitochondria-dependent) [19,31]. SKW6.4 and activated lymphocytes are described as type I cells, while hepatocytes are considered type II cells.

To ensure that our anti-CD95 clone Apo-1 does not induce apoptosis in hepatocytes, we co-incubated SKW6.4 and the hepatic stellate cell line LX-1 with our bsAbs (Figure 5). This resulted in a target cell-mediated depletion of SKW6.4 lymphoma cells ($CD20^+/CD19^+/CD95^+$), while LX-1 cells ($CD20^-/CD19^-/CD95^+$) were unaffected (Figure S2d).

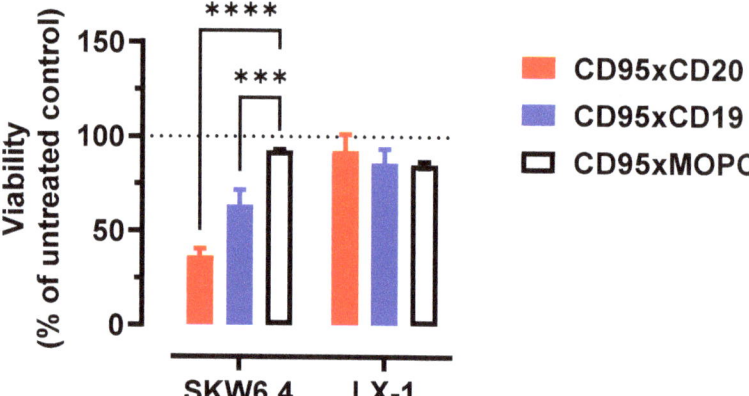

Figure 5. Bispecific anti-CD95 antibodies induce apoptosis in activated lymphocytes (type I cells) but not in hepatocytes (type II cells). SKW6.4 lymphoma cells and LX-1 hepatic stellate cells were co-cultured for 20 h before the depletion of both cell populations was determined by flow cytometry. Statistics were calculated with two-way ANOVA. Treatment versus isotype control. Mean ± SD, $n = 3$. *** $p < 0.001$, **** $p < 0.0001$.

4. Discussion

The selective activation of the CD95 death receptor by bsAbs is a very attractive strategy for depletion of undesired B cells that express CD95. To this end, we developed two antibodies in the IgGsc format targeting the B cell-restricted antigens CD20 and CD19 for target cell-mediated induction of apoptosis. The IgGsc format was chosen for its favorable pharmacokinetic and producibility [24].

CD20 is a rather small antigen (33–35 kDa) and the antibody clone 2H7 binds in close proximity to the cellular membrane to a similar epitope as does rituximab [32]. Herrmann and colleagues reported that anti-CD95 bsAbs induce apoptosis rather in trans than in cis configuration [33]. Therefore, the architecture of CD20 might facilitate bicellular binding of bsAbs and thus creates optimal conditions for CD95 clustering. The combination with its high expression levels on malignant and activated B cells make CD20 a very promising candidate for targeted induction of apoptosis. Our CD95xCD20 bsAb revealed IC_{50} values as low as 25 pM, which was remarkable considering the rather low affinity of the anti-CD20 clone 2H7 as a single chain. The construction of the molecule in a "reversed orientation", with an N-terminal CD20 binder, was not possible as the anti-CD95 clone Apo-1 cannot be expressed as a single chain as some antibodies tend to show high levels of aggregation in this confirmation [23,34]. CD19 expression was much weaker on malignant cells, reducing apoptotic effects.

In a recent publication, we could show that the IgGsc format has a much better pharmacokinetic as compared to our previous Fabsc format [24]. Therefore, we decided to compare both formats with CD95xCD20 specificity in CB17 SCID mice bearing established SKW6.4 tumors. To compensate for Fabsc's lower serum half-life, its total dose was 20-fold higher compared to the IgGsc. Nevertheless, the anti-tumor efficacy of the IgGsc was clearly superior due to its improved serum half-life and, as demonstrated by Zekri et al., due to sustained tumor localization.

A limiting factor for the treatment of lymphomas with our bispecific antibodies of the described kind is loss of CD95 expression or sensitivity [16,17]. The Burkitt lymphoma cell line Raji for example showed high expression levels of CD95 but was still resistant to CD95-mediated apoptosis. The combination with the Bcl-2 inhibitor Venetoclax or Doxorubicin could help restore CD95 sensitivity.

In contrast to malignant cells, normal B cells acquire CD95 expression and sensitivity during the activation [13,14]. This plays a crucial role in regulating the homeostasis of B cell activation, demonstrated by the fact that disorders of CD95-mediated apoptosis can lead to the autoimmune lymphoproliferative syndrome (ALPS) [35,36]. Therefore, bsAbs with CD95xtarget-specificity could be successfully used for the treatment of B cell-mediated autoimmune diseases as these cells should not escape CD95-mediated apoptosis as easily as malignant cells.

Our study confirmed that B cells activated for 7 days are highly sensitive to CD95 signaling. The anti-CD95 bsAbs induced profound B cell depletion and subsequent reduction in IgG and cytokine levels. In contrast to lymphoma cells, the CD95xCD19 construct was also very effective at depleting activated B cells. Since the expression of CD19 on malignant and normal B cells is comparable, this can possibly be explained by a higher sensitivity of normal lymphocytes to CD95-induced cell death and/or the expression of this antigen on antibody-producing plasma cells [37,38]. However, autoantibody production is not the only problem in B cell-mediated autoimmune diseases, as B cell-derived cytokines such as IL-6 can support autoimmunity. Indeed, it has been demonstrated that B cell-derived IL-6 plays an important role in experimental autoimmune encephalomyelitis (EAE) and MS [39]. The secretion of cytokines most likely led to the activation of other lymphocytes in our experiments and explains the "bystander killing" of T and NK cells. In any case, our antibodies showed only minor depletion of resting PBMCs, highlighting to specificity for activated lymphocytes.

Activation of the CD95 death receptor depends on the clustering and immobilization [21]. Immobilization enhances the activity of soluble FasL by several orders of magnitude, but soluble FasL can still induce apoptosis. In principle, our anti-CD95 bsAbs, by inducing "bivalent CD95 stimulation", might also be able to trigger the CD95 death receptor without immobilization in higher concentrations. In patients, this could potentially lead to hepatic damage since hepatocytes are very sensitive to CD95 activation. However, several publications indicate that depending on the antibody clone apoptosis is rather induced in activated lymphocytes (type 1 cells) than in hepatocytes (type II cells) [19,31]. Indeed, we did not observe apoptosis of hepatic stellate cells in the presence of our anti-CD95 (clone Apo-1) bsAbs. Thus, in conclusion, we believe that our novel CD95xCD20 and CD95xCD19 constructs are attractive reagents for treatment of B cell-derived malignancies and autoimmune diseases by targeted induction of apoptosis.

5. Conclusions

In summary, bispecific anti-CD95 antibodies are promising candidates for a more specific depletion of malignant and autoreactive B cells and hold promise to improve the safety and efficacy compared to previously established antibody therapies.

6. Patents

AH is listed as an inventor of the patent application "recombinant bispecific antibody binding to CD20 and CD95", EP2920210B1, applicant Baliopharm AG, Basel, Switzerland.

Supplementary Materials: The following supporting information can be downloaded at: https://www.mdpi.com/article/10.3390/cancers14163941/s1, Figure S1. Biochemical characterization of CD95xMOPC and quantitative analysis of antigen expression on Jurkat and Daudi cells. Figure S2. Antigen expression on resting and activated lymphocytes.

Author Contributions: Conceptualization, G.J., S.H. and L.Z.; methodology and investigation, S.H., M.M.-O., K.T., I.H. and K.N.; validation, J.K., M.P., H.-G.R., T.M., A.H.; formal analysis, H.R.S., G.J., L.Z.; writing—original draft preparation, S.H., L.Z. and G.J.; writing—review and editing, H.R.S., H.-G.R., M.P., J.K. and K.N.; visualization, S.H.; supervision, G.J., H.R.S. and A.H.; project administration, G.J., H.R.S. and A.H.; funding acquisition, A.H., H.R.S., G.J. and H.-G.R. All authors have read and agreed to the published version of the manuscript.

Funding: Funding was provided by the German Cancer Consortium Partner Site Tuebingen (DKTK). This work was funded, in part, by Baliopharm AG.

Institutional Review Board Statement: All animal studies were approved by the animal welfare body at Charles River Discovery Research Services Germany and the local authorities (Study number P500A4A).

Informed Consent Statement: Not applicable. No patient materials were used in this study.

Data Availability Statement: The data presented in this study are available on request from the corresponding author.

Acknowledgments: The authors thank Carolin Walker and Beate Pömmerl for expert technical assistance. We acknowledge the support of the Open Access Publishing Fund of the University of Tübingen. The graphical abstract was created with BioRender.com (accessed on 18 May 2022).

Conflicts of Interest: AH is listed as an inventor of the patent application "recombinant bispecific antibody binding to CD20 and CD95", EP2920210B1, applicant Baliopharm AG, Basel, Switzerland. The other authors declare no conflict of interest.

References

1. Molina, A. A Decade of Rituximab: Improving Survival Outcomes in Non-Hodgkin's Lymphoma. *Annu. Rev. Med.* **2008**, *59*, 237–250. [CrossRef] [PubMed]
2. Lim, S.H.; Levy, R. Translational Medicine in Action: Anti-CD20 Therapy in Lymphoma. *J. Immunol.* **2014**, *193*, 1519–1524. [CrossRef] [PubMed]
3. Faurschou, M.; Jayne, D.R.W. Anti-B Cell Antibody Therapies for Inflammatory Rheumatic Diseases. *Annu. Rev. Med.* **2014**, *65*, 263–278. [CrossRef]
4. Jones, R.B.; Cohen Tervaert, J.W.; Hauser, T.; Luqmani, R.; Morgan, M.D.; Peh, C.A.; Savage, C.O.; Segelmark, M.; Tesar, V.; van Paassen, P.; et al. Rituximab versus Cyclophosphamide in ANCA-Associated Renal Vasculitis. *N. Engl. J. Med.* **2010**, *363*, 211–220. [CrossRef]
5. Abdulahad, W.H.; Meijer, J.M.; Kroese, F.G.M.; Meiners, P.M.; Vissink, A.; Spijkervet, F.K.L.; Kallenberg, C.G.M.; Bootsma, H. B Cell Reconstitution and t Helper Cell Balance after Rituximab Treatment of Active Primary Sjögren's Syndrome. *Arthritis Rheum.* **2011**, *63*, 1116–1123. [CrossRef] [PubMed]
6. Castillo-Trivino, T.; Braithwaite, D.; Bacchetti, P.; Waubant, E. Rituximab in Relapsing and Progressive Forms of Multiple Sclerosis: A Systematic Review. *PLoS ONE* **2013**, *8*, e0066308. [CrossRef]
7. Gottenberg, J.E.; Ravaud, P.; Bardin, T.; Cacoub, P.; Cantagrel, A.; Combe, B.; Dougados, M.; Flipo, R.M.; Godeau, B.; Guillevin, L.; et al. Risk Factors for Severe Infections in Patients with Rheumatoid Arthritis Treated with Rituximab in the Autoimmunity and Rituximab Registry. *Arthritis Rheum.* **2010**, *62*, 2625–2632. [CrossRef]
8. Hoy, S.M. Tafasitamab: First Approval. *Drugs* **2020**, *80*, 1731–1737. [CrossRef]
9. Newman, M.J.; Benani, D.J. A Review of Blinatumomab, a Novel Immunotherapy. *J. Oncol. Pharm. Pract.* **2016**, *22*, 639–645. [CrossRef]
10. Portell, C.A.; Wenzell, C.M.; Advani, A.S. Clinical and Pharmacologic Aspects of Blinatumomab in the Treatment of B-Cell Acute Lymphoblastic Leukemia. *Clin. Pharmacol. Adv. Appl.* **2013**, *5*, 5–11. [CrossRef]
11. Makita, S.; Yoshimura, K.; Tobinai, K. Clinical Development of Anti-CD19 Chimeric Antigen Receptor T-Cell Therapy for B-Cell Non-Hodgkin Lymphoma. *Cancer Sci.* **2017**, *108*, 1109–1118. [CrossRef] [PubMed]
12. Wajant, H. Principles and Mechanisms of CD95 Activation. *Biol. Chem.* **2014**, *395*, 1401–1416. [CrossRef] [PubMed]
13. Sharma, K.; Wang, R.; Zhang, L.; Yin, D.; Luo, X.; Solomon, J.; Jiang, R.; Markos, K.; Davidson, W.; Scott, D.; et al. Death the Fas Way: Regulation and Pathophysiology of CD95 and Its Ligand. *Pharmacol. Ther.* **2000**, *88*, 333–347. [CrossRef]
14. Daniel, P.T.; Krammer, P.H. Activation Induces Sensitivity toward APO-1 (CD95)-Mediated Apoptosis in Human B Cells. *J. Immunol.* **1994**, *152*, 5624–5632. [PubMed]
15. Chen, L.; Park, S.M.; Tumanov, A.V.; Hau, A.; Sawada, K.; Feig, C.; Turner, J.R.; Fu, Y.X.; Romero, I.L.; Lengyel, E.; et al. CD95 Promotes Tumour Growth. *Nature* **2010**, *465*, 492–496. [CrossRef]
16. Xerri, L.; Bouabdallah, R.; Devilard, E.; Hassoun, J.; Stoppa, A.M.; Birg, F. Sensitivity to Fas-Mediated Apoptosis Is Null or Weak in B-Cell Non-Hodgkin's Lymphomas and Is Moderately Increased by CD40 Ligation. *Br. J. Cancer* **1998**, *78*, 225–232. [CrossRef]
17. Plumas, J.; Jacob, M.C.; Chaperot, L.; Molens, J.P.; Sotto, J.J.; Bensa, J.C. Tumor B Cells from Non-Hodgkin's Lymphoma Are Resistant to CD95 (Fas/Apo-1)-Mediated Apoptosis. *Blood* **1998**, *91*, 2875–2885. [CrossRef]
18. Trauth, B.C.; Klas, C.; Peters, A.M.J.; Matzku, S.; Möller, P.; Falk, W.; Debatin, K.M.; Krammer, P.H. Monoclonal Antibody-Mediated Tumor Regression by Induction of Apoptosis. *Science* **1989**, *245*, 301–305. [CrossRef]
19. Ichikawa, K.; Yoshida-Kato, H.; Ohtsuki, M.; Ohsumi, J.; Yamaguchi, J.; Takahashi, S.; Tani, Y.; Watanabe, M.; Shiraishi, A.; Nishioka, K.; et al. A Novel Murine Anti-Human Fas MAb Which Mitigates Lymphadenopathy without Hepatotoxicity. *Int. Immunol.* **2000**, *12*, 555–562. [CrossRef]
20. Galle, P.R.; Krammer, P.H. CD95-Induced Apoptosis in Human Liver Disease. *Semin. Liver Dis.* **1998**, *18*, 141–151. [CrossRef]

21. Schneider, P.; Holler, N.; Bodmer, J.L.; Hahne, M.; Frei, K.; Fontana, A.; Tschopp, J. Conversion of Membrane-Bound Fas(CD95) Ligand to Its Soluble Form Is Associated with Downregulation of Its Proapoptotic Activity and Loss of Liver Toxicity. *J. Exp. Med.* **1998**, *187*, 1205–1213. [CrossRef] [PubMed]
22. Jung, G.; Grosse-Hovest, L.; Krammer, P.H.; Rammensee, H.G. Target Cell-Restricted Triggering of the CD95 (APO-1/Fas) Death Receptor with Bispecific Antibody Fragments. *Cancer Res.* **2001**, *61*, 1846–1848. [PubMed]
23. Nalivaiko, K.; Hofmann, M.; Kober, K.; Teichweyde, N.; Krammer, P.H.; Rammensee, H.-G.; Grosse-Hovest, L.; Jung, G. A Recombinant Bispecific CD20×CD95 Antibody With Superior Activity Against Normal and Malignant B-Cells. *Mol. Ther.* **2016**, *24*, 298–305. [CrossRef] [PubMed]
24. Zekri, L.; Vogt, F.; Osburg, L.; Müller, S.; Kauer, J.; Manz, T.; Pflügler, M.; Maurer, A.; Heitmann, J.S.; Hagelstein, I.; et al. An IgG-based Bispecific Antibody for Improved Dual Targeting in PSMA-positive Cancer. *EMBO Mol. Med.* **2021**, *13*, 1–15. [CrossRef] [PubMed]
25. Hörner, S.; Ghosh, M.; Kauer, J.; Spät, P.; Rammensee, H.; Jung, G.; Pflügler, M. Mass Spectrometry for Quality Control of Bispecific Antibodies after SDS-PAGE In-gel Digestion. *Biotechnol. Bioeng.* **2021**, *118*, 3069–3075. [CrossRef] [PubMed]
26. Van Belle, K.; Herman, J.; Boon, L.; Waer, M.; Sprangers, B.; Louat, T. Comparative in Vitro Immune Stimulation Analysis of Primary Human B Cells and B Cell Lines. *J. Immunol. Res.* **2016**, *2016*, 5281823. [CrossRef]
27. Coloma, M.J.; Morrison, S.L. Design and Production of Novel Tetravalent Bispecific Antibodies. *Nat. Biotechnol.* **1997**, *15*, 159–163. [CrossRef]
28. Liu, A.Y.; Robinson, R.R.; Murray, E.D.; Ledbetter, J.A.; Hellström, I.; Hellström, K.E. Production of a Mouse-Human Chimeric Monoclonal Antibody to CD20 with Potent Fc-Dependent Biologic Activity. *J. Immunol.* **1987**, *139*, 3521–3526.
29. MEEKER, T.C.; MILLER, R.A.; LINK, M.P.; BINDL, J.; WARNKE, R.; LEVY, R. A Unique Human B Lymphocyte Antigen Defined by a Monoclonal Antibody. *Hybridoma* **1984**, *3*, 305–320. [CrossRef]
30. Shen, P.; Fillatreau, S. Antibody-Independent Functions of B Cells: A Focus on Cytokines. *Nat. Rev. Immunol.* **2015**, *15*, 441–451. [CrossRef]
31. Nakayama, J.; Ogawa, Y.; Yoshigae, Y.; Onozawa, Y.; Yonemura, A.; Saito, M.; Ichikawa, K.; Yamoto, T.; Komai, T.; Tatsuta, T.; et al. A Humanized Anti-Human Fas Antibody, R-125224, Induces Apoptosis in Type I Activated Lymphocytes but Not in Type II Cells. *Int. Immunol.* **2006**, *18*, 113–124. [CrossRef] [PubMed]
32. Du, J.; Wang, H.; Zhong, C.; Peng, B.; Zhang, M.; Li, B.; Hou, S.; Guo, Y.; Ding, J. Crystal Structure of Chimeric Antibody C2H7 Fab in Complex with a CD20 Peptide. *Mol. Immunol.* **2008**, *45*, 2861–2868. [CrossRef] [PubMed]
33. Herrmann, T.; Große-Hovest, L.; Otz, T.; Krammer, P.H.; Rammensee, H.G.; Jung, G. Construction of Optimized Bispecific Antibodies for Selective Activation of the Death Receptor CD95. *Cancer Res.* **2008**, *68*, 1221–1227. [CrossRef] [PubMed]
34. Wörn, A.; Plückthun, A. Stability Engineering of Antibody Single-Chain Fv Fragments. *J. Mol. Biol.* **2001**, *305*, 989–1010. [CrossRef]
35. Fisher, G.H.; Rosenberg, F.J.; Straus, S.E.; Dale, J.K.; Middelton, L.A.; Lin, A.Y.; Strober, W.; Lenardo, M.J.; Puck, J.M. Dominant Interfering Fas Gene Mutations Impair Apoptosis in a Human Autoimmune Lymphoproliferative Syndrome. *Cell* **1995**, *81*, 935–946. [CrossRef]
36. Agrebi, N.; Ben-Mustapha, I.; Matoussi, N.; Dhouib, N.; Ben-Ali, M.; Mekki, N.; Ben-Ahmed, M.; Larguèche, B.; Ben Becher, S.; Béjaoui, M.; et al. Rare Splicing Defects of FAS Underly Severe Recessive Autoimmune Lymphoproliferative Syndrome. *Clin. Immunol.* **2017**, *183*, 17–23. [CrossRef]
37. Leandro, M.J.; Cambridge, G.; Ehrenstein, M.R.; Edwards, J.C.W. Reconstitution of Peripheral Blood B Cells after Depletion with Rituximab in Patients with Rheumatoid Arthritis. *Arthritis Rheum.* **2006**, *54*, 613–620. [CrossRef]
38. Yazawa, N.; Hamaguchi, Y.; Poe, J.C.; Tedder, T.F. Immunotherapy Using Unconjugated CD19 Monoclonal Antibodies in Animal Models for B Lymphocyte Malignancies and Autoimmune Disease. *Proc. Natl. Acad. Sci. USA* **2005**, *102*, 15178–15183. [CrossRef]
39. Barr, T.A.; Shen, P.; Brown, S.; Lampropoulou, V.; Roch, T.; Lawrie, S.; Fan, B.; O'Connor, R.A.; Anderton, S.M.; Bar-Or, A.; et al. B Cell Depletion Therapy Ameliorates Autoimmune Disease through Ablation of IL-6-Producing B Cells. *J. Exp. Med.* **2012**, *209*, 1001–1010. [CrossRef]

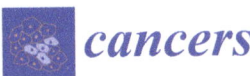

Review

Decoding the Complexity of Immune–Cancer Cell Interactions: Empowering the Future of Cancer Immunotherapy

Kaitlyn Maffuid [1] and Yanguang Cao [1,2,*]

[1] Division of Pharmacotherapy and Experimental Therapeutics, School of Pharmacy, University of North Carolina at Chapel Hill, Chapel Hill, NC 27599, USA; kmaffuid@email.unc.edu
[2] Lineberger Comprehensive Cancer Center, School of Medicine, University of North Carolina at Chapel Hill, Chapel Hill, NC 27599, USA
* Correspondence: yanguang@unc.edu

Simple Summary: Cell-to-cell communication between the immune system and tumors is of the utmost importance; it influences the development of tumors, their growth, and how they respond to treatments. In this article, we provide an overview of why understanding the interactions between immune and tumor cells is so significant for developing anti-cancer therapeutics, particularly cancer immunotherapy. We delve into the methods and tools used to decipher these interactions and discuss the potential impact on the future of cancer treatment. Moreover, we emphasize the power of unraveling these interactions in advancing cancer immunotherapy. We also explore the challenges that can be tackled by gaining insights into these interactions.

Abstract: The tumor and tumor microenvironment (TME) consist of a complex network of cells, including malignant, immune, fibroblast, and vascular cells, which communicate with each other. Disruptions in cell–cell communication within the TME, caused by a multitude of extrinsic and intrinsic factors, can contribute to tumorigenesis, hinder the host immune system, and enable tumor evasion. Understanding and addressing intercellular miscommunications in the TME are vital for combating these processes. The effectiveness of immunotherapy and the heterogeneous response observed among patients can be attributed to the intricate cellular communication between immune cells and cancer cells. To unravel these interactions, various experimental, statistical, and computational techniques have been developed. These include ligand–receptor analysis, intercellular proximity labeling approaches, and imaging-based methods, which provide insights into the distorted cell–cell interactions within the TME. By characterizing these interactions, we can enhance the design of cancer immunotherapy strategies. In this review, we present recent advancements in the field of mapping intercellular communication, with a particular focus on immune–tumor cellular interactions. By modeling these interactions, we can identify critical factors and develop strategies to improve immunotherapy response and overcome treatment resistance.

Keywords: immunotherapy; cell–cell interaction; intercellular labeling; intercellular imaging; bioinformatics; cancer

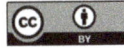

1. Introduction

Intercellular interactions play crucial roles in organism function and development. Cells can interact with each other either directly (in physical proximity) or indirectly (paracrine signaling). These interactions are the basic building blocks of physiological communication and are essential for tissue formation, immune response, homeostasis, and regeneration. In direct cellular communications, contact between cell surfaces can occur via gap junctions, cell adhesion, tunnel nanotubes, and ligand receptor signaling. When cells interact indirectly, cellular information is shared through signaling from extracellular vesicles, cytokines, chemokines, growth factors, metabolites, and exosomes. These intercellular interacting mechanisms contribute to tissue development and physiological functions [1].

A healthy immune system can precisely identify and eliminate precancerous cells, and it eliminates them before they cause any harm, by a process referred to as tumor immune surveillance. Numerous extrinsic and intrinsic factors impair immune–precancerous cell interactions, contributing to tumorigenesis. Once developed, tumor cells evade and disrupt the host immune system, leading to an immune-suppressive tumor microenvironment (TME). The TME is a complex ecosystem comprising tumor cells, immune cells, fibroblasts, extracellular matrices, and signaling molecules. The interaction between the immune cells and cancer cells within the TME evolves and can result in either pro- or anti-tumorigeneses [2]. Restoring the immune function and the network of healthy cell–cell communication within the TME has become a significant component of cancer immunotherapy.

Cancer immunotherapy began in the 1980s with an interferon-α2 inhibitor as the first immunotherapeutic agent approved by the FDA in 1986 [3]. Since then, numerous other immunotherapies have been discovered, including immune checkpoint inhibitors, oncolytic viruses, bispecific T cell engagers, cytokine therapies, and adoptive cell therapies. The central concept of immunotherapy is to restore or reactivate the host anti-tumor immune system [3]. As promising as these immunotherapies are, clinical response varies significantly from patient to patient, primarily because of distinct patterns of immunosuppressive TMEs and different patterns of disruption in cell–cell interactions. About 30–40% of patients respond to immunotherapy, with fewer achieving a durable response [4]. Variability in the TME primarily relates to the different degrees of tumor-infiltrated lymphocytes (TILs) and their functions. Some patients have "hot" tumors, where the tumors have higher TILs, and these patients usually respond well to immunotherapy [5]. On the other hand, some patients have "cold" tumors with poor or almost no TILs, and these tumors often develop resistance to immunotherapy [5]. Elucidating the mechanism of resistance and characterizing the distorted patterns of intercellular interactions between tumor and immune cells within TMEs has become critical for more potent immunotherapies.

Studies over the years have showcased the cell types present in the TMEs associated with positive and negative outcomes of immunotherapy. High $CD8^+$ T cell abundance is often associated with favorable overall survival, whereas increased regulatory T cells are associated with poor overall survival [6,7]. However, a recent pan-cancer analysis showed that high $CD8^+$ abundance is not always associated with a better prognosis, as the spatial cellular assemblies are also crucial [8], which means that different immune cells will have various prognostic factors depending on the location and type of cancer. In addition to PD-L1 expression and tumor mutation burdens, there are still no robust prognostic biomarkers across cancers.

Methods that can characterize the deformed intercellular interactions and identify the cell (sub-) populations that are involved in the interactions are extremely critical for prognosis. Identifying which cell population at which cellular state is associated with positive or negative outcomes in immunotherapy is extremely valuable to patient stratification, prognostic biomarkers, and resistance mechanisms. This review aims to explore the diverse manifestations of cell–cell interactions in the context of cancer, providing an overview of quantitative approaches to assess these interactions. Moreover, it seeks to investigate the potential of leveraging the influence of cell–cell interactions to enhance the efficacy of cancer immunotherapies.

2. Cell–Cell Interactions during Tumorigenesis

The immune system consists of two compartments: innate cells (such as macrophages, neutrophils, dendritic cells, and natural killer cells) and adaptive cells (B cells and T cells). Innate cells rapidly respond to foreign pathogens, presenting antigens to adaptive cells to initiate specific immunological responses. In the context of cancer, antigen-presenting cells detect tumor antigens and present them to naïve lymphocytes. This communication primes and activates lymphocytes, which then migrate to the tumor site. The activated T cells recognize and eliminate tumor cells. The innate and adaptive immune cells collaborate in a process called cancer immunoediting to eliminate tumors. However, if this process is unsuccessful or suppressed, the tumor microenvironment forms.

The progression of the TME towards malignancy can be understood within the framework of cancer immunoediting. Cancer immunoediting refers to the dynamic interplay between the host immune system and the tumor cells, whereby immune mechanisms either restrain or promote tumor development. This process can be divided into three distinct phases: elimination, equilibrium, and escape [9].

During the elimination phase, innate and adaptive immune responses collaborate to recognize and eliminate malignant cells. The innate immune system, including dendritic cells and antigen-presenting cells, primes and activates T cells by presenting tumor antigens. These activated T cells are then mobilized to directly interact with cancer cells, leading to their destruction [9]. However, tumors can evade elimination by exploiting immune checkpoints, such as PD-1/PD-L1 and CTLA-4, which act as brakes on T cell activity. When T cells engage with cancer cells bearing PD-L1 or CTLA-4, inhibitory signals are transmitted, causing T cell exhaustion and inactivation [9].

Tumors that successfully evade elimination enter the equilibrium phase, during which they remain dormant but develop resistance mechanisms against immune surveillance [9]. This resistance is mediated by immunosuppressive cell types, including tumor-associated macrophages (TAMs), myeloid-derived suppressor cells (MDSCs), cancer-associated fibroblasts (CAFs), and regulatory T cells (Tregs) [10]. These cells actively communicate with other components of the TME, dampening T cell activation, modulating effector cell function, and promoting tumor progression. Of special significance, CAFs and TAMs play pivotal roles in carcinogenesis and the maturation of TMEs [10]. CAFs can promote tumor growth, angiogenesis, the invasion of tumor cells into surrounding tissues, and the modulation of the tumor response to immunotherapy [11–13]. They also secrete various signaling molecules and cytokines that can modulate immune responses and create an environment favorable for tumor growth. The equilibrium phase sets the stage for the subsequent escape phase, characterized by clinically detectable tumor growth and the need for therapeutic intervention [9,10].

Effective immunotherapy can revert tumors to the elimination phase, where the suppressive mechanisms are counteracted, leading to the elimination of the tumor [9]. However, a partial response to immunotherapy may shift the tumor back into the equilibrium phase, enabling the emergence of resistant clones and eventually leading to the escape phase, signifying acquired resistance to immunotherapy [9]. In cases where immunotherapy fails to induce a response, the tumor demonstrates innate resistance to treatment [9].

Understanding the intricate dynamics of cancer immunoediting and intercellular interactions between tumor and immune cells is crucial for the development of effective therapeutic approaches aimed at restoring immune control over tumors and achieving durable clinical responses.

3. Cell–Cell Interactions Are the Pharmacological Basis of Immunotherapy

Almost all types of immunotherapies involve direct cell–cell interactions for antitumor effect. One of the key cell–cell interactions during immunotherapy is the interaction between T cells and tumor cells. T cells can recognize and target tumor cells through the recognition of specific antigens presented by the tumor cells. However, tumors can evade T cell recognition by downregulating antigen presentation or by producing immune-suppressive molecules. Cell–cell interactions are the pharmacological basis of immunotherapy (Figure 1). The most successful immunotherapy—immune checkpoint inhibitors—have been approved for over 19 types of cancer treatment [14]. Blocking the immune checkpoint, CTLA-4 or PD-1/PD-L1, can restore the function of TILs for cytotoxic effects, which entail direct physical and functional contact between TILs and tumor cells. TILs, once engaged with target cells, can secrete perforin and granzyme B for cytotoxic effects [15].

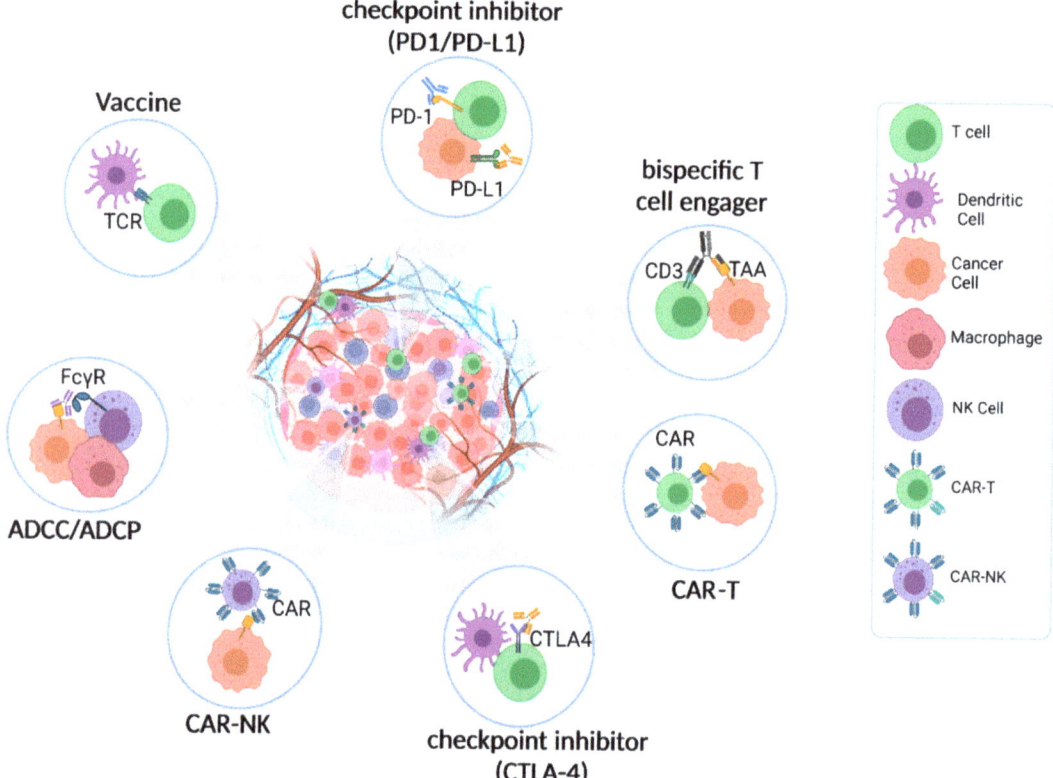

Figure 1. Cell–Cell interactions are the pharmacological basis of immunotherapy. The primary pharmacological mechanism of immunotherapy entails the activation or engagement of diverse immune cell populations to identify and eradicate cancer cells. This crucial process heavily relies on the dynamic interplay between immune cells and cancer cells within the TME. Within the TME, immune cells, including T cells, natural killer (NK) cells, dendritic cells (DCs), and macrophages, establish various types of interactions with cancer cells. These interactions encompass intricate molecular signaling pathways, direct cell-to-cell contact, and the exchange of soluble factors. The ultimate objective of immunotherapeutic approaches is to either alleviate immune suppressive interactions within the TME or activate immune effector functions, thereby unleashing the anti-cancer pharmacological effects of immunotherapy.

Another mechanism in which immune cells can have a cytotoxic effect on cancer cells is the process of antibody-dependent cellular cytotoxicity (ADCC) [15,16]. In ADCC, tumor-specific monoclonal antibodies (mAbs) recognize tumor-selective antigens on the surface of cancer cells. The Fc receptor expressed by the effector immune cell binds the Fc portion of the antibody attached to the cancer cells. Upon binding, the immune cell secretes proteins and enzymes, inducing cancer cell lysis. Many IgG-based targeted therapies, such as rituximab and trastuzumab, can trigger antibody-dependent cellular cytotoxicity (ADCC) through interactions between Fc and Fcγ receptors expressed on effector cells, initiating direct cell–cell interactions and cytotoxicity [16].

Another therapeutic approach that utilizes antibodies is bispecific T cell engagers (BiTEs) [17]. BiTEs are characterized by having two different antigen-binding sites in a single molecule, with one site binding to T cell receptors to activate cytotoxic T lymphocytes, and the other site binding to tumor-specific antigens (TSAs). The engagement between cytotoxic T lymphocytes and tumor cells triggered by BiTEs leads to the elimination of the tumor cells. Examples of BiTEs include CD3 and 4-1BB, which activate cytotoxic T lymphocytes, and target tumor-associated antigens (TAA), such as CD19 and CD20. BiTEs redirect cytotoxic T lymphocytes to specifically recognize and engage tumor cells, initiating cell–cell contact, known as the immunological synapse, and inducing cytotoxicity [17,18].

Chimeric antigen receptor (CAR) cell therapies represent a novel immunotherapeutic approach that signifies a significant advancement in personalized cancer treatment [19]. This approach involves genetically modifying T cells or natural killer (NK) cells to express synthetic receptors (CARs) that can bind to tumor antigens [19]. This genetic modification enables the redirected T or NK cells to specifically recognize cancer cells and initiate immune responses against them.

Oncolytic virus therapy holds promise as an immunotherapy approach that involves T cell activation and cell–cell interactions. This therapy utilizes either genetically engineered or naturally occurring viruses that can selectively replicate within cancer cells and kill them while sparing non-cancerous cells [20,21]. Upon administration, the oncolytic virus activates the immune system, leading to the recruitment of natural killer (NK) cells and CD8$^+$ T cells to the tumor site. This process results in the reduction in regulatory T cells (T$_{regs}$) and facilitates an effective immune response against the cancer cells [20,21].

In summary, intercellular interactions between effector cells (such as cytotoxic T lymphocytes and NK cells) and tumor cells have emerged as crucial steps for the efficacy of immunotherapies. Therapeutic approaches such as BiTEs, CAR cell therapies, and oncolytic virus therapies exploit these interactions to enhance the immune response against cancer cells, and they hold promise for the improvement of cancer treatment outcomes.

4. Experimental and Modeling Systems for Studying Cell–Cell Interactions

The intricate interplay between immune cells and structural components within the TME significantly influences patient outcomes, therapeutic response, and disease progression [22]. While existing data shed light on the communicative relationships between immune cells and tumor cells within the TME, there remains a substantial knowledge gap with regard to the intra-patient and intra-cancer types of communication. Consequently, the TME and its diverse cellular components have emerged as an enticing landscape for the research aiming to discover novel therapeutic strategies and optimize patient management [22].

To investigate and elucidate the intricate cellular interactions within the TME, numerous methodologies and systems have been developed (Figure 2). These approaches encompass in vitro and in vivo models, employing molecular analysis techniques, proximity labeling methods, and bioinformatic approaches [22,23]. Understanding the composition of distinct cell types within different TMEs and patient contexts is pivotal for advancing therapeutic interventions and identifying prognostic biomarkers. In this section, we delve into various experimental techniques and modeling systems for the comprehensive study of cell–cell interactions, encompassing experimental modeling systems, microscopy/imaging, proximity labeling, and bioinformatic approaches.

The study of cell–cell interactions employs various in vitro experimental systems, including two-dimensional (2D) cell culture and three-dimensional (3D) methods such as spheroids and organoids, as well as tissue samples (Table 1). Traditional 2D culture using primary cells and cell lines has long been considered a gold standard in cell culture due to its cost-effectiveness, long-term culture viability, low maintenance requirements, and user-friendly nature [24]. However, 2D culture falls short in mimicking the natural tissue structure, and it lacks biologically relevant cell–environment interactions when investigating complex environments like TME or normal tissue structures. To address this limitation, 3D cell culture techniques have revolutionized in vitro methodologies by providing more physiologically relevant options [24]. Organoids and spheroids have gained popularity as they enable the comparison of in vivo organs in vitro. Organoids, derived from stem cells or patient tumor cells, are three-dimensional tissue cultures that replicate the morphological and genetic features of the original tumor, allowing for patient-specific models and in vitro representations of the TME [25]. However, organoids have limitations, such as high patient variability, absence of specific essential cellular components, challenging culture maintenance, and higher costs [25]. On the other hand, spheroids are simpler three-dimensional clusters of cells derived from various cell types, including tumor tissues and hepatocytes [26]. They do not require scaffolding to form 3D cultures but rely on cell adhesion. However, spheroids lack the ability to self-assemble or regenerate, making them less desirable compared to organoids [26]. Both models enable three-dimensional assessment of tumors in vitro, providing improved translational models for clinical applications. Tissue biopsy slices are also valuable for identifying the spatial distribution and location of cells within the TME or normal tissues. However, the slicing process introduces variability in cell distribution due to the method employed [27].

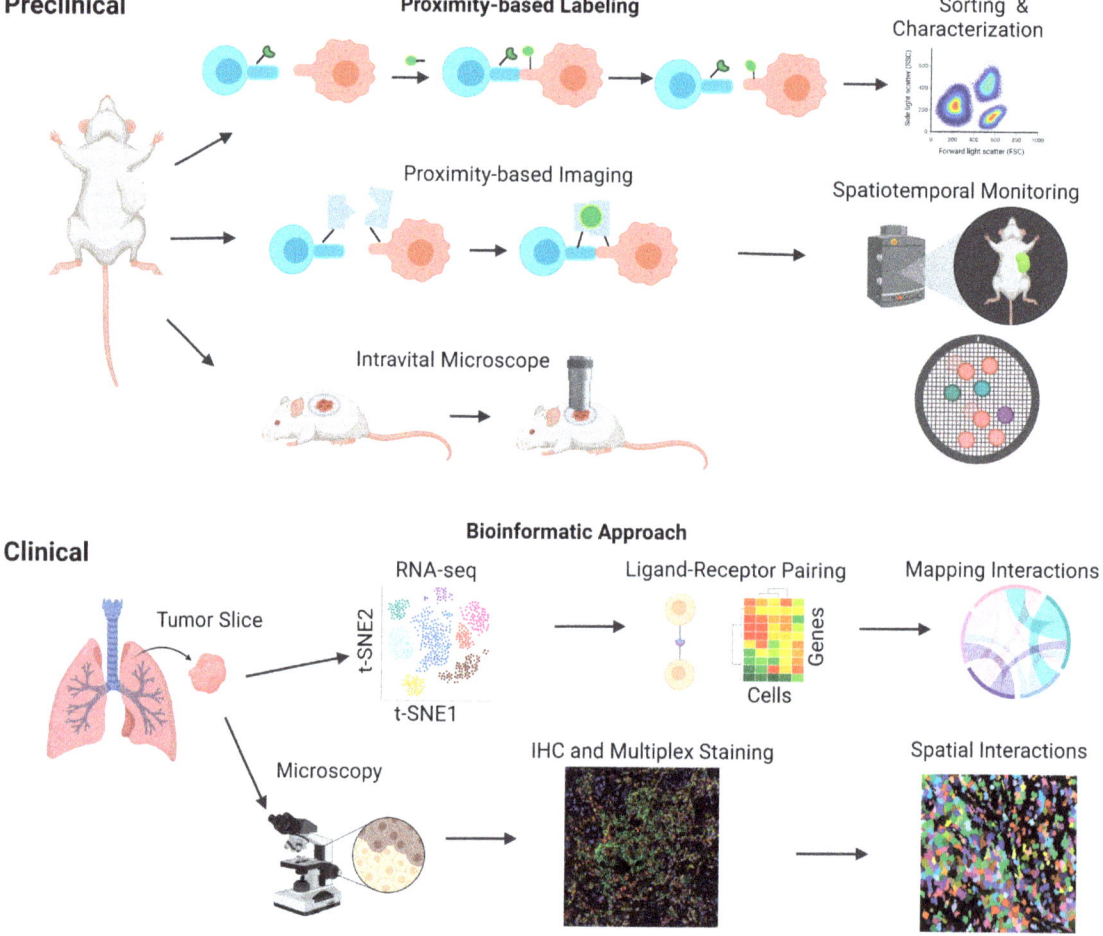

Figure 2. Human and murine methods to study cell–cell interactions. Schematic overview of the current human and murine methods for studying intercellular interactions. Human samples, obtained primarily from tissue biopsies and blood samples, serve as valuable resources for investigating these interactions. Two key techniques employed in human models are single-cell RNA sequencing (scRNA-seq) and immunohistochemical staining (IHC). scRNA-seq enables the analysis of ligand–receptor interactions, facilitating the mapping of diverse cell–cell interactions. On the other hand, IHC provides spatial information, allowing for the identification of cell locations and their physical

proximity to one another. In addition to the techniques utilized in human models, other innovative methods have been developed to study intercellular interactions. These include proximity-based intercellular labeling approaches such as LIPSTIC and EXCELL, which enable the identification of neighboring cells and the assessment of their interactions. Proximity-based intercellular imaging approaches such as confocal microscopy and CODEX offer further insights into intercellular communication by visualizing the spatial relationships between cells. Furthermore, intravital microscopy has emerged as a powerful tool for the real-time monitoring of lymphocyte localization and movement within tumor microenvironments.

Table 1. Experimental modeling systems for intercellular interactions.

Model System	Sample	Method Description	Reference
2D cell culture	Cells	Cells grow in a monolayer if adherent or suspended in a culture flask. These cultures are a straightforward, cost-effective, and low-maintenance approach. Within the controlled environment, it is possible to investigate the interactions between different cell lines and observe their behavior and responses to treatments.	[24]
3D cell culture	Cells	Cell growth and interactions occur in 3D space, where cells interact with their surrounding environment and neighboring cells. Two approaches: scaffold-based methods using hydrogels or structural scaffolds and scaffold-free techniques (spheroids).	[24]
Spheroids	Cells	Organoids, also known as multicellular spheroids, are self-assembled structures that mimic the physiological environment and interactions found in vivo. They provide a more physiologically relevant context, allowing the investigation of intercellular interactions and responses within a 3D microenvironment resembling in vivo conditions.	[25]
Organoids	Patient-derived cells and tissues	Primary patient-derived microtissues grown in a 3D extracellular matrix that represents in vivo physiology and genetic diversity, allowing the investigation of intercellular interactions and responses in a patient-specific manner.	[26]
Tissue Slices	Tumor Tissue	Tumor biopsy taken from patients or xenograft models, stained to assess tumor morphology and spatial location of cells.	[27]
Animal models	Tumor Tissue	Compatible with intravital and intercellular imaging/labeling techniques, as well as other genetic systems designed to detect cell–cell interactions upon contact or external stimulation, including UV or fluorescent light.	[28]

Nevertheless, in vitro systems lack the host tissue contexture and immune system, which are critical components for studying cell–cell interactions. Cell–cell interactions rely heavily on the tissue contexture, and techniques that support in vivo investigations have the potential to unveil novel modes of cell–cell interactions and their impact on tumor response to therapies. In vivo systems with an intact host immune system, such as syngeneic mouse models, are useful for studying the TME since the host immune system can interact with the TME [28,29]. However, a drawback of in vivo models lies in the fact that the interacting immune system being studied is often the host mouse immune system, which differs significantly from the human immune system, especially concerning cellular interactions [28].

Furthermore, tumor xenograft models using cell lines often undergo substantial genetic changes, fail to recapitulate the natural tumor structure, and may lead to mouse-specific tumor evolution [29]. While mice are the preferred experimental model for immunologists, there are significant differences between mice and humans, particularly in innate and adaptive immunity, leading to challenges in translating findings to humans [30]. The low success rate of clinical trials, which is less than 15%, can be attributed, in part, to the inadequate modeling of human diseases in animals and the limited predictability of animal models [31]. Future advancements in ex vivo models and platforms, such as microfluidics, hold promise with regard to the use of patient-derived human samples to study cell–cell interactions, leading to better clinical translation.

5. Proximity-Based Labeling Approaches for Studying Cell–Cell Interactions

Intercellular proximity labeling approaches have revolutionized the study of cell–cell interactions by providing spatially resolved information. These methods involve the tagging or labeling of proteins or other molecules that are in proximity to a specific cell type or surface marker [32] (Table 2). By identifying and analyzing the labeled molecules, researchers can gain valuable insights into the neighboring cell types and their interactions. In the context of studying the TME, proximity labeling approaches play a crucial role. Understanding the interactions between cancer cells and immune cells within the TME is essential for developing effective immunotherapies. By labeling and tracking immune cells that have come into proximity or contact with tumor cells, we can investigate the molecular features of immune cells and assess how these cells influence the composition and function of the TME.

Unlike the IHC or fluorescent staining approaches, proximity labeling techniques can go beyond a time-frozen snapshot, helping to identify and track cells and providing a more dynamic approach to cell–cell interactions. This becomes important when studying where immune cells go after interacting with cancer cells and how that cellular movement affects the composition of the TME. To ensure the applicability of proximity labeling approaches in both in vivo and in vitro environments, it is essential that these methods are non-disruptive and non-toxic to cells. This consideration ensures that the labeled cells maintain their physiological properties and behave naturally during the experimental process. By utilizing labeling techniques that are minimally invasive and compatible with live cell imaging, researchers can gain a comprehensive understanding of cell–cell interactions in the TME.

Table 2. Proximity-based labeling approaches for studying cell–cell interactions.

System	Scale	Application	Method	Reference
EXCELL	In vitro	Labeling Imaging	EXCELL (enzyme-mediated intercellular proximity labeling) is a method that utilizes a variant of SrtA, mgSrtA, to enable the non-specific labeling of cell surface proteins containing a monoglycine residue at the N-terminus. Unlike other methods, EXCELL does not require pre-engineering of acceptor cells and was applied in in vitro studies.	[33]
G-BaToN	In vitro In vivo Ex vivo	Labeling Imaging	G-BaToN is a versatile system for physical contact labeling between cells. Sender cells express surface-bound GFP, while receiver cells carry a synthetic element that selectively binds to GFP. Upon cell contact, GFP is transferred from sender to receiver cells, leading to fluorescence labeling of the receiver cells. This method requires pre-engineering of both sender and receiver cells and can be used for in vitro and ex vivo studies.	[34]
LIPSTIC	In vitro	Labeling	LIPSTIC (Labelling Immune Partnerships by SorTagging Intercellular Contacts) is a proximity-dependent labeling method that employs bacterial sortase (SrtA) to detect receptor–ligand interactions between cells. It involves the attachment of biotin to cell surface proteins, which can be detected using flow cytometry. LIPSTIC can be used in both in vitro and in vivo settings by pre-engineering the cells on both sides of the interaction.	[35]
FucoID	In vitro Ex vivo	Labeling	FucoID is a method for identifying antigen-specific T cells using interaction-dependent fucosyl biotinylation. This technique enables the isolation of endogenous tumor antigen T cells from tumor digests without prior knowledge of the tumor-specific antigens and has been used for ex vivo studies.	[36,37]

Table 2. Cont.

System	Scale	Application	Method	Reference
PUP-IT	In vitro	Labeling	PUP-IT (pupylation-based interaction tagging) is a method used to identify membrane protein interactions. In this approach, a small protein tag, Pup, is applied to proteins that interact with a PafA-fused bait, enabling transient and weak interactions to be enriched and detected by mass spectrometry. PUP-IT enables the identification and analysis of protein–protein interactions occurring at the membrane level.	[38]
2CT-CRISPR	In vitro Ex vivo	Genetic influence	Two-cell type CRISPR assay. This assay can genetically manipulate T cells to interact with cancer cells ex vivo to determine the genes that influence T cell effector function on cancer cells.	[39]
TRACC	In vitro	Labeling Imaging	TRACC (Transcriptional Readout Activated by Cell–Cell Contacts) is a system that utilizes light gating to detect cell–cell contacts based on transcriptional activity (TF). Cells are engineered to express a light-responsive TF that regulates the expression of a reporter gene. When two cells come into contact, a light signal is applied to activate the TF, resulting in the activation of the reporter gene and subsequent detection of the cell–cell contact, monitoring cell–cell interactions in a controlled and dynamic manner.	[40]
Cherry-niche	In vivo	Labeling Imaging	Cherry-niche is an innovative method that allows cells expressing a fluorescent protein to selectively label their surrounding cells in the tumor niche. This technique involves generating cancer cells capable of transferring a liposoluble fluorescent protein to their neighboring cells within the tumor microenvironment.	[41]
Caged luciferins	In vitro In vivo	Imaging	Caged luciferins are utilized for bioluminescent activity-based sensing. Activator cells expressing β-galactosidase catalyze the cleavage of caged luciferin, known as Lugal, resulting in the release of D-luciferin. The liberated D-luciferin can then enter nearby reporter cells, where it serves as a substrate for the luciferase enzyme, leading to the production of light and allowing for the identification and visualization of cells that are in close proximity to the sender cells.	[42]
SynNotch-activated MRI	In vivo	Imaging	The SynNotch system is utilized to induce the expression of an MRI contrast agent in recipient cells when they interact with sender cells expressing the corresponding synthetic notch receptor, enabling the detection and visualization of cell–cell communication events in real time.	[43]
CLIP	In vivo	Labeling Imaging	CLIP (cre-induced intercellular labeling protein) secretes a membrane-permeable fluorescent protein (mCherry) from a donor cell that can mark neighboring receptor cells. This method can label both direct cell contact receptor cells and receptor cells at a close-range distance.	[44]

Two prominent intercellular proximity labeling methods, EXCELL and LIPSTIC, employ the Staphylococcus aureus enzyme Sortase A (SrtA) to measure cell–cell interactions. LIPSTIC (Labeling Immune Partnerships by SorTagging Intercellular Contacts) enables the identification of ligand–receptor interactions between immune cells and their target cells [33,35]. Cells expressing SrtA on their surface covalently attach biotin molecules to neighboring surface proteins upon cell–cell contact [45]. The interacting cells are then exposed to a streptavidin-conjugated fluorescent dye, allowing for quantification of the interaction. LIPSTIC offers an unbiased approach for identifying ligand–receptor interactions and allows for the study of interaction dynamics over time. However, it relies on the genetic modification and the expression of both donor and receiver cells, limiting its application to specific cell types or tissues [35]. EXCELL (enzyme-mediated intercellular proximity labeling) represents a recent development; it uses an SrtA variant, mgSrtA, enabling promiscuous labeling of various cell surface proteins containing a monoglycine residue at the N-terminus [33]. Unlike LIPSTIC, EXCELL does not require genetic modification of the receiver cells, and it supports the identification of novel cellular interactions, including the subtype identification of TILs interacting with tumor cells. For both approaches, the biotin-labeled proteins can then be isolated and identified using streptavidin-based purification methods such as flow cytometry, and these labeled cells could then be subjected to further molecular characterization.

GFP-based Touching Nexus or G-baToN harnesses the trogocytosis communication of cells to transfer GFP from a donor cell to an acceptor cell [34]. However, the G-baToN approach requires the donor and receiver cells to both be transfected, which does not support the identification of unknown or novel CCIs [34]. FucoID has several advantages over other proximity labeling approaches. It enables the labeling of glycoproteins, which are an important class of proteins involved in many biological processes [36,37]. Additionally, the fucose tag is relatively small, and it interferes minimally with the function of the labeled proteins, which can reduce the likelihood of introducing artifacts into downstream analyses. FucoID can also be combined with other techniques, such as single-cell RNA sequencing, to gain a deeper understanding of the molecular mechanisms underlying intercellular communication. However, FucoID also has some limitations. It is dependent on the expression level and accessibility of the cell surface marker of interest, which may limit its application to certain cell types or tissues. Additionally, the labeling efficiency of FucoID may be affected by the density of glycoproteins on the cell surface and the availability of fucose residues. Careful experimental design and validation are necessary to ensure the accuracy and specificity of the results obtained using FucoID [36,37].

A subsequent method that is able to detect membrane proteins through proximity labeling is population-based interaction tagging (PUP-IT) [38]. In this system, the small protein tag Pup is weakly attached to proteins or prey interacting with the gene *PafA* or bait [38]. PUP-IT was utilized to label the interaction between CD28-expressing Jurkat T cells and CD80/86-expressing Raji B lymphocytes. PUP-IT CD28 extracellular Jurkat T cells were able to label the Raji B cell in vitro [38]. However, for this interaction to be observed both cells needed to be modified with the prey or bait genes. PUP-IT is also classified as a "weak" interaction and may not be suitable for long-term tracking [38]. This highlights that PUP-ID needs some knowledge of ligand–receptor interactions before using.

2CT-CRISPR assay is a novel and interesting approach for identifying genes that are essential for effector T cell function in tumors. In the 2CT-CRISPR assay, human T cells were represented as effectors, and melanoma cells were represented as targets [39]. The purpose of this assay was to determine whether genetically manipulating the immune cell would influence the tumor cell during ligand–receptor interactions [39]. A recombinant TCR-engineered CD8$^+$ T cell was used to target a specific antigen (NY-ESO-1) that can mediate tumor size in melanoma patients. The 2CT method was used to control the selection pressure and killing effects shown by the T cell as well as to modulate the effector to target ratio. Furthermore, the 2CT method was used in combination with a CRISPR-Cas9 library that held over 100,000 single-guide RNAs which impaired effector function in T cells. The 2CT method allowed for the analysis of genes necessary for immunotherapy, specifically those that target effector T cell function. The 2CT method has exciting translation and clinical opportunities to uncover genes in immunotherapy-resistant patients [39].

Other proximity-based methods for studying cell–cell interactions include TRACC (Transcriptional Readout Activated by Cell–Cell Contacts) and SynNotch-activated MRI (magnetic resonance imaging), both of which exploit specific receptor–ligand interactions between two interacting cells to facilitate labeling and detection [40,43]. TRACC utilizes a g-protein-coupled receptor with a light-sensitive domain to detect cell–cell interactions using a transcriptional readout [40]. This approach allows for the visualization and identification of cell populations involved in the interaction of interest. SynNotch-activated MRI combines synthetic biology and imaging techniques to detect cell–cell interactions [43]. It involves the engineering of cells expressing a synthetic Notch receptor that can be activated upon interaction with a specific ligand presented by neighboring cells. Upon activation, the engineered cells produce a contrast agent detectable by MRI, enabling the visualization and tracking of the interacting cell populations [43].

Most proximity-based methods are dependent on cell–cell contact and interaction. Cherry-niche, caged luciferins, and CLIP (cre-induced intercellular labeling protein) are three approaches that do not solely rely on direct cell–cell contact for labeling [41,42,44]. In the Cherry-niche method, cells are engineered to express the enzyme Cherry-tagged ligase, which can attach a fluorophore to nearby cells expressing a complementary Cherry-tagged receptor [41]. This proximity labeling occurs within a specific microenvironment or niche defined by the presence of the ligase and receptor [41]. Caged luciferins, on the other hand, involve the use of caged luciferin molecules that can be activated by specific enzymes or stimuli produced by engineered cells [42]. Upon activation, the caged luciferins produce luminescent signals that can be detected and used to identify neighboring cells in the vicinity [42]. CLIP has an interesting methodology in that it can label cells that are in direct contact as well as those that are not in direct contact but are in proximity to each other [44]. This method involves the engineering of both the donor and receiver cells, where the donor cell secretes a lipid-soluble tag containing mCherry that labels the recipient cells [44]. These approaches provide additional tools for studying cell–cell interactions, offering different mechanisms for labeling and detection beyond direct cell–cell contact.

In summary, intercellular proximity labeling or imaging approaches offer significant potential for elucidating the intricate cellular interactions and communication networks within the TME. These methods have been successfully employed in various research areas, including the investigation of tumor metastasis [37,41], T cell priming [35], cell migration [35], tumor–immune cell interactions [37], cellular therapy [37], and the examination of interactions between neurons and glioma cells [40]. As these techniques continue to advance, it is anticipated that their application will expand further, enabling a broader understanding of the factors and mechanisms that impede the pharmacological effects of immunotherapies. Overall, intercellular proximity labeling approaches can provide valuable insights into the complex cellular interactions and communication networks in the TME, which can inform the development of more effective cancer immunotherapies.

6. Bioinformatic Techniques for Inferring Cell–Cell Interactions

Enzyme-based intercellular proximity labeling approaches are predominantly employed in experimental systems. However, with the growing availability of large clinical datasets, bioinformatic methods have gained significance in the study of cell–cell interactions and the identification of novel interactions. In clinical settings, bioinformatics methods play a crucial role in inferring intercellular interactions or communication by examining the coordinated expression patterns of ligand–receptor pairs' cognate genes. Ligand–receptor analysis has emerged as a valuable approach for investigating intercellular communication, particularly in the context of cancer immunotherapy. This approach enables the identification of the specific ligand–receptor pairs involved in immune cell interactions with cancer cells or the TME (Table 3).

This approach proves to be especially valuable in deducing intercellular interactions that are not solely reliant on cell-to-cell contact. This is evident when immune cells and cancer cells release diverse cytokines, chemokines, and growth factors that govern immune reactions and inflammation. These signaling molecules and their corresponding receptors may be modulated based on environmental cues. Through these bioinformatics methods, we can deduce the likelihood of intercellular interactions based on their ligand–receptor profiles; this is potentially pivotal in forecasting patient prognosis and treatment outcomes.

The analysis of ligand–receptor interactions primarily relies on single-cell RNA sequencing (scRNA-seq) or bulk RNA-seq data. The procedure typically involves the following steps:

Data preprocessing: This step involves normalizing, quality controlling, and filtering of gene expression data to ensure data integrity and reliability.

Gene set selection: A specific set of ligand and receptor genes is chosen based on prior knowledge or by utilizing databases such as CellPhoneDB or Interactome INSIDER.

Calculation of ligand–receptor expression: The expression levels of ligand and receptor genes are calculated for each cell or cell type within the dataset, regardless of whether the data are scRNA-seq or bulk RNA-seq.

Ligand–receptor interaction analysis: Interactions between ligands and receptors are predicted by assessing the co-expression patterns of ligand and receptor genes across different cells or cell types. Several methods, including CellPhoneDB, scRNA-seq-based ligand–receptor pair analysis (sLRPA), and LigandNet, are available for performing this analysis.

Table 3. Bioinformatic techniques for inferring cell–cell interactions.

Platform	Data Source	Method	Reference
CellTalkDB	scRNA-seq	Manually curated database of ligand–receptor pairs from both human and mouse samples.	[46]
iTalk	scRNA-seq	Identifying and illustrating alterations in intercellular signaling network. R package made to analyze and visualize ligand–receptor pair.	[47]
PyMINeR	scRNA-seq	Python maximal information network exploration resource. Fully automates cell type-specific identification, and pathways as well as in silico detection of autocrine and paracrine signaling networks	[48]
CellChat	scRNA-seq	Open source R package that is able to visualize, analyze, and deduce intercellular communications from a data input. Uses mass action models and differential expression analysis to deduce cell state-specific signaling communications. Also provides visualization outputs to compare intercellular communication methods.	[49]
CellPhoneDB	scRNA-seq	Identifies biologically relevant interacting ligand–receptor pairs. Cells with the same cluster are pooled together as one cell state. Ligand–receptor interactions are derived based on the expression of a receptor of one state and a ligand of the other state.	[50]
Giotto	scRNA-seq	Open source spatial analysis platform that contains two modules, Giotto analyzer and Giotto viewer, which are both independent and fully integrated. Analyzer provides instructions about steps in analyzing single-cell expression data, and the viewer provides an interactive view of the data.	[51]
ICellNET	RNA-seq, scRNA-seq, and microarray	Transcriptomic-based framework that integrates a database of ligand–receptor interactions, communication scores, and connections of cell populations of interest with 31 human reference cell types and three visualization methods.	[52]
SingleCellSignalR	scRNA-seq	Open source R platform. Relies on a database of known ligand–receptor interactions called LR*db*.	[53]
CCC Explorer	Transcriptome profiles	Java-based software. Uses a computational model to look at cell–cell communications ranging from ligand–receptor interactions to transcription factors and target genes.	[54]
NicheNet	Gene expression data	Open source R platform. Uses a database of ligand–receptor interactions to identify ligand–receptor interactions that could drive gene expression changes	[55]
SoptSC	RNA-seq	Similarity matrix-based optimization for single-cell data analysis. Uses a cell-to-cell similarity matrix via gene marker identification, lineage reference, clustering, and pseudo-temporal ordering. From this information, it predicts cell–cell communication networks.	[56]
SpaoTSC	scRNA-seq	Spatially optimal transporting of the single cells. The method has two major components: (1) constructing spatial metric for cells from scRNA-seq data and (2) reconstructing the cell–cell communication networks from the data and identifying relationships between genes from intercellular relationships. Uses python.	[57]
scTensor	scRNA-seq	Open source R package. Instead of looking at one-to-one cell–cell interactions, this software focuses on many-to-many cell–cell interactions. scTensor looks at a three-way relationship (hypergraph) between ligand expression, receptor expression, and ligand–receptor pairs.	[58]

Visualization and interpretation: The results of the analysis are visualized using heatmaps, networks, or other visualization techniques. These results can be interpreted to identify the specific ligand–receptor pairs that may be involved in intercellular communication and to gain insights into the underlying biological processes.

Bioinformatic methods offer valuable tools for inferring intercellular interactions and communication based on transcriptome data. These approaches provide valuable insights into the intricate network of cell–cell interactions in the context of cancer immunotherapy. Notably, ligand–receptor analysis holds promise for the identification of predictive biomarkers for immunotherapy response and the monitoring of treatment efficacy.

Nevertheless, it is important to acknowledge the limitations of these bioinformatic methods in inferring intercellular interactions. Firstly, their predictions solely rely on gene expression data and overlook additional factors like post-translational modifications or protein localization that can influence interactions. Secondly, these methods hinge upon existing knowledge of ligand–receptor pairs, which may be incomplete or imprecise. Thirdly, the biological relevance of the predictions is not guaranteed, necessitating experimental validation. Lastly, technical artifacts such as batch effects, sequencing depth, and normalization methods can influence the accuracy and reproducibility of the results. Considering these limitations, it is crucial to exercise caution and combine bioinformatic predictions with experimental validation to ensure the reliability and significance of the findings. Continued advancements in bioinformatic techniques and complementary experimental approaches will enhance our understanding of intercellular interactions and their role in cancer immunotherapy.

7. Potential Questions to Be Addressed by These Approaches

A wide array of scientific questions concerning cancer immunotherapy could be answered by utilizing these cell-cell interactions techniques. These questions include:

What are the subpopulations of immune cells interacting with the tumor cell during immunotherapy?

What are the molecular features of these interacting immune cells, and how are the molecular features related in response to immunotherapy?

Do the effector cells that have interacted with the tumor cells migrate across tumor metastatic lesions?

Ultimately, the answers to these questions can uncover the pharmacological actions of cancer immunotherapy and reveal the underlying molecular mechanism of resistance.

8. Concluding Remarks

The TME represents an intricate network comprising diverse cell types engaged in communication; it plays a pivotal role in shaping the tumor landscape. Effective communication between immune cells and cancer cells holds great significance in the determination of the patients' responses to immunotherapy, and it contributes to treatment resistance and interpatient variability in the responses. The investigation of cell–cell communication in immune cells under normal and pathological conditions provides crucial insights into the mechanisms of cancer immunotherapy, patient responses, disease progression, and TME status. Various experimental and computational approaches exist for elucidating pathological intercellular interactions, both directly and indirectly, with the aim of identifying the communicating cell populations. Comprehensive understanding, modeling, and the discovery of cell–cell interactions within the TME hold immense potential for the identification of the critical factors and strategies influencing immunotherapy response, treatment resistance, and TME status.

In recent times, advances in imaging, microscopy, cellular engineering, and bioinformatics have emerged as powerful tools for the unraveling of novel mechanisms and cellular relationships, thereby paving the way for improved immunotherapy options for patients. By leveraging these methodologies synergistically, it becomes possible to bridge existing knowledge gaps and gain a comprehensive understanding of treatment resistance and to design more potent cancer immunotherapies.

Author Contributions: Conceptualization, Y.C.; investigation, Y.C. and K.M.; resources, Y.C.; data curation, Y.C. writing—original draft preparation, K.M. and Y.C.; writing—review and editing, Y.C.; visualization, Y.C.; supervision, Y.C.; project administration, Y.C.; funding acquisition, Y.C. All authors have read and agreed to the published version of the manuscript.

Funding: This research was funded by National Institute of General Medical Sciences, R35 GM119661.

Conflicts of Interest: The authors declare no conflict of interest.

References

1. Armingol, E.; Officer, A.; Harismendy, O.; Lewis, N.E. Deciphering cell-cell interactions and communication from gene expression. *Nat. Rev. Genet.* **2021**, *22*, 71–88. [CrossRef]
2. Anderson, N.M.; Simon, M.C. The tumor microenvironment. *Curr. Biol.* **2020**, *30*, R921–R925. [CrossRef]
3. Eno, J. Immunotherapy through the years. *J. Adv. Pract. Oncol.* **2017**, *8*, 747–753.
4. Ma, W.; Gilligan, B.M.; Yuan, J.; Li, T. Current status and perspectives in translational biomarker research for PD-1/PD-L1 immune checkpoint blockade therapy. *J. Hematol. Oncol.* **2016**, *9*, 47. [CrossRef]
5. Lanitis, E.; Dangaj, D.; Irving, M.; Coukos, G. Mechanisms regulating T-cell infiltration and activity in solid tumors. *Ann. Oncol.* **2017**, *28*, xii18–xii32. [CrossRef] [PubMed]
6. Saleh, R.; Elkord, E. FoxP3+ T regulatory cells in cancer: Prognostic biomarkers and therapeutic targets. *Cancer Lett.* **2020**, *490*, 174–185. [CrossRef]
7. Blessin, N.C.; Li, W.; Mandelkow, T.; Jansen, H.L.; Yang, C.; Raedler, J.B.; Simon, R.; Büscheck, F.; Dum, D.; Luebke, A.M.; et al. Prognostic role of proliferating CD8+ cytotoxic Tcells in human cancers. *Cell. Oncol.* **2021**, *44*, 793–803. [CrossRef] [PubMed]
8. Zuo, S.; Wei, M.; Wang, S.; Dong, J.; Wei, J. Pan-Cancer Analysis of Immune Cell Infiltration Identifies a Prognostic Immune-Cell Characteristic Score (ICCS) in Lung Adenocarcinoma. *Front. Immunol.* **2020**, *11*, 1218. [CrossRef]

9. O'Donnell, J.S.; Teng, M.W.L.; Smyth, M.J. Cancer immunoediting and resistance to T cell-based immunotherapy. *Nat. Rev. Clin. Oncol.* **2019**, *16*, 151–167. [CrossRef]
10. Schreiber, R.D.; Old, L.J.; Smyth, M.J. Cancer immunoediting: Integrating immunity's roles in cancer suppression and promotion. *Science* **2011**, *331*, 1565–1570. [CrossRef]
11. Liu, T.; Han, C.; Wang, S.; Fang, P.; Ma, Z.; Xu, L.; Yin, R. Cancer-associated fibroblasts: An emerging target of anti-cancer immunotherapy. *J. Hematol. Oncol.* **2019**, *12*, 86. [CrossRef]
12. Hanley, C.J.; Thomas, G.J. Targeting cancer associated fibroblasts to enhance immunotherapy: Emerging strategies and future perspectives. *Oncotarget* **2021**, *12*, 1427–1433. [CrossRef]
13. Pei, L.; Liu, Y.; Liu, L.; Gao, S.; Gao, X.; Feng, Y.; Sun, Z.; Zhang, Y.; Wang, C. Roles of cancer-associated fibroblasts (CAFs) in anti-PD-1/PD-L1 immunotherapy for solid cancers. *Mol. Cancer* **2023**, *22*, 29. [CrossRef]
14. Twomey, J.D.; Zhang, B. Cancer Immunotherapy Update: FDA-Approved Checkpoint Inhibitors and Companion Diagnostics. *AAPS J.* **2021**, *23*, 39. [CrossRef]
15. Zhang, Y.; Zhang, Z. The history and advances in cancer immunotherapy: Understanding the characteristics of tumor-infiltrating immune cells and their therapeutic implications. *Cell. Mol. Immunol.* **2020**, *17*, 807–821. [CrossRef]
16. Gómez Román, V.R.; Murray, J.C.; Weiner, L.M. Antibody-Dependent Cellular Cytotoxicity (ADCC). In *Antibody Fc*; Academic Press: Cambridge, MA, USA, 2014; pp. 1–27.
17. Zhou, S.; Liu, M.; Ren, F.; Meng, X.; Yu, J. The landscape of bispecific T cell engager in cancer treatment. *Biomark. Res.* **2021**, *9*, 38. [CrossRef]
18. Liu, C.; Zhou, J.; Kudlacek, S.; Qi, T.; Dunlap, T.; Cao, Y. Population dynamics of immunological synapse formation induced by bispecific T cell engagers predict clinical pharmacodynamics and treatment resistance. *eLife* **2023**, *12*, e83659. [CrossRef]
19. Pan, K.; Farrukh, H.; Chittepu, V.C.S.R.; Xu, H.; Pan, C.-X.; Zhu, Z. CAR race to cancer immunotherapy: From CAR T, CAR NK to CAR macrophage therapy. *J. Exp. Clin. Cancer Res.* **2022**, *41*, 119. [CrossRef]
20. Shalhout, S.Z.; Miller, D.M.; Emerick, K.S.; Kaufman, H.L. Therapy with oncolytic viruses: Progress and challenges. *Nat. Rev. Clin. Oncol.* **2023**, *20*, 160–177. [CrossRef]
21. Cao, G.-D.; He, X.-B.; Sun, Q.; Chen, S.; Wan, K.; Xu, X.; Feng, X.; Li, P.-P.; Chen, B.; Xiong, M.-M. The oncolytic virus in cancer diagnosis and treatment. *Front. Oncol.* **2020**, *10*, 1786. [CrossRef]
22. Dominiak, A.; Chełstowska, B.; Olejarz, W.; Nowicka, G. Communication in the cancer microenvironment as a target for therapeutic interventions. *Cancers* **2020**, *12*, 1232. [CrossRef] [PubMed]
23. Shelton, S.E.; Nguyen, H.T.; Barbie, D.A.; Kamm, R.D. Engineering approaches for studying immune-tumor cell interactions and immunotherapy. *iScience* **2021**, *24*, 101985. [CrossRef] [PubMed]
24. Kapałczyńska, M.; Kolenda, T.; Przybyła, W.; Zajączkowska, M.; Teresiak, A.; Filas, V.; Ibbs, M.; Bliźniak, R.; Łuczewski, Ł.; Lamperska, K. 2D and 3D cell cultures—A comparison of different types of cancer cell cultures. *Arch. Med. Sci.* **2018**, *14*, 910–919. [CrossRef]
25. Yuki, K.; Cheng, N.; Nakano, M.; Kuo, C.J. Organoid models of tumor immunology. *Trends Immunol.* **2020**, *41*, 652–664. [CrossRef] [PubMed]
26. Białkowska, K.; Komorowski, P.; Bryszewska, M.; Miłowska, K. Spheroids as a Type of Three-Dimensional Cell Cultures-Examples of Methods of Preparation and the Most Important Application. *Int. J. Mol. Sci.* **2020**, *21*, 6225. [CrossRef]
27. Mao, Y.; Wang, X.; Huang, P.; Tian, R. Spatial proteomics for understanding the tissue microenvironment. *Analyst* **2021**, *146*, 3777–3798. [CrossRef]
28. Zhong, W.; Myers, J.S.; Wang, F.; Wang, K.; Lucas, J.; Rosfjord, E.; Lucas, J.; Hooper, A.T.; Yang, S.; Lemon, L.A.; et al. Comparison of the molecular and cellular phenotypes of common mouse syngeneic models with human tumors. *BMC Genom.* **2020**, *21*, 2. [CrossRef]
29. Taylor, M.A.; Hughes, A.M.; Walton, J.; Coenen-Stass, A.M.L.; Magiera, L.; Mooney, L.; Bell, S.; Staniszewska, A.D.; Sandin, L.C.; Barry, S.T.; et al. Longitudinal immune characterization of syngeneic tumor models to enable model selection for immune oncology drug discovery. *J. Immunother. Cancer* **2019**, *7*, 328. [CrossRef]
30. Richmond, A.; Su, Y. Mouse xenograft models vs GEM models for human cancer therapeutics. *Dis. Model. Mech.* **2008**, *1*, 78–82. [CrossRef]
31. Mestas, J.; Hughes, C.C.W. Of mice and not men: Differences between mouse and human immunology. *J. Immunol.* **2004**, *172*, 2731–2738. [CrossRef]
32. Arnol, D.; Schapiro, D.; Bodenmiller, B.; Saez-Rodriguez, J.; Stegle, O. Modeling Cell-Cell Interactions from Spatial Molecular Data with Spatial Variance Component Analysis. *Cell Rep.* **2019**, *29*, 202–211.e6. [CrossRef] [PubMed]
33. Ge, Y.; Chen, L.; Liu, S.; Zhao, J.; Zhang, H.; Chen, P.R. Enzyme-Mediated Intercellular Proximity Labeling for Detecting Cell-Cell Interactions. *J. Am. Chem. Soc.* **2019**, *141*, 1833–1837. [CrossRef] [PubMed]
34. Tang, R.; Murray, C.W.; Linde, I.L.; Kramer, N.J.; Lyu, Z.; Tsai, M.K.; Chen, L.C.; Cai, H.; Gitler, A.D.; Engleman, E.; et al. A versatile system to record cell-cell interactions. *eLife* **2020**, *9*, e61080. [CrossRef] [PubMed]
35. Pasqual, G.; Chudnovskiy, A.; Tas, J.M.J.; Agudelo, M.; Schweitzer, L.D.; Cui, A.; Hacohen, N.; Victora, G.D. Monitoring T cell-dendritic cell interactions in vivo by intercellular enzymatic labelling. *Nature* **2018**, *553*, 496–500. [CrossRef] [PubMed]
36. Liu, Z.; Li, J.P.; Chen, M.; Wu, M.; Shi, Y.; Li, W.; Teijaro, J.R.; Wu, P. Detecting Tumor Antigen-Specific T Cells via Interaction-Dependent Fucosyl-Biotinylation. *Cell* **2020**, *183*, 1117–1133.e19. [CrossRef] [PubMed]

37. Qiu, S.; Zhao, Z.; Wu, M.; Xue, Q.; Yang, Y.; Ouyang, S.; Li, W.; Zhong, L.; Wang, W.; Yang, R.; et al. Use of intercellular proximity labeling to quantify and decipher cell-cell interactions directed by diversified molecular pairs. *Cancer* **2022**, *8*, eadd2337. [CrossRef]
38. Liu, Q.; Zheng, J.; Sun, W.; Huo, Y.; Zhang, L.; Hao, P.; Wang, H.; Zhuang, M. A proximity-tagging system to identify membrane protein-protein interactions. *Nat. Methods* **2018**, *15*, 715–722. [CrossRef]
39. Patel, S.J.; Sanjana, N.E.; Kishton, R.J.; Eidizadeh, A.; Vodnala, S.K.; Cam, M.; Gartner, J.J.; Jia, L.; Steinberg, S.M.; Yamamoto, T.N.; et al. Identification of essential genes for cancer immunotherapy. *Nature* **2017**, *548*, 537–542. [CrossRef]
40. Cho, K.F.; Gillespie, S.M.; Kalogriopoulos, N.A.; Quezada, M.A.; Jacko, M.; Monje, M.; Ting, A.Y. A light-gated transcriptional recorder for detecting cell-cell contacts. *eLife* **2022**, *11*, e70881. [CrossRef]
41. Ombrato, L.; Nolan, E.; Kurelac, I.; Mavousian, A.; Bridgeman, V.L.; Heinze, I.; Chakravarty, P.; Horswell, S.; Gonzalez-Gualda, E.; Matacchione, G.; et al. Metastatic-niche labelling reveals parenchymal cells with stem features. *Nature* **2019**, *572*, 603–608. [CrossRef] [PubMed]
42. Porterfield, W.B.; Jones, K.A.; McCutcheon, D.C.; Prescher, J.A. A "Caged" Luciferin for Imaging Cell-Cell Contacts. *J. Am. Chem. Soc.* **2015**, *137*, 8656–8659. [CrossRef] [PubMed]
43. Wang, T.; Chen, Y.; Nystrom, N.N.; Liu, S.; Fu, Y.; Martinez, F.M.; Scholl, T.J.; Ronald, J.A. Visualizing cell-cell communication using synthetic notch activated MRI. *Proc. Natl. Acad. Sci. USA* **2023**, *120*, e2216901120. [CrossRef]
44. Zhang, S.; Zhang, Q.; Liu, Z.; Liu, K.; He, L.; Lui, K.O.; Wang, L.; Zhou, B. Genetic dissection of intercellular interactions in vivo by membrane-permeable protein. *Proc. Natl. Acad. Sci. USA* **2023**, *120*, e2120582120. [CrossRef] [PubMed]
45. Chen, L.; Cohen, J.; Song, X.; Zhao, A.; Ye, Z.; Feulner, C.J.; Doonan, P.; Somers, W.; Lin, L.; Chen, P.R. Improved variants of SrtA for site-specific conjugation on antibodies and proteins with high efficiency. *Sci. Rep.* **2016**, *6*, 31899. [CrossRef] [PubMed]
46. Shao, X.; Liao, J.; Li, C.; Lu, X.; Cheng, J.; Fan, X. CellTalkDB: A manually curated database of ligand-receptor interactions in humans and mice. *Brief. Bioinform.* **2021**, *22*, bbaa269. [CrossRef]
47. Wang, Y.; Wang, R.; Zhang, S.; Song, S.; Jiang, C.; Han, G.; Wang, M.; Ajani, J.; Futreal, A.; Wang, L. iTALK: An R Package to Characterize and Illustrate Intercellular Communication. *BioRxiv* **2019**, 507871. [CrossRef]
48. Tyler, S.R.; Rotti, P.G.; Sun, X.; Yi, Y.; Xie, W.; Winter, M.C.; Flamme-Wiese, M.J.; Tucker, B.A.; Mullins, R.F.; Norris, A.W.; et al. PyMINEr Finds Gene and Autocrine-Paracrine Networks from Human Islet scRNA-Seq. *Cell Rep.* **2019**, *26*, 1951–1964.e8. [CrossRef]
49. Jin, S.; Guerrero-Juarez, C.F.; Zhang, L.; Chang, I.; Ramos, R.; Kuan, C.-H.; Myung, P.; Plikus, M.V.; Nie, Q. Inference and analysis of cell-cell communication using CellChat. *Nat. Commun.* **2021**, *12*, 1088. [CrossRef]
50. Efremova, M.; Vento-Tormo, M.; Teichmann, S.A.; Vento-Tormo, R. CellPhoneDB: Inferring cell-cell communication from combined expression of multi-subunit ligand-receptor complexes. *Nat. Protoc.* **2020**, *15*, 1484–1506. [CrossRef]
51. Dries, R.; Zhu, Q.; Dong, R.; Eng, C.-H.L.; Li, H.; Liu, K.; Fu, Y.; Zhao, T.; Sarkar, A.; Bao, F.; et al. Giotto: A toolbox for integrative analysis and visualization of spatial expression data. *Genome Biol.* **2021**, *22*, 78. [CrossRef] [PubMed]
52. Noël, F.; Massenet-Regad, L.; Carmi-Levy, I.; Cappuccio, A.; Grandclaudon, M.; Trichot, C.; Kieffer, Y.; Mechta-Grigoriou, F.; Soumelis, V. ICELLNET: A transcriptome-based framework to dissect intercellular communication. *BioRxiv* **2020**. [CrossRef]
53. Cabello-Aguilar, S.; Alame, M.; Kon-Sun-Tack, F.; Fau, C.; Lacroix, M.; Colinge, J. SingleCellSignalR: Inference of intercellular networks from single-cell transcriptomics. *Nucleic Acids Res.* **2020**, *48*, e55. [CrossRef] [PubMed]
54. Choi, H.; Sheng, J.; Gao, D.; Li, F.; Durrans, A.; Ryu, S.; Lee, S.B.; Narula, N.; Rafii, S.; Elemento, O.; et al. Transcriptome analysis of individual stromal cell populations identifies stroma-tumor crosstalk in mouse lung cancer model. *Cell Rep.* **2015**, *10*, 1187–1201. [CrossRef] [PubMed]
55. Browaeys, R.; Saelens, W.; Saeys, Y. NicheNet: Modeling intercellular communication by linking ligands to target genes. *Nat. Methods* **2020**, *17*, 159–162. [CrossRef]
56. Wang, S.; Karikomi, M.; MacLean, A.L.; Nie, Q. Cell lineage and communication network inference via optimization for single-cell transcriptomics. *Nucleic Acids Res.* **2019**, *47*, e66. [CrossRef]
57. Cang, Z.; Nie, Q. Inferring spatial and signaling relationships between cells from single cell transcriptomic data. *Nat. Commun.* **2020**, *11*, 2084. [CrossRef] [PubMed]
58. Tsuyuzaki, K.; Ishii, M.; Nikaido, I. Uncovering hypergraphs of cell-cell interaction from single cell RNA-sequencing data. *BioRxiv* **2019**, 566182. [CrossRef]

Disclaimer/Publisher's Note: The statements, opinions and data contained in all publications are solely those of the individual author(s) and contributor(s) and not of MDPI and/or the editor(s). MDPI and/or the editor(s) disclaim responsibility for any injury to people or property resulting from any ideas, methods, instructions or products referred to in the content.

MDPI
St. Alban-Anlage 66
4052 Basel
Switzerland
www.mdpi.com

Cancers Editorial Office
E-mail: cancers@mdpi.com
www.mdpi.com/journal/cancers

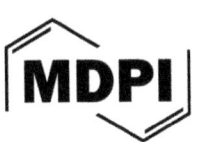

Disclaimer/Publisher's Note: The statements, opinions and data contained in all publications are solely those of the individual author(s) and contributor(s) and not of MDPI and/or the editor(s). MDPI and/or the editor(s) disclaim responsibility for any injury to people or property resulting from any ideas, methods, instructions or products referred to in the content.